CAT/2C

EXPLORATIONS IN SOCIOLOG

British Sociological Association conference

Sami Zubaida (editor)	1	*Race*
Richard Brown (editor)	2	*Knov ... ...u Cultural Change*
Paul Rock and Mary McIntosh (editors)	3	*Deviance and Social Control*
Emanuel de Kadt and Gavin Williams (editors)	4	*Sociology and Development*
Frank Parkin (editor)	5	*The Social Analysis of Class Structure*
Diana Leonard Barker and Sheila Allen (editors)	6	*Sexual Divisions and Society: Process and Change*
Diana Leonard Barker and Sheila Allen (editors)	7	*Dependence and Exploitation in Work and Marriage*
Richard Scase (editor)	8	*Industrial Society: Class, Cleavage and Control*
Robert Dingwall, Christian Heath, Margaret Reid and Margaret Stacey (editors)	9	*Health Care and Health Knowledge*
Robert Dingwall, Christian Heath, Margaret Reid and Margaret Stacey (editors)	10	*Health and the Division of Labour*
Gary Littlejohn, Barry Smart, John Wakeford and Nira Yuval-Davis (editors)	11	*Power and the State*
Michèle Barrett, Philip Corrigan, Annette Kuhn and Janet Wolff (editors)	12	*Ideology and Cultural Production*
Bob Fryer, Alan Hunt, Doreen MacBarnet and Bert Moorhouse (editors)	13	*Law, State and Society*
Philip Abrams, Rosemary Deem, Janet Finch and Paul Rock (editors)	14	*Practice and Progress: British Sociology 1950–1980*
Graham Day, Lesley Caldwell, Karen Jones, David Robbins and Hilary Rose (editors)	15	*Diversity and Decomposition in the Labour Market*
David Robbins, Lesley Caldwell, Graham Day, Karen Jones and Hilary Rose (editors)	16	*Rethinking Social Inequality*

*Gareth Rees, Janet Bujra, Paul Littlewood, Howard Newby and Teresa L. Rees (editors) — 19 *Political Action and Social Identity: Class, Locality and Ideology*

*Howard Newby, Janet Bujra, Paul Littlewood, Gareth Rees, Teresa L. Rees (editors) — 20 *Restructuring Capital: Recession and Reorganization in Industrial Society*

*Sheila Allen, Kate Purcell, Alan Waton and Stephen Wood (editors) — 21 *The Experience of Unemployment*

*Kate Purcell, Stephen Wood, Alan Waton and Sheila Allen (editors) — 22 *The Changing Experience of Employment: Restructuring and Recession*

*Jalna Hanmer and Mary Maynard (editors) — 23 *Women, Violence and Social Control*

*Colin Creighton and Martin Shaw (editors) — 24 *The Sociology of War and Peace*

*Alan Bryman, Bill Bytheway, Patricia Allatt and Teresa Keil — 25 *Rethinking the Life Cycle*

*Patricia Allatt, Teresa Keil, Alan Bryman and Bill Bytheway — 26 *Women and the Life Cycle*

*Ian Varcoe, Maureen McNeil and Steven Yearley (editors) — 27 *Deciphering Science and Technology: The Social Relations of Expertise*

*Maureen McNeil, Ian Varcoe and Steven Yearley (editors) — 28 *The New Reproductive Technologies*

*David McCrone, Stephen Kendrick and Pat Straw (editors) — 29 *The Making of Scotland: Nation, Culture and Social Change*

*Stephen Kendrick, Pat Straw and David McCrone (editors) — 30 *Interpreting the Past, Understanding the Present*

*Helen Corr and Lynn Jamieson — 31 *Politics of Everyday Life: Continuity and Change in Work and the Family*

*Lynn Jamieson and Helen Corr — 32 *State, Private Life and Political Change*

**Published by Macmillan*

The New Reproductive Technologies

Edited by

Maureen McNeil
University of Birmingham

Ian Varcoe
University of Leeds

and

Steven Yearley
Queen's University, Belfast

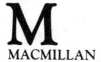

MACMILLAN

First published 1990

Published by
THE MACMILLAN PRESS LTD
Houndmills, Basingstoke, Hampshire RG21 2XS
and London
Companies and representatives
throughout the world

Printed in Hong Kong

British Library Cataloguing in Publication Data
The new reproductive technologies.—(Explorations in
sociology; 28).
1. Man. Reproduction. Scientific innovation. Social
aspects
I. McNeil, Maureen II. Varcoe, Ian III. Yearley,
Steven IV. Series
362.1′042
ISBN 0–333–46559–8 (hardcover)
ISBN 0–333–46560–1 (paperback)

Series Standing Order

If you would like to receive future titles in this series as they are
published, you can make use of our standing order facility. To place a
standing order please contact your bookseller or, in case of difficulty,
write to us at the address below with your name and address and the
name of the series. Please state with which title you wish to begin your
standing order. (If you live outside the United Kingdom we may not
have the rights for your area, in which case we will forward your order
to the publisher concerned.)

Customer Services Department, Macmillan Distribution Ltd
Houndmills, Basingstoke, Hampshire, RG21 2XS, England.

This book is dedicated to the memory of
David Robbins (1946–86)

Contents

List of Figures   viii

Foreword   ix

Notes on the Contributors   xii

1   Reproductive Technologies: A New Terrain for the
    Sociology of Technology   1
    Maureen McNeil

2   Whose Mind Over Whose Matter? Women, *In Vitro*
    Fertilisation and the Development of Scientific Knowledge   27
    Cristine Crowe

3   The Normalisation of a New Reproductive Technology   58
    Annette Burfoot

4   The Depersonalisation of Women through the
    Administration of '*In Vitro* Fertilisation'   74
    Deborah Lynn Steinberg

5   The Management of Uncertainty in Obstetric Practice:
    Ultrasonography, *In Vitro* Fertilisation and Embryo
    Transfer   123
    Frances V. Price

6   Recreating the Family? Policy Considerations Relating to
    the 'New' Reproductive Technologies   154
    Erica Haimes

7   Conflicting Concerns: The Political Context of Recent
    Embryo Research Policy in Britain   173
    Edward Yoxen

8   Deconstructing 'Desperateness': The Social Construction
    of Infertility in Popular Representations of New
    Reproductive Technologies   200
    Sarah Franklin

Bibliography   230

Index   250

List of Figures

3.1 Citation analysis: Robert G. Edwards, 1975–86, rate of citation   63

3.2 Citation analysis: Robert G. Edwards, 1975–86, impact factor of journals   65

Foreword

The British Sociological Association annual conference on science, technology and society, held at Leeds in 1987, attracted some 100 papers on a wide variety of topics. All, however, had the question of the social relations of science and technology at their centre. In this respect, they more than fulfilled the expectations that had emerged in the planning of the meeting.

The conference had been designed to draw together research being conducted in different, and sometimes disparate, quarters. To this end, the headings under which discussion took place were suitably inclusive. In the event discussion appeared to return to some key issues: technological risks and hazards, the state and legal frameworks regulating technology, the role of the mass media and of experts. In addition, a number of fundamental conceptual debates recurred: what are the boundaries between nature and society, between, for example, biology and social relations, between the 'given' and the culturally constructed? More broadly, the whole issue of the dialectic between social relations and innovation ran throughout the conference. In addition, there was a range of questions about the origins of innovation: why do certain technologies absorb the energies of scientists and engineers and not others, and how are those technologies shaped by the societies that spawn them?

When, as organisers of this conference, we discovered that we had been presented with a cluster of contributions on a particular set of technological innovations and relations which explored this range of issues, it seemed something of a gift from the gods (or goddesses). The papers on reproductive technologies proved remarkable in seeming to reflect these concerns in a particularly intense way. The new reproductive technologies emerged as a rich case study – exemplar even – of what the sociology of science and technology is, properly conceived, and what it might achieve. It seemed wise not to let pass the opportunity of presenting this to a wider public.

The fact that reproductive technologies emerged as a key topic was the result of several factors. First of all, widespread interest in the topic was not surprising given the fact that there had been considerable technological innovation in the field since the 1970s. Of course, such developments, in turn, invite investigations and call out for social explanations. Second, there has been much public attention given to these developments. The contributors to this volume are responding to this, as well as to the innovations themselves.

Moreover, these technologies matter because they are the crux of a number of social issues in Western societies. This is the third reason why they capture the imagination of sociologists and become the objects of their investigation. Michelle Stanworth argues that current controversies over sexuality, parenthood, reproduction and the family lie behind the concern about these technologies. We would add to this that these technologies also intersect with recent debates about the power, role and regulation of expertise – particularly medical and scientific expertise (Stanworth, 1987a). Indeed, in Britain at least, some of the most heated public controversies about experts have centred on their role in regulating and 'policing' sexuality, parenthood and the family. In this respect, the debates about the investigation and handling of the sexual abuse of children (exemplified in the recent Cleveland cases) and those about reproductive technologies have much in common. This focus on expertise and the examination of various facets of the power and position of scientific and medical experts is at the core of this volume. (As, indeed, it is that of its companion volume, Varcoe *et al.*, *Deciphering Science and Technology*, London, Macmillan, 1990.)

So, this book was by no means a gift of the gods or goddesses. True to our sociological colours, we would insist that it is the product of complex social forces. Perhaps that is also why it was through these studies that the issues discussed at the conference came to be focused most completely. Energy had been invested. And so, the various issues, dimensions and fields (medicine, gender issues, the media, state and social control) all found treatment. All these aspects had been covered. And so, the new reproductive technologies appeared as a model. In this 'single' technology the various pieces of our original jigsaw seemed to fall into place.

Innovation is taking place at a rapid rate in the reproductive field. It is quite clear that a variety of ethical questions – of disclosure, of the ethics of scientific research, etc. – have arisen. Definitive or consensual answers have not yet been found. A complex 'politics' of concern and lack of it, is being enacted. Certainly legal and administrative arrangements have yet to be finalised. We believe that the sociologist, like the philosopher, the medical scientist, the lawyer, as well as those who are directly involved, has a distinctive contribution to make to the unfolding debate. Clarifying and analysing the social processes surrounding *in vitro* fertilisation and other techniques is a necessary counterweight to certain moral and even 'purely logical' or legal analyses, not least because of its reflexivity: its attention to where the sociological analyst stands in the processes under examination. More important, however, is the attention given to experience through the careful recording of subjects' thoughts and feelings, which are too often imputed or inferred from abstract principles. We would maintain that the detailed ethnography, as well as the bringing to bear of the resources and traditions of social research, is, in this respect, of no little consequence.

In these and other respects this volume represents our hopes for what sociology can offer in the current dilemmas about reproductive technologies and our sense of the possibilities for the whole field of the sociology of technology.

MAUREEN MCNEIL, *Birmingham*
IAN VARCOE, *Leeds*
STEVEN YEARLEY, *Belfast*

Notes on the Contributors

Annette Burfoot is a PhD research student with the Science Policy Research Unit at the University of Sussex. Her research project, 'The Politics of Innovation', examines the socio-economics of the new reproductive technologies.

Christine Crowe is completing her doctoral thesis in sociology at the University of New South Wales, Australia. She has conducted research on the development of *in vitro* fertilisation and embryo research in both Australia and the United Kingdom. She is a member of FINRRAGE (Feminist International Network of Resistance to Reproductive and Genetic Engineering).

Sarah Franklin is a research student in cultural studies at the University of Birmingham. Her previous work was in anthropology and women's studies, and she is currently completing an ethnographic study of women's experiences of new reproductive technologies.

Erica Haimes is a lecturer in sociology at Stirling University. She is co-author, with Noel Timms, of *Adoption, Identity and Social Policy* (1985). Her current research is an investigation of the social construction of families through policy-making on the new reproductive technologies.

Maureen McNeil is a lecturer in the Cultural Studies Department of the University of Birmingham. She is the author of *Under the Banner of Science: Erasmus Darwin and His Age* (1987) and editor of *Gender and Expertise* (1987). Her research and teaching are centred on (but not restricted to) science, technology and popular culture, and gender relations and science and technology.

Frances V. Price is a Senior Research Associate in the Child Care and Development Group, Department of Paediactrics and Social and Political Sciences Committee of the University of Cambridge. She is currently writing up a study involving the parents of triplets, quadruplets and higher-order multiple birth children born in the United Kingdom (which is one of a series of integrated studies of the same population). She is also involved in the first phase of the ESRC research initiative 'The Public Understanding of Science', in which her specific research concern is diagnostic obstetric ultrasonography.

Deborah Lynn Steinberg is co-editor, with Patricia Spallone, of *Made to Order: The Myth of Reproductive and Genetic Progress* (1987). She has been active in the Women's Reproductive Rights Movement for many years and has been a researcher in the Women Health and Reproductive Rights Information Centre in London. She has published and spoken widely about the subject of reproductive and genetic engineering. She is currently working on her doctoral thesis at the Department of Cultural Studies, University of Birmingham.

Edward Yoxen worked in the Department of Science and Technology Policy at the University of Manchester from 1976 to 1988. There he taught courses on the history and politics of modern biology. He is the author of *The Gene Business* (1983) and *Unnatural Selection?* (1986). He now works on forecasting the future of health care at the Centre for the Exploitation of Science and Technology, Manchester.

1 Reproductive Technologies: A New Terrain for the Sociology of Technology

Maureen McNeil

It is an established assumption within some quarters of the sociology of technology (see Touraine, 1971; Bell, 1973; Gorz, 1982) that Western societies are becoming 'post-industrial' or 'leisure' societies. Such claims are based, to some degree, on assessments of the social implications of a particular set of technological changes in the mode of production. The essays in this book are concerned with a different set of transformations in technology – those in the domain of human reproduction. Some would say that the technological innovations in this realm in recent years have constituted a 'reproductive revolution', ushering in a new era which might be labelled 'the age of the test-tube-baby' or 'the age of biotechnology'. My own sense of the continuities in the history of medical and scientific interventions into reproduction make me cautious about such judgements.[1] In any case, it is useful to situate this collection of essays alongside the controversies about the 'post-industrial' or 'leisure' society. This can help to illustrate the project of this book and to locate it within the sociology of technology more generally.

Comparisons with studies of post-industrialism are used in the first part of this chapter to help sketch the features of this relatively new field of study – the sociology of reproductive technologies. The second part considers some of the distinctive problems encountered by those working in this field. The third and final section introduces the specific content of this volume.

The Future

It is common in the Western world to link technology and the future. Technology is for us a powerful signifier of novelty, of progress, of 'the new'. As we are reminded over and over again by advertisers, to invest in technology is to invest in the future. Being associated with

1

the latest model of transport hardware (car, plane or even high-speed train) suggests that we are 'forward looking' – orientated towards the future. High-technology purchases promise to take us into the twenty-first century.

We live in a culture in which a major source of our fascination with technological innovations is their promise of an imaginative and material link to the future. For example, the entire genre of science fiction as a cultural form has evolved from this association.[2] This facet of the cultural perception of technology draws upon the myths of progress which so preponderate in Western science generally (Pollard, 1968; Whitehead, 1975). In turn, this set of future associations contributes to technological determinism – the popular belief that technology changes and determines the features of our lives. This view lies behind the cultivation of the expectation that we never just purchase a piece of technology – we are buying a transformed life.

Social studies of technology have, to some extent, mirrored this social pattern. It is no coincidence that perhaps one of the major schools of 'future studies' within sociology grew out of interpretations of the patterns of technological innovation from the 1960s onwards. The view that we were living in a 'post-industrial' society was linked by some commentators to the assessment that technological change had become qualitatively and quantitatively sufficient to transform the nature of work and economic lives in the Western world (for example, see Gorz, 1982).[3] The thesis proposed that our society was evolving into 'one in which the dominant activity is not the production of goods but the production of services, and in which knowledge, rather than capital or labour, is the key resource' (MacKenzie and Wajcman, 1985, p. 25). Although there were variations amongst the positions taken by commentators, in general, the popular link between technological innovation and the future was intensified and given a sociological gloss through this thesis.

Here was the academic equivalent of the popular assumption that buying a piece of technology was opening the way to a future-orientated life-style. In this sense, post-industrialism was a fitting ideological commentary on contemporary consumerism: it confirmed what the consumer was expected to believe: that technology was going to transform our lives dramatically and definitively. In this sense, it was very technologically determinist.

Of course, in this and other instances, sociologists of technology are themselves responding to social changes in which they themselves, as well as the technologies they study, must be located. For example, it could be argued that, as a result of recent changes in reproductive technologies, they are bearing witness to a profound alteration in the definition and understanding of technology. Nevertheless, social researchers are not merely passive recorders; they are active contributors to the social processes with which they are concerned. This means that they themselves help to shape the wider social understandings of, and attitudes towards, technology.

I have noted that this association of new technologies with the future is commonplace in contemporary Western culture. In the case of reproductive technologies, the link between technology and the future has a double valency. The purpose of these technologies is quite literally to realise the biological future, the next generation. It is this double association with the future – technological and generational – which might account for some of the popular interest in them. In recent years, new reproductive technologies have often been represented in the popular media as the leading edge of scientific and technological development. This fascination with the technologies of inner space seems to have usurped the appeal of technologies of outer space in the popular imagination.

Production and Reproduction: the Politics of Location
Thus, social researchers concerned either with the 'post-industrial' society or with recent innovations in reproductive technologies are dealing with the link between technologies and the future. In both cases, the term 'revolution' slips easily off the tongue and popular predictions of dramatic changes in our modes of life abound. However there are significant differences between the two fields, in terms of both content and focus. The main focus for many theorists of post-industrialism (Touraine, 1971; Gorz, 1982) or the leisure society was the displacement of the (predominantly male) factory worker because of innovations in production (MacKenzie and Wajcman, 1985, p. 5). In contrast, the innovations in reproductive technologies are mainly directed towards women within their child-bearing years, and this book, like much of the research in this field is, for the most part (though not exclusively), concerned with them.

It will be obvious to the readers of this volume that there are also notable analytical differences between the recent research on reproductive technologies and that of the post-industrial theorists. Generally the authors in this collection have tried to avoid formulations which see technological innovations as *causing* a new form of society. This is largely owing to the influence of a body of detailed research –

mainly by feminists – in the history of obstetrics and gynaecology (see especially Ehrenreich and English, 1976a; Ehrenreich and English, 1976b; Gordon, 1977; Ehrenreich and English, 1979). This work has heightened awareness of the continuities between recent innovations and more long-term trends in social relations (particularly concerning gender) in these bio-medical fields. In general, such historical sensitivity was not so well developed amongst post-industrial commentators and this may have been a factor which drew some of them into forms of technological determinism (MacKenzie and Wajcman, 1985, pp. 4–5).

In contrast, the best feminist history and sociology of science, technology and medicine has disavowed technological determinism in another respect. The push within it has been towards the identification of agency. This has involved both the delineation of the role of experts and the tracing of patterns of female opposition and resistance.

It is also striking that the researchers contributing to this book are far from sanguine about the changes they are investigating. By way of contrast, there was more optimism amongst post-industrial theorists about implications of technological change. This may reflect the fact that some of the former group, like many other contemporary students of the social dimensions of technological change, have been swayed by the ecology and anti-nuclear movements, particularly in the wake of disasters such as Bhopal and Chernobyl. Secondly, and probably more significantly, virtually all of the contributors to this volume have been alerted by feminism to the suspect pedigree of science and technology in mediating power relations between men and women. Science and technology, as they are well aware and as has now been well documented, have been major tools of patriarchal domination (Easlea, 1980; 1981; Sayers, 1982; Harding, 1986).

As suggested above, sociologists since the 1960s have been speculating about the future of manual labour. Given their own position in the division of labour, it is perhaps not surprising that some of them were not pessimistic about the displacement (literally, and in terms of social and political function) of such workers. The prediction that society was being transformed into 'one in which . . . knowledge, rather than capital or labour is the key resource' (MacKenzie and Wajcman, 1985, p. 25) was unlikely to disturb them.

Whereas much of this work was undertaken by men, it is significant that a great deal of the research in the sociology of reproductive technologies field has been undertaken by women – a fact reflected in

the list of contributors to this book. In writing about medical practices surrounding conception and birth, women investigating reproductive technologies are entering a world which may easily include
them. In investigating reproductive technologies, they are not re-
searching some distant others, but often see themselves as (or,
indeed, are experiencing themselves to be) part of the group under
scrutiny.[4] In addition, a number of the researchers working in this
field have been active in various campaigns on behalf of women's
reproductive rights. These factors have contributed to their scepticism about the benevolence of technological change. Yet, none of
this should be taken as an indication that only women should be
concerned with the new reproductive technologies.

From Technologies of Production to Technologies of Reproduction
Some claims that Western societies are becoming leisure or post-
industrial societies are based on the notion that technologies of
production determine the nature of society. Like many of their
Marxist predecessors, post-industrial theorists felt that social analysts
should be watching technological changes as the key feature of the
mode of production. In contrast with Marxists, however, they argued
that, henceforth, it would be the production of services and knowledge, rather than goods, which would dominate.

The post-industrial thesis fitted easily into the conventional history
and sociology of technology which has been constructed primarily as
the study of technologies of production. This has been true from Karl
Marx to Lewis Mumford, through to Harry Braverman and more
recent labour process analysts. Since these three figures have probably been the most influential theorists in the social study of technology, much of the theoretical framework for this field of sociological research has been developed in relation to technologies of
production. This state of the art is reflected in a recent anthology in
which there are as many articles in the section on 'the technology of
production' as there are in the two other sections (on domestic and
military technologies) combined (MacKenzie and Wajcman, 1985;
see also Bijker, Hughes and Pinch, 1987).

The sociology of technology has not only been characteristically
linked to production, it has also been identified with the study of paid
employment in the public realm.[5] This precluded much attention to
the labour or technologies of reproduction (including biological
reproduction, and the production and consumption which occurs in
the home). These trends have been attributed to 'the gender bias of

both the sociology of work and the history of technology' (MacKenzie and Wajcman, 1985, p. 174). As this quotation suggests, the orientation of much of the sociological analysis of technology has been towards production, paid labour and the public sphere. This has gone hand-in-hand with the neglect of gender relations. The result has been that aspects of women's relationship to technology have been denied or ignored. So, for example, knitting (MacKenzie and Wajcman, 1985, p. 22), the baby bottle (Cowan, 1979, p. 52) and hairdressing (Linn, 1987, p. 134) have been pretty much excluded from the history and sociology of technology. However, this is not just a matter of women's absence or of inattention to 'their' technologies. The exclusion of gender relationships from historical and sociological studies of technology impoverished such work. Amongst the 'founding fathers' (Marx, Mumford, Braverman) only Harry Braverman brought them under scrutiny in his examination of the technological transformations taking place in the modern office (see Braverman, 1974). Moreover, Braverman by no means made gender relations a primary element in his studies and there are profound limitations in his research in this respect (see Barker and Downing, 1980).

The only exception was the study of domestic technologies which began over twenty years ago, and has burgeoned since the late 1970s (see especially Ravetz, 1965; Cowan, 1979; 1983; Zimmerman 1983, pp. 77–144; Cowan, 1980; Davidson, 1986). Such research has challenged the main orientation towards paid, productive labour in the public domain within the sociology of technology.[6] In some cases there have been adaptations of established sociological analyses of paid work to accommodate domestic technologies. In others there have been new frameworks constructed to interpret such technologies and corresponding social relations.

More recently, winds of change have been blowing in this field from a number of directions. Gender has been definitively placed on the agenda by those constructing new frameworks for interpreting technology in Western societies (Cowan, 1979; Merchant, 1980; Cockburn, 1981). Cynthia Cockburn's insightful reconstruction of Mumford's history of technology brought attention to the key role of technology in the reproduction of sexual divisions (Cockburn, 1981). Her study of the print industry showed convincingly that technology mediates gender relations even in single-sex workplaces (Cockburn, 1983). Her focus has been on technology as crucial, not only to the power relations between employer and employee, but also to those between men and women. Hence, the genderless perspectives of the 'founding fathers' of the social studies of technology have been dislodged or, at least, challenged.

Likewise, there has been a shift from investigations of the 'public' domain of technologies associated with paid employment to the more 'private' technologies of the domestic sphere. Certainly students of the sociology of technology will increasingly have to come to grips with home computers, videos and other 'personal', domestic technologies, and their gender relations. In this sense, the topic of this book – reproductive technologies – is at the centre of a number of shifts within the sociology of technology.

This is not to say that the sociology of reproductive technology has appeared *ex nihilo* in the 1980s. Demography and population studies are well-established fields of social research. In addition, general histories of contraception (including Himes, 1970) have been available for some time. Some histories of contraceptive practices and abortion (including McLaren, 1984) have given attention to the way technologies fit into these accounts. But feminists have transformed research on the prevention of reproduction, by highlighting the power relations such practices mediate (see Gordon, 1977; Greenwood and King, 1981; Petchesky, 1986). In its most sophisticated forms, as in Rosalind Petchesky's *Abortion and Woman's Choice* (1986), feminist analysis has opened up what appear as strictly technical issues to show their full social and political significance.

The investigation of the management of labour and childbirth has constituted another prominent thread of feminist interpretations of the history of science and technology. The tracing of the attacks on midwifery and the growing ascendancy of, mainly, male doctors in this domain has provided the background for much of the current work on technological interventions into labour and childbirth (Ehrenreich and English, 1976b; Oakley, 1976; Donnison, 1977; Ehrenreich and English, 1979; Easlea, 1980). Ann Oakley's studies of pregnancy and childbirth in contemporary Britain have appeared simultaneously with much of this historical work. They have influenced both contemporary research and wider public discussions (Oakley, 1976; 1979; 1980; 1981a; 1984). Built upon a base of empirical investigation and personal experience, this research also challenged some assumptions about the subjective–objective divide, thereby, once again, questioning the researcher's role (see note 4; Oakley 1981b). There have been a number of other explorations of the management of labour and childbirth with similar orientations to that of Oakley (Brighton Women and Science Group, 1980; Roberts,

1981b; Rakusen and Davidson, 1982; Rothman, 1987). Most of these have given considerable attention to the role of technological innovation in women's changing experiences of pregnancy and childbirth.

In addition, there has been continuity between sociological research and particular campaigns for women's control of labour and childbirth. Sheila Kitzinger's work, as a campaigner for more 'natural childbirth' is a case in point (Kitzinger, 1987). This is also true of the struggles of some female practitioners against the increasing reliance on high-technology medicine in antenatal care and deliveries (see Harrison, 1982; Savage, 1986). Once again, feminist investigations in this field have challenged conventional boundaries dividing research, the personal and the political.

It is only recently that social studies of technology have addressed the full range of reproductive technologies. As recently as 1985, social research on reproductive technologies was referred to in a chapter entitled 'Other Areas of Study', rather than in a substantive section of a survey of social studies of technology (MacKenzie and Wajcman, 1985, pp. 305–7). In this respect, the present book is a contribution to a relatively new, but growing, field within social studies of technology. During the last few years there have been some important feminist accounts of the new reproductive technologies (Arditti, Duelli Klein and Minden, 1984b; Corea, 1985; Corea, Duelli Klein *et al.*, 1985; Stanworth, 1987c; Spallone and Steinberg, 1987). These books have all, in somewhat different ways, surveyed the field and range of reproductive technologies and identified their significance to patriarchal social relations. They were important in focusing attention, not on the technology *per se*, but on the sexual politics in which it was embedded. In this sense they have drawn upon, and been complementary to, more general studies of the politics of reproduction (Daly, 1979; O'Brien, 1981; Homans, 1985).

Recently, there has been some attempt to make distinctions within the field of reproductive technologies by emphasising the specific nature of each technology and the differing positions of women in relationship to them. Most notably, Michelle Stanworth frames the collection of articles she has edited by arguing that these two sets of differences are fundamental to understanding reproductive technologies (Stanworth, 1987b, p. 3). There has been no consensus on this issue amongst the many researchers in this area, and the contributors to the present volume are no exception. My own position would be to recognise specificity, while maintaining that we must not lose sight of the connections either amongst the technologies or amongst women's experiences of them. Many of the articles in this book begin with a particular technology in a manner that recognises its specificity while locating it within the broader context in which these technologies are interrelated. For example, Frances Price shows how the use of ultrasonography has become not only a technology of antenatal care, but also of infertility 'treatment' (two of Stanworth's discrete categories of reproductive technologies) (Stanworth, 1987b, pp. 10–11). In all cases, the situation of individual women is related to the broader framework of patriarchal social relations.

Thus far my concern has been to show how studies of reproductive technologies relate to the broader field of social studies of technology as a whole. I want to turn my attention now to the special problems faced by those working on these particular technologies.

Individualism and Choice

One reason the investigation of the social dimensions of reproductive technologies proves so difficult is that, in the Western industrial world, their realm of operation is associated with the paramount spheres of perceived individuality and privacy – sexuality and the family. Some of the concern about the new reproductive technologies undoubtedly results from the prospect of technologies impinging on what have been regarded as very private domains. Heterosexual intercourse is 'private' in three ways: sexually, in its connections with procreation, and with ownership (patriarchal property rights).

In reality, heterosexual reproduction has never been removed from the public sphere. The individual and the social, the private and the public are not easily separable. Moreover, as Rosalind Petchesky argues, there is something deeply biologistic about the notion that our individuality is posited at conception (Petchesky, 1986, pp. 342–6). This view denies the importance of long-term social processes which form the individual. And yet, in the contemporary Western world, the notion that heterosexual reproduction is a private, very personal matter and a primary source of individuality has considerable purchase.

Despite its limitations, the language of individual rights, particularly in matters relating to women's control over their bodies, has often been employed by feminists. 'A woman's right to choose' was used in both Britain and America in the 1970s as the slogan for abortion rights campaigns (Greenwood and Young, 1976; Petchesky, 1986). Subsequently, it came to be associated with a much wider range of claims for women's reproductive freedoms. Demands for individual rights have played an important role in the women's movement in the West, as they had in the American civil rights movement. Implicitly, in using such a slogan, feminists were calling, and continue to call, the bluff of many of their opponents. For, although right-wing theorists and politicians consistently applaud and support a politics of individual rights, they, together with many doctors and scientists, deny its validity in relationship to women's reproductive freedoms.

Nevertheless, there has always been some ambivalence within feminism about the use of the language of rights. So, on the one hand, as suggested above, the assertion of a woman's right to choose was a radical rallying call. On the other hand, the slogan has been taken, by some, as an endorsement for an exclusively liberal, individualistic approach to issues of reproduction. The language of rights is, after all, the language of bourgeois liberalism. As such, it can reinforce rather than transform the established social order (Petchesky, 1986, p. 7). There is potentially something asocial about the focus on '*a woman*'s right to choose'. It begs the questions of *who* has the right to such choices, thereby ignoring how race, class and sexual orientation influence the possibility of choice.

The language of individual choice also infuses the language of consumerism. In this sense, situating reproductive rights and technologies within a framework of individual choice makes it easier to regard them as consumer goods (Overall, 1987, p. 170). Such constructions are particularly evident with new reproductive technologies such as *in vitro* fertilisation. As in all consumerist frameworks, choice is restricted to what the market produces in the way of goods and services. As in most Western markets, these are designed mainly by white, middle-class men. With the development of reproductive technologies, women's reproductive rights have increasingly been presented as involving the purchase of consumer goods or services; that is, they have been increasingly 'commodified'.

Recently feminists have confronted some of the limitations in such a conceptual foundation for their struggles for reproductive freedoms. Essentially this has amounted to a recognition of the difference between choice and freedom.[7] I have already alluded to the growing awareness of the political origins and limitations of this conceptual framework. Like much in the bourgeois world, this framework has been identified with illusions and links to the 'future promise' of technology mentioned previously. So, some analysts have demonstrated how the promise of enhanced choice may indeed disguise restrictions (Rowland, 1985; Overall, 1987, p. 198). Of course, this is particularly relevant in relation to the new technologies. For example, as some commentators have pointed out, 'developments' in treatments for infertility may make it difficult for some women to accept their childlessness and stop seeking treatment (Pfeffer and Woollett, 1983).[8]

In addition, there have been attempts to examine the substance of the slogan 'a woman's right to choose'. While it was important for Adrienne Rich, in her extremely influential *Of Woman Born* (first published in 1976), to turn this phrase into a rallying call for increased choice for women in the field of reproduction, it was hard to know precisely what was being called for (Overall, 1987, p. 198; see also Crowe, 1987). There have been many reassessments of the phrase 'reproductive choice' (see Rothman, 1984; Overall, 1987, pp. 124, 198). As these reflections have emphasised, quantitative increases in the number of options open to women do not necessarily guarantee the qualitative improvement of their lives. Making choices, as Barbara Katz Rothman argues, involves stresses and costs (Rothman, 1986).

There has also been a much stronger sense of the social and political location of all choices: 'The concept of choice cannot operate outside of [*sic*] the social structures in which it is embedded'. This means that: 'Our actions are constrained and shaped by the forces of economics, social ideology, personal psychology, and power structures' (Corea *et al.*, 1987, p. 7). But feminists have also become aware that there is differential access to choices 'depending on a woman's race, class, age, marital status, sexuality, religion, culture, and sometimes disability' (Corea *et al.*, 1987, p. 8). Michelle Stanworth questions another dimension of the concept – its presumption about the idealistic, asocial nature of knowledge: 'even our notions of what is "satisfactory"', she suggests, 'would be shaped partly by our knowledge of existing or potential alternatives' (Stanworth, 1987a, p. 12). These elaborations make it clear that an individual woman cannot be idealistically abstracted or deterministically separated from her social setting.

Many feminists have incorporated long-standing reservations about the concept of choice into their reflections on reproduction. Barbara Katz Rothman suggests that the prospect of individual choice implies individual responsibility, and some women, in some circumstances, might not want to choose, know, and/or control aspects of their reproductive capacities. In this sense, to adopt such a framework is to reinforce and re-emphasise certain features of the characteristic attitude of Western science in relationship to the body, particularly the female body. In other words, that it is to be disciplined and controlled for the use of others, particularly men. Likewise, other feminists have shown that, in our culture, 'Women lose control rather than gain choice' (Corea *et al.*, 1987, p. 7; Rowland, 1987, p. 80). They have documented the way in which, under the guise of being given more choice, women are becoming subject to greater medical control and that there is no straight play-off between choice and control.

It has also been pointed out that rights are far too easily translated into responsibilities, or imperatives. Petchesky, for instance, warns that the absolute assertion of women's rights to reproductive choice can be turned back against them to reinforce the view that this is their special 'biologically destined' province and mission (Petchesky, 1986, p. 7). In the hands of some doctors, scientists and politicians, it is relatively easy for alleged concern for what women want to become the justification for 'antifeminist policies' (Overall, 1987, p. 202; see also Crowe, Price, Steinberg in this volume).

Finally, some feminists have posed some serious questions about the individualism of the language of reproductive choices. Should women in the Western world have the 'right' to a child 'of their own flesh and blood' in any circumstances? For example, are they justified in expressing this right through the use of drugs provided by companies which are implicated in the compulsory sterilisation of women in Third World countries (Mies, 1987, p. 43)? Posing such questions not only highlights the individualistic and idealistic basis of the language of choice, but also its Western, commercialised myopia.

In short, the social researcher comes up against the tightly woven fabric of the individualism in which reproductive technologies are located. Here I am borrowing Jan Zimmerman's metaphor when she refers to these technologies being 'dressed in the silken folds of "individual rights"' (Zimmerman, 1986, p. 27). This is encountered as both a conceptual and practical problem for researchers. To undertake investigations of such technologies requires the challenging of the conventions about them, insisting on their social nature. But, it can also involve, in the course of the research, stepping into what are often regarded as private domains.

The political implications of the recent feminist questioning about the framework of 'reproductive choices' are often contradictory (see Zimmerman, 1986, p. 24). Nevertheless, as I have shown, addressing this framework of individual choice has cleared the way for more comprehensive social analyses of reproduction and its technologies in the contemporary West.

The Problems of Biology

Opening up the social dimensions of contemporary reproductive technologies brings us to the thorny problem of what is meant by biology. The problem begins as an epistemological and linguistic one. In common usage, the term biology refers *both* to the study or science of the human body *and* to its structure and functions. In short, the term denotes both the science and its object of study. This is in significant contrast to the term 'sociology', for example, which refers to the systematic study of the clearly discrete object – society. This use of the term 'biology' makes it difficult to separate ontology from epistemology when it comes to human bodies. This double significance of the term can be confusing and it often deters us from thinking about the social construction of biological knowledge.[9]

Likewise it is precisely this difficulty which has plagued women in their interactions with medical and biological experts. On the one hand, there has been a sustained effort to bring attention to women's medical needs – to have their bodies taken seriously. However, often the only way of voicing these has been through the language and conceptual frameworks provided by the biomedical sciences themselves.[10] This is the hidden crux of the history of feminist *Biological Politics* as documented by Janet Sayers (1982). She is quite right to insist that women have needed and continue to need to take their bodies seriously. Hence, one-half of her book documents instances of feminist politics which have been based on claims about the functions (or malfunctions) of women's bodies. The other half is devoted to feminist challenges to scientific and medical expertise and to the constraints implicit in the ways in which the sciences have constructed, defined and dictated treatments of women's bodies. In any particular instance, it is very difficult to prise open the distinction between *women*'s biology, in the sense of the actual nature of women's bodies, and *scientific* biology, in the sense of the socially-constructed and value-laden knowledge systems of the scientific experts who describe, diagnose and treat women (Overall, 1987, p. 5).

As Michelle Stanworth has suggested, the so-called new reproductive technologies with which this book is concerned have made us more aware of the often obscured social dimensions of biology (Stanworth, 1987b, p. 2). However, there has certainly been no automatic increase in the awareness of the social construction of reproduction with recent technological innovation. Indeed, there continues to be considerable confusion about the realm of reproduction. For example, many of the 'new' reproductive technologies (for example, some forms of infertility treatment) are by no means new (Duelli Klein, 1985). Moreover, my preceding analysis would suggest that there are no 'biological givens' easily separable from the social realm. Similarly, the term 'technology' has often been used rather imprecisely to include practices such as surrogacy and self-insemination that, in some instances, require virtually no technology.

Some of these problems are illustrated when Stanworth goes on to elaborate her point: 'in practices such as surrogacy, the gulf between "biological motherhood" and "social motherhood" is vividly exposed, provoking new personal and legal choices; fewer and fewer female and male infertilities are now "final" in the physiological sense; fewer genetic abnormalities are undetectable'. She describes this as 'altering the boundaries between the biological and the social' (Stanworth, 1987b, p. 2). Indeed, her whole analysis is premised on the notion that there are definite boundaries between the biological and the social. But, 'infertilities' and 'genetic abnormalities' are not only biological states, they are also social categories. There must be some assessment about what conditions are undesirable before any judgement can be made about what constitutes a 'genetic abnormality'.[11] As has been indicated above, this field is particularly thorny precisely because the social element cannot be neatly sifted out of biology.

This book tackles these issues in presenting a series of case studies of contemporary reproductive science and technology. The authors explore diverse facets of one particular focus of these technologies – infertility. Infertility is at the centre of an elaborate set of social relations, some of which are sketched in this volume. In considering it we are dealing with a concrete instance of the difficulties I have been discussing. Implicated in the definition and diagnosis of this medical condition is a whole set of social conditions, including the beliefs and values which sustain the 'need' for a baby (Overall, 1987, pp. 160–72, 197–211) in our society, which are often ignored in the attention given to recent technological innovations. In dealing with infertility, women are facing the socially sustained need for a baby, as well as having to cope with a condition of their bodies. (Indeed, as Deborah Lynn Steinberg points out in Chapter 4, because the label 'infertile' is often used in relationship to couples, rather than women specifically, there may not even be any 'condition' of a woman's body with which to deal.)

Recently there have been key social and political movements which have focused on the body. The women's health movement has probably been the most important influence, as a crucial conscious-ness raiser for many women in Europe and America (McNeil, 1987a, pp. 23–8; O'Sullivan, 1987). *Our Bodies Ourselves*, which first appeared in the USA in 1971 and which subsequently was translated into many languages, was the key text of this movement (Boston Women's Health Collective, 1978). It both contributed to, and reflected a growing bodily awareness amongst women in the Western world. Women's movement analyses of, and campaigns against, male violence have also been important in this respect (see Hanmer and Maynard, 1987; Hanmer and Saunders, 1984; Rhodes and McNeill, 1985).

In addition, the ecology movement and the increasing general awareness of health issues (not to mention their commercialisation) have also been influential. Conceptually, the broadening of the definition of materialism beyond its original Marxist economistic parameters (see Timpanaro, 1980) can also play a role in bringing more attention to the body. Hence, there have been a number of influences drawing social researchers towards work on the body (Turner, 1984).

Perhaps the most significant theoretical figure in this trend has been Michel Foucault. Foucault was particularly interested in the regimes of truth, control, regulation and discipline which have been established around the body (see especially Foucault, 1982; Foucault, 1980a, pp. 55–62; but also Foucault, 1973). Some of his research dealt with the two levels of the regulation of individual bodies and of population generally. One of the attractions of his work has been the fact that it provides a way of discussing biology as a discipline which constructs knowledge of the body. He challenged the notion that there is a set of objects of study for any science which precede the system of knowledge in which they figure (Foucault, 1970; Foucault, 1972; Foucault, 1980b). He thereby addressed himself directly to the nub of the difficulty confronting those investigating biology and the technologies associated with it, deconstructing the accepted bound-aries between the 'biological' and the 'social'; the 'natural' and the 'cultural'. In this book, Sarah Franklin uses and develops Foucault's notion of discourse theory fruitfully to delineate the social conven-tions surrounding accounts of infertility.

A major problem with Foucault's work and that of some of his followers is the fact that it does not take sufficient account of gender. Indeed, some would maintain that it has encouraged too much generalised discussion of regimes of regulation of *the* body, without specifying key differences amongst bodies, belonging differently as they do, to women and men, or black people and white people (Bland, 1981). In contrast, many feminists have demonstrated the ways in which women's bodies have been sites of oppression and resistance (Ehrenreich and English, 1976a; Sayers, 1982; Birke, 1986). Certainly, the full integration of a gender perspective into social research on the body is crucial in the study of reproductive technologies.

Nevertheless, even for those sensitised by feminism to gender relations, there remain certain dangers in the current concern with women's bodies. There is the possibility that the generalised discussion of *the* body will be replaced by a similarly generalised discussion of the social relations of *women*'s bodies without sufficient attention being given to other social divisions (including race and class) amongst women. Also, without an awareness of the peculiar ontological claims implicit in the common use of the term 'biology' as outlined above, biological determinism can easily creep into such analyses. Finally, there is the possibility that such work can simply reinforce the identification of women with nature – again a version of holding together some familiar and problematic dichotomies: for example, women with bodies and nature; men with mind and culture (see Brown and Jordanova, 1981).

The chapters in this volume are situated against this background of the particular problems biology and its associated technologies pose for the social researcher. However, as I have indicated in my rather cursory sketch, there have been some new directions emerging from this field. The political attention given to 'the body' by new social and political movements and the theoretical framework provided by Foucault are instances of these (even if, as I have indicated, they have problems of their own). Although there can be no definitive resolution of the particular difficulties inherent in social research about biological science and technology, the researchers in this volume and elsewhere are beginning to grasp this nettle.

The Media Dimension

There is a third peculiarity of these technologies which also merits consideration and that is the media attention they have received. In this respect, new reproductive technologies have shared the stage

with recent developments in microelectronics. It is instructive to
contrast the more restrained and sober coverage of the latter with
that given to reproductive technologies. This media coverage, it
could be argued, has challenged, or at least should challenge, the
framework for the sociology of technology in a number of respects. It
is important for at least three reasons. First and foremost, it raises the
issue of representations of technology. Second, it requires a methodological shift within the field. And, finally, it involves some fundamental questions about popular culture and technology.

In their investigations of new reproductive technologies contemporary researchers are confronted with social constructions, dissemi-
nated by the popular media, of what these innovations are. Terms
like 'test-tube babies', 'scientific miracle', 'revolution in reproductive
technologies' are representative versions of the social significance of
these innovations. This adds an additional dimension through which
these technologies are socially and culturally mediated. Hence those
working on reproductive technologies are likely to be more exposed
than researchers on other topics in the sociology of technology to
definite media views regarding their topics.

The extensive media coverage surrounding these technologies has
potentially some contradictory implications for those engaged in the
sociological analysis of them. It is difficult to gauge the impact this
has had. For example, the term 'test-tube baby' has slipped into
common parlance and it takes a real effort for analysts to step back
from it and explore its assumptions (see Stanworth, 1987b). Likewise, it is possible for media versions to be encountered as a set of
particular representations of these technologies: for example, the
Sun or 'Panorama's' specific interpretations. This self-consciousness
about representations can contribute to greater sensitivities about the
way in which we constantly 'meet' technologies through representations of them (oral accounts of those engaged with them, written
technical specifications, and so on).[12]

The attention given to the new reproductive technologies in the
media has been complemented by a considerable exposure to pic-
tures of the foetus. This has been characterised as the recent appearance of the foetus in 'full public view' (Overall, 1987, p. 40). Rosalind
Petchesky contends that the picture of the 'de-contextualised' foetus,
that is, images of it seemingly outside the uterus, have been powerful
tools in discouraging concern for women in recent debates about
pregnancy, abortion and related issues (Petchesky, 1987, p. 78).
Even *Marxism Today* used such an image on its front cover (January

1988 issue), while opposing the parliamentary bill (the Alton Bill) which was drawn up to restrict abortion rights in Britain.

It is important to juxtapose Petchesky's argument with the media coverage of the new reproductive technologies in order to clarify an important feature of the contemporary context for social studies in this field. There has been extensive exposure to foetus and baby images in association with reproductive technologies. In some ways, the media and social researchers could be seen as responding to the same stimulus – innovations in reproductive technology. However, it is important to note that one of the results of this encounter has been the media's production of a very specific set of visual images which have, in turn, in some ways influenced sociological investigations in this field.[13]

The skills of the social analyst of technology have been challenged once again by this new field. Sarah Franklin's use of 'discourse' and 'narrative' analysis in this volume is an example of this. Researchers like her have drawn in an exciting and constructive way on theories of representation to enrich the resources of the social studies of technology. In particular, the analysis of visual materials could become more prominent in the sociology of technology. Some earlier work on the visual dimensions of the history of medicine has pioneered similar uses of media studies and of art history (see Mort, 1980). Certainly, it would seem likely that future research on reproductive technologies will have to extend in these directions.

Reproductive technologies and their media exposure have brought sociologists into the world of popular culture. This means that the range of research has to be extended and its nature changed. On the one hand, there is still important work to be done on the world of experts: on the origins of particular artefacts, on experts' practices, procedures and publications (such as the *Lancet*). Annette Burfoot's research on citation indices and Frances Price's on risk assessment in ultrasound are valuable attempts to look at the career structure and practices emerging in connection with the new reproductive technologies. Similarly, Christine Crowe looks at the kinds of experiments undertaken by a major figure in the field of *in vitro* fertilisation (IVF): Robert Edwards. But the social studies of these technologies must not focus only on the scientific and medical communities. To comprehend the social meanings of these technologies, there must be a qualitatitve improvement in the understanding of their role and construction in popular culture. This could involve studying the popular press and women's magazines. It also means that it is important to comprehend not only what Robert Edwards thinks, but also what women undergoing IVF and those reading about it in women's magazines think of multiple births.

In the case of the media dimensions of the new reproductive technologies, I have been elaborating a theme that emerged earlier in my examination of the peculiar problems of individualism and biology facing the sociologist of technology in this field. These problems, I have suggested, are also challenges which have the potential to enrich and enlarge social studies of technology more generally. In the case of each of these problems, I have sketched some new directions which have emerged as they have been confronted. I have also tried to provide what I consider to be crucial background to current work in this field – including the chapters in this volume. I now want to look in more detail at the contents of this book.

This Volume: Immediate Background

In the first two parts of this chapter I have established the context for the following essays by providing my own interpretation of both the features and problems of the sociology of reproductive technologies. I have drawn attention to some of the recent social and political forces which have influenced and, in turn, been influenced by, research on the sociology of technology. In both sections, I have suggested ways in which new work in this field could stretch and transform the parameters of the sociology of technology as a whole. Let us now consider the specific contents of this volume.

Which Reproductive Technologies?
Reproductive technologies have been defined as 'all forms of biomedical intervention and "help" a woman may encounter when she considers having – or not having – a child' (Arditti, Duelli Klein and Minden, 1984a, p. 1). Although I have already acknowledged the fact that it is something of a misnomer, the term 'new' reproductive technologies has been used in this volume to designate a range of innovations (defined as the introduction of new practices or the extension of their use) in this sphere in recent years. These include artificial insemination, *in vitro* fertilisation, amniocentesis, embryo transfer and freezing, ultrasonography, sex pre-selection, gamete intrafallopian transfer, chorionic villus sampling and laparoscopy. (And this is by no means an exhaustive list.) However, the main focus of the following chapter is *in vitro* fertilisation. There are at

least two justifications for this focus: (1) *in vitro* fertilisation is one of the most extensively used and publicised 'new' reproductive technologies, and (2) it provides the basis for other new technological practices (including ultrasonography, laparoscopy, embryo transfer, embryo freezing, and so on).

Although it might have been desirable to have more extensive coverage of the full range of technologies, as suggested, there have been advantages to having a special focus on IVF. However, there is one absence which merits comment. Many collections on reproductive technologies have included articles on surrogacy (see Arditti, Duelli Klein and Minden, 1984b; Stanworth, 1987a). Surrogacy was also a crucial topic considered by the Warnock Committee which was established by the British government to investigate developments in human fertilisation and embryology in 1982 (Warnock, 1985). Few commentators draw attention to the fact that surrogacy, in itself, requires no technological intervention (for a notable exception to this, see Overall, 1987, p. 11). Of course, some feminists have linked surrogacy with the new reproductive technologies because it is identified with changing expectations about motherhood. In addition, there is some justification for considering them together because they involve similar legal problems.

Surrogacy (together with self-insemination) was one of the practices which alarmed members of the Warnock Committee. With a minority dissension, they recommended that it should be outlawed (Warnock, 1985, pp. 42–7, 87–9). In part, the strong response against surrogacy within the Committee reflected the fact that, in its commercialised forms, it was regarded as a form of prostitution and baby-selling. It disturbed established notions of motherhood (Zipper and Sevenhuijsen, 1987). However, the inclusion of surrogacy, without comment, under the label 'reproductive technologies' also tells us much about the power of medical expertise in this domain. The Warnock Committee generally reacted negatively to reproductive practices – including surrogacy and self-insemination – which did not involve the intervention of scientific or medical experts. In other words, 'artificial' modes of reproduction were condoned in so far as they were under the supervision of such experts. Hence, including surrogacy (and, indeed, self-insemination) with the rubric of reproductive technologies suggests the strong push (within the Warnock Committee and elsewhere) to make scientific and medical experts the exclusive regulators of all 'artificial' modes of procreation.

Thus, recent debates in Britain about surrogacy indicate the centrality of medical and scientific expertise to any consideration of contemporary reproductive technologies. This is a main focus of the chapters in this book. The first four contributions explore the emergence of the scientific and medical institutions of the new reproductive technologies, in particular those relating to IVF. The last three move outside the institutions of scientific medicine. However, somewhat predictably, in the examinations of legal institutions and media provided in this volume, medical and scientific experts are shown to be powerful and dominant figures.

The Immediate Focus of this Volume
The chapters in this volume arise from a specific context. Although there is some consideration of the situation in Australia and the United States (and occasional references to European developments), the analyses mainly focus on Britain. In examining reproductive technologies it is imperative to consider their international dimensions. For example, the banning of the use of the dangerous contraceptive injection, Depo Provera, in the USA must be juxtaposed with its export to Third-World countries (Bunkle, 1984). Moreover, as suggested earlier, it is important to see the concern about infertility in the West against the backdrop of increasing population controls in other parts of the world. For this reason, it is appropriate that there have been a number of feminist anthologies on reproductive technologies which have been international in orientation (Arditti, Duelli Klein and Minden, 1984b; Corea *et al.*, 1985; Spallone and Steinberg, 1987). Nevertheless, such international reviews cannot devote much attention to the way particular societies grapple with new reproductive practices. So, there are advantages to be gained from the specificity of the present volume.

The New Reproductive Technologies: Institutionalisation within Scientific Medicine
Chapters 2 and 3 deal with aspects of the careers of the pioneers of IVF and the establishment of this field of technology and scientific knowledge. Chapter 2 provides an account of the way scientific knowledge emerged from the social context of the early practice of IVF. Christine Crowe considers different facets of the careers of pioneers in the development of IVF and how these influenced the forms of the subsequent treatment. Her examination of the concept of 'pre-embryo' is a valuable case-study of the social construction of scientific knowledge in the field of reproductive technologies.

By using citation indices, and by looking at the establishment of professional groupings and evidence of commercialisation, Annette Burfoot documents the emergence of IVF as a new field of medical science. Burfoot's research is situated within the growing literature on male medical hierarchies and on the social control of female reproduction. Her contribution illuminates the professional dimensions of the extended use of new technologies of reproduction. Ultrasound, amniocentesis, Caesarean sections and so on are amongst those techniques which began as unusual practices and have become increasingly commonplace (Spallone and Steinberg, 1987, p. 5).

Chapters 4 and 5 look at what the newly institutionalised practices of IVF involve. Deborah Lynn Steinberg examines the language and conceptual frameworks of IVF practitioners. She shows how the linguistic erasure of women reflects and contributes to their concomitant procedural subordination. This work is part of the documentation of the significant linguistic shifts that have accompanied these technological innovations. Elsewhere, Françoise Laborie has outlined the different meanings of the term 'pregnancy' which have emerged with these developments (Laborie, 1987, p. 49). *The Third Report of the Voluntary Licensing Authority* similarly proffers the following definition of pregnancy (for use in measuring the success rate of IVF), explaining that 'a more precise definition of pregnancy' was required: 'This was defined as the presence of the fetal heart on ultrasound' (VLA, 1988, p. 18). Such definitions focus attention on the achievement of medical experts, on a technical goal, rather than on women's experience of pregnancy. This definition of pregnancy is another example of the linguistic shifts which, as Steinberg demonstrates, make women's experiences invisible.

Frances Price writes, in part, about the relationship between external regulation (or lack of it) and the practices internal to medicine. Her chapter addresses the regulation of uncertainty in the use of two reproductive technologies – ultrasonography and IVF and embryo transfer (ET). She supports her discussion through reference to the double standard which currently exists in Britain, whereby chemical innovations, in contrast to other technological innovations, are subjected to extensive testing prior to their use in treatment. Although she examines two very different technologies – ultrasonography, which has been designated as non-invasive, and IVF and ET, which are invasive technologies – she underlines the uncertainties surrounding both. She highlights a complex picture of the internal dimensions of scientific medicine, including its divisions of labour and the hermetic nature of the doctor–patient relationship, which make the regulation of uncertainty a problematic goal.

The New Reproductive Technologies: Outside the Institutions of Science and Medicine
The remaining chapters in the volume address the question of how other social institutions in Britain have dealt with recent developments in reproductive technology. Erica Haimes explores aspects of the conventions surrounding the reproductive technologies, including the prohibitions surrounding information on donors involved in artificial insemination. Edward Yoxen continues the examination of issues of regulation, looking at the social forces which have inhibited the construction of legal regulations of embryo research. The final chapter looks at media representations of IVF.

The popular image of a 'revolution' in reproductive technologies may discourage researchers from investigating how they relate to other social practices. However, Erica Haimes's chapter draws some interesting comparisons between adoption and IVF regulations. These help to show the social interests at stake in the negotiation of parental rights in relation to IVF. She indicates how the structural, ideological and genetic forms of the nuclear family are challenged and yet revalued through different forms of IVF. The convention of withholding information about the donor she shows to be part of the reinforcement of the ideological hold of traditional nuclear family forms.

In considering the emergence of social concern about embryo research, Edward Yoxen observes a hesitancy to construct legal structures of regulation. His chapter explores the social and political context of the response to embryo research in Britain. He points out that government reaction to such research has been slow. His account exposes the conflicting moral ideologies which have framed this issue in the United Kingdom. He argues that concern about the fate of the embryo in such research has served, to a considerable extent, as a foil for anti-abortion pressure groups.

As indicated above, the media coverage of the new reproductive technologies has been extensive and sensational. Sarah Franklin tries to get behind the images of 'miracle babies' by using discourse and narrative analysis. This enables her to sketch the protection of existing social conventions in the telling of the story of IVF. With the exception of Petchesky's (1987) work on foetal imagery, there has been little detailed work on the popular representation of these technologies. Franklin's essay offers a framework for further research in this field.

Methodologies
Exploration of a variety of research methods and much innovation is required fully to comprehend the social dimensions of contemporary new reproductive technologies. Contributors to this volume have used such tools as discourse and narrative analysis (Franklin), analyses of citation indexes (Burfoot), linguistic analysis (Steinberg), and content analysis (Yoxen). Christine Crowe and Frances Price have used interview and ethnographic materials drawn from their research with women undergoing 'treatment'. This methodological eclecticism is a reflection of the variety and richness of research in this area. In this sense, this book is a very exciting beginning.

A Missing Dimension – Political Economy
It is notable, and deserving of comment, that none of the chapters pursues a political economy perspective. It is clear that we need to know much more about the relationship between genetic engineering and the new reproductive technologies (Minden, 1984; Murphy, 1984; Spallone and Steinberg, 1987). The links between the pharmaceutical industry and new obstetric and gynaecological practices which Burfoot begins to explore in this volume are obviously also crucial. Perhaps more immediately, popular debate about, and official investigations of, the new reproductive technologies, in Britain at least, suggest that there is much to be clarified. For the Warnock Committee and some of the popular press, for example, commercialisation was and is a major issue. (As indicated above, this was one of the sources of the objections to surrogacy.) Yet the terms of reference of that Committee precluded any consideration of the fact that reproductive technologies are already firmly embedded in a complex political economy. The *Warnock Report* and the subsequent reports of the Voluntary Licensing Authority fail to consider the role of the pharmaceutical companies in recent developments. Nor is there anything more than a cursory acknowledgement of the significance of privatised medicine in this sphere (VLA, 1988). This is despite the fact that there are few other areas of medical care in which privatised medicine is utilised so extensively. Overall, there has been little attempt to tackle the more fundamental aspects of the commodification of bodies and of reproduction involved in recent innovations in

reproduction in Britain. As was suggested in the second part of this chapter, both the individualisation of choice and the commodification of these technologies make it difficult to comprehend their significance.

The tone of the chapters in this volume is critical. None of the contributors would want to deny that the birth of a child, facilitated by new technologies, brings considerable joy to some women and men, but they would want to insist that this is only one part of a broader social picture. They themselves are concerned by some of the more neglected features of the panorama associated with the new reproductive technologies. This volume by no means constitutes the final word on the 'new' reproductive technologies. Instead, it provides some fresh perspectives on these, while inviting much more rigorous thinking about them and about the sociology of technology as a whole.

Notes

I am grateful to the following people for their help in the drafting and re-drafting of this chapter: Christine Crowe, Sarah Franklin, John Gabriel, Erica Haimes, Deborah Lynn Steinberg, Ian Varcoe, Steve Yearley.

1. I generally avoid the term 'test-tube baby' because, as some of the contributors to this volume make clear (see, for example, Steinberg), it is profoundly ideological, denying the agency of women in reproduction.
2. Other instances of this connection can be found in feminist work; see particularly the titles of Jan Zimmerman's books (1983; 1986).
3. Many analysts failed to note the very different conditions of 'Third-World' countries and, hence, generalised about global shifts towards post-industrialism. For a useful review of the debates about post-industrialism see Badham, 1984; Kumar, 1986.
4. It is perhaps not insignificant that some of the most interesting work on feminist methodologies in social research has emerged from studies of women's interactions with the medical profession. See Oakley, 1981b; Roberts, 1981b. For broader examinations of the ways in which feminists have challenged some of the conventions regarding objectivity in social research, see Roberts, 1981a; Stanley and Wise, 1983.
5. I am grateful to Ian Varcoe for reminding me that there could be complex debates about which technologies are 'productive'. These might mirror the debates which have been conducted (with particular reference to domestic labour) about which sorts of labour are 'productive'. In this chapter, I have adopted the convention (used by MacKenzie and Wajcman, 1985) of labelling all technologies associated with the production

and distribution of goods as 'productive'. I am also avoiding questions about how comprehensive the use of the term 'reproductive' technology might be. (For example, should it include all technologies associated with health care?)

6. There has been an extensive debate about whether domestic labour is 'productive' or 'unproductive' labour, which is not my main concern here. Many of the contributions to this debate have been assembled in Malos, 1980.

7. Indeed prevalent market philosophies encourage the cultivation of choice of consumer goods, while advocating curtailment of certain kinds of freedoms (of speech and political organisation).

8. There is, of course, a compulsiveness which comes into play in other areas of medical treatment as well (for example, cancer treatment). In other words, within the regimes of contemporary Western medicine, individuals can find it difficult to stop treatment. (I am grateful to Steve Yearley for bringing this point to my attention.) However the compulsiveness surrounding infertility treatment is different in that it does not involve a life-threatening condition.

9. I am grateful to Sarah Franklin for the discussions from which this point emerged.

10. Emily Martin's work is an interesting exception to this, in its attention to the distinctive way in which different groups of women (in her studies, middle- and working-class women) perceive their bodies and construct descriptions of them (Martin, 1987).

11. The designation of socially desirable and undesirable states takes a negative form in eugenics, the 'science' of improving human stock by giving '"the more suitable races or strains of blood a better chance of prevailing speedily over the less suitable"' (Francis Galton, quoted in Kevles, 1986, p. ix). The eugenic dimensions of the 'new' reproductive technologies have been a matter of considerable concern, although this is not a topic handled extensively in the present volume (see Spallone and Steinberg, 1987; especially Spallone, 1987, 177–80).

12. My argument here about technologies and their representations is similar to that made about representations of science by Steve Woolgar (1988).

13. Even feminists have entered into this practice. For example, a recent collection of essays by feminists on reproductive technologies uses an ultrasound image of a human foetus on its cover (see Stanworth, 1987c).

2 Whose Mind Over Whose Matter? Women, *In Vitro* Fertilisation and the Development of Scientific Knowledge
Christine Crowe

Introduction

This chapter is concerned with the development of scientific knowledge as a social activity. Specifically, the recent formulation of scientific knowledge of early cell differentiation represented in the term 'pre-embryo' is investigated. I examine the circumstances giving rise to the perception and articulation of the concept 'pre-embryo', and outline how this particular interpretation of perceived events 'in nature' is being incorporated as knowledge within the scientific community. That is, I examine the social infrastructure which gave rise to the expression and incorporation of this concept. In so doing, I show the connection between particular goals and interests relating to experimentation on embryos derived from women's eggs,[1] and the development of the concept 'pre-embryo' within science.

Concepts do not, of course, present themselves to the researcher already packaged and ready to be employed in scientific explanation. Particular knowledge relating to what are considered to be the 'natural sciences' can be understood as the expression of one particular interpretation of a phenomenon taking place 'in nature', rather than as merely a description of such events. As a social activity, the development of scientific knowledge is a process whereby the activities of communities give meaning and legitimation to newly introduced concepts.

The social setting for the development of scientific knowledge is intrinsic to the practice known as scientific 'research'. Culture is not a 'backdrop' which provides only the historical setting, and which serves to highlight the scientists as *'dramatis personae'*, centre stage in this knowledge creation. It enters into and shapes the research itself.

This chapter examines such issues relating to scientific knowledge through a specific case study. I take as my example the development of what is known as 'embryo research'.[2] Included in this is an investigation of circumstances surrounding the possible legislation in Britain of a fourteen day time-limit for such research, and the coining and institutionalisation of the term 'pre-embryo'.

I begin with an account of the development of *in vitro* fertilisation (IVF). As I illustrate, the development of current IVF practices involves the maturation of many eggs within a woman's body. These practices have brought about the possibility of experimentation on embryos developed from women's eggs. My account begins with a description of current IVF procedures which would confront an individual woman entering such a programme, and is followed by an account of the history of these procedures. In the light of these procedures, I have tried to illustrate the kind of connection that exists between the 'treatment' each woman receives on an IVF programme and the use of women as a group in the development of the techniques. The constitution of IVF as a research area itself, the material for experimentation, methods employed, and criteria upon which judgements are made are culturally specific. Examination of the history of development and legitimation of IVF as a 'research' area may reveal the social forces present at the time of innovation, as well as the values inherent in its design. I then consider how the perception of IVF as being a medical/scientific concern, introduced as a 'treatment for infertility', makes it possible for its practitioners to become the arbiters of values and standards relating to women's reproduction and motherhood.

After showing IVF's primary orientation towards experimentation on embryos derived from women's eggs, I consider the development of the term 'pre-embryo'. I propose that the evolution of this term is indicative of this facilitation of experimentation, and that this imperative has framed IVF and the 'treatment' of infertility. In the second section of the chapter I examine the context of the development of the concept 'pre-embryo'. I suggest that the enunciation of perceived qualitative differences in embryo development between day fourteen and day fifteen after fertilisation (as illustrated in the 'pre-embryo'/embryo distinction) arose as a result of negotiation between interest groups with particular goals and objectives related to embryo research. This negotiation was focused on the decision for a time-limit on embryo research.

IVF: The Technical Procedure

The birth of the first baby born from an egg fertilised *in vitro* took place in Great Britain in 1978. Depending upon research facilities available, the expertise of the practitioners, and legislation pertaining to the procedure, IVF techniques may vary. The technical aspects of the most commonly known IVF procedure, first developed by Robert Edwards and Patrick Steptoe in Britain, involve a woman undergoing superovulation, intensive monitoring of her hormone levels during her menstrual cycle, and a laparoscopic procedure to remove any eggs which may have developed during the cycle.[3]

From the first day of her menstrual cycle a woman undergoing an IVF procedure begins to take tablets of clomiphene citrate, a synthetic hormone,[4] or has injections of organically produced hormones.[5] These hormones stimulate her ovulation, the ripening of several eggs and bursting of follicles, releasing up to twenty-two eggs per IVF cycle (Bruel and Kjaer, 1986). As Renate Klein and Robyn Rowland (Klein and Rowland, 1988) have shown, accounts vary as to the dosage and length of time these drugs are given. It is often recommended that they be taken for five days.[6]

Blood tests may be taken every day to measure a woman's oestrogen level. By measuring the levels of hormones circulating in her body, practitioners may be able to estimate how many eggs are developing. Ultrasound may also be used to monitor the development of her eggs; high-frequency sound waves are bounced off her ovaries and images are transferred to a screen. The size of the developing ovarian follicle may give an indication to the practitioner of when ovulation will take place. A woman may also undergo a pelvic examination to determine the time of her ovulation. Samples of her cervical mucus and tissue from her vaginal wall are taken, examined and assessed. She may have further blood tests to confirm that her eggs are still developing. Practitioners are aiming at precise timing. The eggs must be mature enough, so that they can be fertilised, yet not so mature as to have already left her ovary. The presence of certain hormones detected by blood tests can indicate that a woman is about to ovulate.[7]

Around day thirteen or fourteen of her cycle a woman is admitted to the hospital or clinic in anticipation of undergoing a laparoscopic procedure some time in the following forty-eight hours. Blood samples are taken regularly. Again, monitoring is vital for practitioners as the timing of the laparoscopic procedure (to collect the woman's eggs) must be ascertained. A woman may spontaneously release her own hormone to stimulate ovulation, in which case the laparoscopy will take place at a time dictated by her own cycle rather than being induced by drugs. Practitioners may inject a hormone (HCG – human chorionic gonadotrophin, see note 5) which stimulates her ovulation. The laparoscopic procedure is then scheduled for approximately thirty-five hours later.

As suggested above, the most commonly used IVF procedure involves a laparoscopy. This is a surgical procedure which requires a woman to undergo a general anaesthetic. The surgeon makes an incision in the woman's abdomen, which has been filled with carbon dioxide gas to allow easier access to her internal organs. A long, thin optical tool, a laparoscope, is inserted so that the surgeon can view the woman's ovaries and control the 'collection' of her eggs. When, and if, the surgeon locates any follicles containing mature eggs, a second incision is made in her abdomen below the first; forceps are then used to hold the ovary in place while her eggs are 'collected'. The surgeon then passes a hollow needle through the woman's abdomen and punctures her follicles containing eggs. The follicular fluid containing her eggs is sucked into a syringe and the needle is removed from her abdomen. Any eggs collected are taken to a laboratory for inspection. The laparoscopic procedure takes about thirty minutes.

Corea and Ince have outlined the ways in which 'success' rates at some IVF clinics have been 'managed' (Corea and Ince, 1987, pp. 133–45). Various criteria and definitions have been used to determine 'success rates' of IVF. Definitions of 'pregnancy' and actual 'attempts' at IVF may vary, for example, and give a misleading indication of the chances of woman actually going home with a baby as a result of this procedure. The chances of a woman becoming a biological mother as a result of IVF are 7.4 per cent in Australia and 8.6 per cent in the United Kingdom (Klein and Rowland, 1988; VLA, 1988).[8] Moreover, figures can be misleading even when given in terms of 'live births'. Since, in this case, the number of *live births* rather than women's *deliveries* is cited, the relatively high number of *multiple* births occurring as a result of IVF practices in effect inflates the figures. In one study, for example, 24 per cent of *deliveries* were *multiple* births (Laborie, 1987, pp. 48–57). The chances of an individual woman becoming a biological mother would, in effect, be much less than the 'success' rate claimed by the clinic. In other words, the 'success' rate stated in terms of births rather than deliveries is constructed in relation to the clinic itself, but does not give a woman about to enter an IVF programme an accurate indication of *her* chances of becoming a biological mother as a result of the procedure.

After being aspirated from the ovary, the eggs are inspected in the laboratory. If any are considered suitable for fertilisation, they are placed in an incubator and kept at temperatures and pressures which are thought to approximate conditions within a woman's body. They are kept in a culture medium for five or six hours, approximately the length of time considered necessary for sperm to go through a woman's cervix, uterus and fallopian tube, before fertilisation.

Sperm are prepared by a process of washing and using a centrifuge. This process is designed to replicate in some way the processes taking place during the sperm's passage through the woman's cervix, uterus and fallopian tube. The most 'suitable' sperm are placed in a Petri dish containing eggs. When, and if, any eggs are fertilised they are left in a culture medium for approximately forty-eight hours.

Usually three fertilised eggs, between two and eight cells in development, are placed in the woman's uterus. The surgeon guides a catheter containing the fertilised eggs through her cervix and flushes them into her uterus. The woman usually lies on her back for the next twelve hours. This is thought by practitioners to facilitate fertilisation. She is then released from hospital and goes home to await the outcome of this procedure.

Steps in the Development of IVF

I have described the IVF procedure in considerable detail because an understanding of the intricacies involved can facilitate an appreciation of the kinds of practices at issue. The development of the IVF and Embryo Transfer (ET) procedure by Patrick Steptoe and Robert Edwards in Britain was the culmination of work in two areas of research: genetics and gynaecology. Robert Edwards obtained his first degree in zoology. He later completed his postgraduate studies in genetics at Edinburgh University. During this time he gained knowledge of genetic inheritance, embryology, animal breeding and the evolution and growth of cells. Edwards's doctoral thesis was on the development of haploid embryos in mice.[9] Specifically, he wished to investigate the ways in which mouse embryos would be altered if the sperm used to fertilise their eggs were made inactive. He wished to conduct experiments using embryos resulting from fertilisation where the twenty-three chromosomes from the sperm did not contribute to the development of an embryo.

The procedure for obtaining such embryos required artificial insemination (AI) of female mice at the time of ovulation. Precise timing was required for fertilisation to occur. Edwards wished to facilitate his experimentation by being able to predict when the female mice would be likely to conceive. He injected female mice with hormones to induce ovulation. This was intended to make their reproductive cycles more convenient for experimentation (that is, the mice ovulated during daylight hours rather than at night, the usual time for ovulation in mice). These injections brought about hyperstimulation of ovaries in mature female mice. Subsequently, many more embryos developed in each mouse than would otherwise be possible. Edwards's priorities were apparent:

> We had not merely discovered a means of obtaining as many eggs as any research scientist may require – not just ovulation to order, foetuses when needed, day and night – but there were other exciting prospects: what about effecting superovulation in farm animals? How valuable that might be! And what about human beings? Those women who had difficulty in having children – could not they be helped? (Edwards and Steptoe, 1980, p. 38)

From his experience working with haploid mice embryos Edwards believed that differences in development of embryos had their beginnings in the earliest stages of growth. He stated: 'I needed human [*sic*] eggs though, not mouse eggs, to prove my point' (Edwards and Steptoe, 1980, p. 38).[10]

Edwards ascertained that eggs of mice could reach maturity in a culture medium. This knowledge later led to experiments on women's eggs. If women's eggs did not have to be 'collected' at the time of maturation, fertilisation of women's eggs *in vitro* was made more feasible. Edwards would not have to wait for the eggs to develop within a woman's body. At this point he writes: 'Surely the whole field then was within my grasp – cows, sheep, monkeys – and man [*sic*] too, if only I could get their eggs?' (Edwards and Steptoe, 1980, p. 39).[11] He obtained women's eggs at this stage with the help of gynaecologists who would inform him of their intention to perform ovariectomies and hysterectomies. Edwards required eggs from part or whole ovaries. He would attend the surgery 'clutching my glass sterile pot – the receptacle for that precious bit of superfluous ovarian tissue'. As he perceived it, he was 'merely there for some spare eggs, for a piece of ovary that had to be removed anyway' (Edwards and Steptoe, 1980, p. 42). It is important to note at this point that one of the conditions which enabled Edwards to obtain women's eggs for experimentation was the fact that women were perceived by medical practitioners as requiring removal of parts of their reproductive organs. The extensive use of this surgery has been questioned by many authors (Donovan, 1976; Macklin and Gaylin, 1981; Clarke, 1984; Corea, 1984).

For Edwards this method of obtaining women's eggs proved time-consuming and unreliable. It eventually proved unsuccessful as a reliable method of egg collection. He writes: 'Human [*sic*] eggs were still slow coming my way . . . if only human eggs had come my way more freely' (Edwards and Steptoe, 1980, pp. 50–1). However, despite the inconvenience, he persisted with this method. Meanwhile, he also continued his experiments on the ovaries of monkeys, cows, sheep and pigs, as these eggs were easier for him to obtain. Edwards carried out further experiments on women's eggs at Johns Hopkins University in Baltimore, USA. Here he had access to a supply of women's ovarian tissue which had been sent for pathologist's exam-ination. Experiments at this stage did not result in fertilisation of a woman's egg. Edwards then thought that sperm may have to mature in a woman's reproductive system before fertilisation. He wrote: 'So we collected living spermatozoa from the cervix of some . . . patients [that is, women] soon after they had sexual intercourse with their husbands. These spermatozoa are transferred to the oocytes [eggs] in the laboratory' (Edwards and Steptoe, 1980, p. 54). Fertilisation did not take place as a result of these experiments. Edwards concluded that a woman's cervix is not the place where sperm mature.

Edwards conducted further experiments to ascertain where sperm matured. He collected women's eggs, and sperm, and placed them in the fallopian tubes of rabbits and rhesus monkeys. These eggs were later removed from the animals to see if any had fertilised. These attempts at fertilisation of women's eggs also 'failed'.

To test whether a woman's uterus was the site of sperm matu-ration, Edwards devised an experiment in which each woman volun-teer had a receptacle, which held sperm, and which was able to absorb fluids from her reproductive system, placed in her uterus. The receptacle remained in her uterus overnight and was removed and examined the following morning. Again, fertilisation of women's eggs did not occur. As the preceding experiment had enabled Ed-wards to ascertain that a woman's cervix is not the site of sperm maturation, he then supposed that a woman's fallopian tube might be the location of this process.

It was at this time that Edwards came into contact with Patrick

Steptoe, a gynaecologist who had published a paper on the use of the laparoscope. Steptoe informed Edwards when he was going to perform the type of surgery on women which would make their ovarian tissue available for experimentation. Edwards would then gather the eggs and place them in culture to mature. Steptoe obtained sperm by asking women who were going to have a hysterectomy to have intercourse with their husbands the night before surgery. Steptoe would first perform a laparoscopy on these women to collect the matured sperm from their fallopian tube. He would then perform the hysterectomy.

Fertilisation of women's eggs *in vitro* was achieved with the development of a culture fluid in which sperm could mature. Although fertilisation did take place at this stage, the fertilised eggs did not develop. The next step in the development of the IVF procedure involved taking *already* matured eggs from women rather than maturing their eggs in culture medium. Edwards considered it necessary to take eggs which had been matured in women's bodies; he believed that eggs matured in culture medium, although being fertilised, would not result in viable embryos.

So far I have outlined the need for pieces of women's reproductive organs to be used in experiments during the development of IVF. Women's ovarian tissue had been required as a source of eggs; their reproductive tract (cervix, uterus or fallopian tube) had been needed for those experiments relating to sites of sperm maturation. Women's whole bodies were used at this point as sites of egg *maturation* as well as collection. A laproscope was devised to suck women's eggs from their ovarian follicles during a laparoscopy performed by Steptoe. As Edwards writes: 'The volunteer patients [that is, women] would have to be given hormones to impose some control over the menstrual cycle and to stimulate the ripening of the eggs in the ovary' (Edwards and Steptoe, 1980, p. 87).

Women undergoing this procedure were given hormones in various dosages to bring about ovarian hyperstimulation. Gaining control of a woman's reproductive cycle proved to be difficult. The amounts of hormones given to women to bring about further hyperstimulation were increased over a period of time. At this stage of IVF experimentation *no* fertilised eggs were being transferred to a woman's uterus. Women underwent the preliminary stages of what would later be the IVF procedure; they would undergo superovulation and a laparoscopy at a time when the procedure was entirely experimental and there was no possibility of producing a live baby as a result.

In 1971, the first egg fertilised *in vitro* was placed in a woman's uterus. This did not result in a pregnancy. Indeed, no pregnancy took place for several years. One of the perceived 'problems' was the lack of 'receptivity' of a woman's uterus after superovulation.[12] Further experiments were conducted to ascertain the dosages of drugs which would counteract the unwanted effects of the superovulatory drugs. Edwards writes: 'Since we had *taken over* the first part of the menstrual cycle of our patients by giving them fertility drugs it would be worthwhile *continuing to support it later on* with hormones – that is to say, after laparoscopy . . . But which hormones to give?' (Edwards and Steptoe, 1980, p. 123, my emphasis). The manipulation of women's reproductive cycles was phrased in terms of these cycles being 'taken over' and needing 'support' as a result of the initial manipulation. The assumption in this case is that women's cycles are a resource for scientific investigation and have a separable existence, phrased in terms of function, from the experiences of the women themselves. Women were given dosages of HCG. This was not 'successful' in bringing about implantation as it disturbed the woman's oestrogen and progesterone levels. Additions of oestrogen- and progesterone-like substances were made to the HCG to no avail. Injections of 'extra powerful hormones' (Edwards and Steptoe, 1980, p. 127) were given: 'We prescribed more progesterone, more oestrogen, or related compounds for our patients after we had replanted their embryos' (Edwards and Steptoe, 1980, p. 124). Although a few women did become pregnant using these high-dosage hormones, no woman had a full-term pregnancy. As Edwards writes: 'as far as I was concerned it was goodbye to the fertility drugs . . . there was *no alternative* but to collect the single egg ripening naturally within the mother' (Edwards and Steptoe, 1980, p. 138, my emphasis).[13]

Leslie Brown, mother of the first baby born from an egg fertilised *in vitro*, became pregnant as a result of a *single* mature egg being removed from her body, fertilised *in vitro*, and placed in her uterus. From 1971 to 1977 women were given various dosages of hormones to stimulate superovulation. Such hormones are now used routinely in IVF procedures. Superovulation is part of the IVF procedure even though IVF using a woman's single egg, developed without superovulation, has obviously been 'successful'.[14] Moreover, no mention of the possible effects of these hormones is made by Edwards and Steptoe.[15]

IVF practitioners consider ovarian hyperstimulation necessary in order to take more than one egg per IVF cycle from a woman. All eggs are fertilised;[16] usually three of these are placed in the woman's uterus. Hence, IVF is oriented towards the creation of many more embryos than are actually placed in a woman's uterus. A small number of women may, as a result of the IVF procedure, produce a live baby. In many cases there are more eggs brought to maturation and taken from a woman than there are fertilised eggs placed in a woman's uterus. This necessarily results in a 'surplus' of eggs. The term 'spare embryos' is used to describe those fertilised eggs not placed in a woman's uterus. The term itself implies that these fertilised eggs, since they are 'spare', are at the disposal of scientists and are, therefore, available for experimentation. Certainly, when one objective incorporated into the IVF procedure is to secure as many eggs as possible for fertilisation, the concomitant objective is the production of extra embryos for experimentation.

Significance of the Way IVF Developed

So far I have located the development of IVF in the context of the research interests of the developers. Edwards was interested in gaining access to women's eggs for experiments on early cell differentiation. Steptoe's development of the laparoscopic technique, which enabled him to carry out laparoscopies for the length of time necessary to gather a woman's eggs from her ovaries, gave Edwards and Steptoe access to eggs which had matured within a woman's body. The development of IVF involved, in the first place, the use of women's bodily parts as material for experimentation: ovarian tissue, secretions from her reproductive tract, and the use of her reproductive tract as the site for experiments relating to sperm maturation. Fertilisation had, at this point, taken place with women's eggs which had matured *in vitro*. However, there was no subsequent development of eggs fertilised this way. At this stage in the history of IVF, women's eggs matured in their bodies were necessary for further experiments on embryos. As Edwards writes: 'We had to ask Patrick's infertile patients [that is, women], those desperate for help and willing to undergo many trials in the hope of one day having their own babies, to cooperate' (Edwards and Steptoe, 1980, p. 88). Thus women who themselves had no prospect of having a baby from this technique were, in effect, being asked to 'donate' their bodies for 'scientific progress'. The orientation towards embryo experimentation served to override considerations of the way this objective comes about.

In the development of IVF, the authority of the scientific enterprise gives legitimacy, or at least an implication of reasonableness, to such research. An examination of scientific practices and the 're- search' methods employed reveals some of the specific cultural el- ements of the scientific enterprise. Through the examination of the steps in the developments of IVF, the activities of, and methods employed by, the innovators, have been identified. These methods were in the process of becoming acceptable practices within science and medicine. As Deborah Steinberg shows in Chapter 4, and as my account reinforces, the IVF procedure is primarily experimental. In the development and implementation of IVF, women's bodies were needed as sites for experimentation.

With the development of the IVF procedure women have become a resource for egg maturation, as well as test sites for the further developments of IVF. I have moved back and forth, from the history of the development of certain procedures, to their installation as a routine part of current infertility 'treatment'. This, together with my account of current procedures, and with Edwards's and Steptoe's account, highlights several features of IVF. It suggests the ways in which treatment evolved, and in which it remains orientated towards the facilitation of experimentation on women's eggs. It also underlines how the practices were made routine and given legitimacy, irrespective of their effect on women or the likelihood of their efficacy.

Women and IVF: A Technological Fix

Having outlined the history and nature of IVF procedures, I now examine and assess the 'problem' they purport to 'solve'. The mean- ing of reproduction is culturally specific. Definitions of 'mother', 'father' and 'family', for example, vary with cultures and in different historical periods. A woman enters an IVF programme in the hope of becoming a mother. One of the preconditions for the implementation of the IVF procedure is a society in which the term 'mother' usually applies to a woman whose primary relationship to a child is biologi- cal. In such a society women who are unable to form this exclusive relationship are termed 'childless'. Adrienne Rich questions this assumption:

> What makes us mothers? The care of small children? The physical changes of pregnancy and birth? The years of nurture? What of the woman who, never having been pregnant, begins lactating when she adopts an infant? . . . What of the woman who . . . has practically raised her younger sisters and brothers? (Rich, 1977, p. 255)

I propose that IVF is a technological fix for the social condition of 'childlessness' rather than for the biological condition of infertility. IVF is not a 'treatment' for infertility. The small percentage of women who do become biological mothers as a result of this procedure will not have regained their fertility. Indeed, they will need medical/scientific intervention to attempt any subsequent pregnancies. As a technological fix, IVF is a particular attempt to find a 'solution' to the 'social problem' of 'childlessness'.[17] The perceived solution is then applied without attempting to deal with the cause.

With the implementation of the IVF procedure, the issue of the social construction and the social meaning of motherhood is not addressed. Instead, the concept of motherhood as the biological production of a baby is enhanced. The reinforcement of this definition may make it more difficult to envisage or realise potential shifts in relationships to children such as co-parenting or community responsibility for child care. This perception of a woman's 'childless' condition is made visible within a certain social context – that of the 'nuclear family'. IVF is currently available to those women who are married (or, at least, in what practitioners of IVF consider to be a 'stable', monogamous, heterosexual relationship). The nuclear family as the locus of socially-sanctioned procreation is thereby reinforced. IVF practices effectively reinforce the conceptualisation of 'childlessness' exclusively in terms of a biological inability to reproduce.

There are reasons other than biological ones which may preclude a woman's reproducing. For example, given the present social circumstances in which there is a general lack of community responsibility for child care, a woman may feel that the demands made on her in having a child would restrict her realisation of positive personal and social identity in other ways (such as career, for example). A woman may wish to reproduce but be constrained by her economic circumstances. A lesbian has to consider, amongst other things, whether she will be able to keep her child if she has one. My point here is that IVF does not address itself to the social construction of 'childlessness' beyond the specific parameters of biological inability.

The location of infertility and fertility solely within the discussion of biological relationships exemplifies dominant values around the nuclear family and sexuality. Marriage and the social structure of the nuclear family are based on heterosexist ideological presumptions about the relationship between sexuality and reproduction. IVF attempts to 'produce' a child through the bonding of heterosexuallylinked partners. Hence, it strengthens particular values by structuring marriage and heterosexuality into the scientific practices themselves. In this case the practices incorporated in the IVF procedure exemplify the symbiotic relationship between scientific activity and certain social sanctions. IVF not only reflects normative structures relating to reproduction in society, but reinforces such structures by specifically expressing a set of *social* conditions necessary for biological reproduction.

Criteria for Selection for Treatment
A further illustration of this reproduction of specific social structures and relations is found in the criteria used by IVF practitioners to select suitable women for 'treatment'. Social criteria, such as being heterosexual, married (or what practitioners consider to be the equivalent) and having the financial capacity to undertake IVF are amongst the conditions for eligibility.

Psychological criteria are also applied to women entering an IVF programme. Most women enter a programme with the knowledge that this may be their 'last chance' to have a biologically-related child with a particular man. Knowing that there is only one chance of obtaining a sought-after goal provokes anxiety in any situation. For IVF practitioners, a woman's desire for a child must be apparent but not 'too apparent'. Edwards has described women seeking his assistance as 'desperate for help' (Edwards and Steptoe, 1980, p. 88). Nevertheless, psychological criteria for selection involve a 'realistic appreciation of IVF . . . because of the difficulties that may be encountered' (Wood, 1982, p. 20). A woman is assumed to be 'desperate' enough to undergo the rigours of the procedure, yet not to be 'too desperate', as this might lead to an 'unrealistic' appreciation of the difficulties she may encounter. I am not saying here that women undergoing IVF are, indeed, 'desperate'. Rather, I am referring to the way women must be perceived by IVF practitioners in order to be accepted on a programme.

When women on such a programme spoke to me about their experiences, I gathered that for the women concerned a 'realistic appreciation' of IVF involves compliance with the demands of the procedure, and an acceptance of 'failure' which involves as little emotional disturbance (for the doctor) as possible (Crowe, 1987, pp. 84–97; Crowe, 1988). Women were very perceptive as to what was really required of them: to appear concerned but not 'overly concerned' about their situation, to be co-operative, to be 'reasonable' about 'failure', and not to upset the doctors. Women believed that their access to IVF depended upon their being perceived this way. One woman participating in an IVF programme stated: 'Patients feel that they're under a lot of pressure *not* to "crack up", and they have to be "suitable", and if you showed any signs of emotional distress you'd be "out".' Another woman said: 'You couldn't really say what you wanted to say because you could feel the repercussions coming from it . . . it might affect your position in the queue.'

The criteria by which women are selected for IVF exemplify not only the location of reproduction within specific *social* structures but an evaluation of the *personal* qualities necessary for a woman to enter the programme. Such precepts imply not only an evaluation of which individual woman is suitable for motherhood, but which qualities, social and psychological, are preferred.

Medical indications for acceptance on IVF were originally specifically related to women with blocked or damaged fallopian tubes. A woman had to ovulate regularly, have no abdominal adhesions, and have ovaries which were accessible for 'egg collection'. Currently, the range of indications for 'treatment' are expanding. In one study, 12 per cent of women on IVF were diagnosed as having idiopathic infertility (where no cause is found after medical investigation) (Laborie, 1987, p. 51). In 11 per cent of the cases the woman was herself fertile; her *husband*'s infertility was, in these cases, considered a medical indication for *her* receiving IVF. 'Infertility', whether originating in a woman's own fertility problems, or those of her husband, requires that *she* undergo IVF.

The IVF procedure has developed as a medical/scientific activity. I have shown that this has militated against discussion of the social significance of the practices involved. IVF is being introduced and made routine and the continuation of the practice of the procedure gives it an air of legitimacy. I now consider one particular example of this legitimation – the advocacy of a fourteen day time-limit for embryo experimentation in Britain and the concomitant emergence of the term 'pre-embryo'. In order to understand these developments it is necessary to look at the Warnock Committee.

The Warnock Report and the 'Problem of Legislation'
In July 1982, the British government established a Committee of Inquiry into Human Fertilisation and Embryology. The terms of reference of this Committee of Inquiry were: 'To consider recent and potential developments in medicine and science related to human

fertilisation and embryology; to consider what policies and safeguards should be applied, including consideration of the social,
ethical and legal implications of these developments; and to make
recommendations' (Warnock, 1985, p. 4). This Committee was chaired
by Dame (now Baroness) Mary Warnock, a philosopher, Senior
Research Fellow at Oxford, and Mistress of Girton College, Cambridge. Members of the Committee were professionals in disciplines
which included law, medicine, theology, natural science and social
science. Two years later this Committee published, in what is now
known as the *Warnock Report*, the results of its deliberations.[18] It is
important to note the Committee's recommendation relating to experimentation on embryos developed from women's eggs: 'No live
human embryo derived from in vitro fertilisation, whether frozen or
unfrozen, may be kept alive, if not transferred to a woman, beyond
fourteen days after fertilisation, nor may it be used as a research
subject beyond fourteen days after fertilisation' (Warnock, 1985,
p. 66, my emphasis).

The method of approaching the issues involved is demonstrated in
the setting out of the *Warnock Report* itself. Of the thirteen chapters,
eight are devoted to the discussion of reproductive technology such
as IVF under the heading of 'Techniques for the Alleviation of
Infertility'. The issue of embryo research, where the decision for the
time-limit for such research is discussed, is in a chapter entitled
'Scientific Issues'. The Committee's 'method of working' further
illustrates the extent to which the group perceived IVF and embryo
research as a medical/scientific problem which entailed medical/
scientific solutions. The work was divided into two sections: one
section related to infertility, the other concerned 'the pursuit of
knowledge' (Warnock, 1985, p. 5).[19]

Several groups submitting proposals to the Committee opposed
embryo research at any stage after fertilisation. Organisations such as
SPUC (Society for the Protection of Unborn Children), LIFE, and
CARE amongst others advocate that legislation should 'protect
rights of unborn children'.[20] Mary Warnock, however, defined the
question of embryo research as: 'How is it right to treat the human
embryo?' (Warnock, 1985, p. 60) rather than whether or not the
embryo was alive or human. As she states: 'In practical terms, a
collection of four or sixteen cells was so different from a full human
being . . . that it might quite legitimately be treated differently . . .
Specifically we argued that . . . it might legitimately be used as a
means to an end that was good for other humans' (Warnock, 1985,

p. xv). A majority of the Committee agreed that embryo research should, indeed, continue. The reasons stated for continuation are themselves set within the context of the medical/scientific frame of reference: 'advances in the treatment of infertility . . . could not have taken place without such research; and that continued research is essential, if advances in . . . medical knowledge are to continue' (Warnock, 1985, p. 64).

As I have indicated previously, both the setting out of, and the issues raised in the Report exemplify current medical/scientific interpretations and formulations of the issues involved. In accepting and adopting this particular perception, the criteria for making any judgements concerning embryo research were more likely to be based on information which was intelligible within that frame of reference. The Committee's decision as to which issues were to be addressed and what weight was to be given to various submissions on the issue of embryo research defines the debate as a medical/scientific one.

A majority on the Committee felt that research on embryos was necessary to further scientific research. At the same time, they wished to acknowledge the special status of the embryo because it was derived from 'the human species': 'We recommend that the embryo of the human species should be afforded some protection in law' (Warnock, 1985, p. 63). As Mary Warnock has stated, the question for most of the Committee was never one of what value to place on human life in general, but what value should be placed on 'human life at its *very earliest* stage of development' (Warnock, 1985, p. xv, my emphasis).[21] Consequently, a definition of 'very early' was required (Warnock, 1985, p. xv).

The Negotiation of a Decision: Setting a Time-limit for Embryo Research

A majority of the Committee maintained that: 'the timing of the different stages of development is critical; once the process had begun, there is *no particular part of the developmental process that is more important than another*; all are part of a continuous process' (Warnock, 1985, p. 65, my emphasis). Nevertheless, opinions varied as to what particular 'stage' of development should be adopted as a time-limit for embryo research, and various criteria were suggested. For example, the Committee considered as a possible criterion the perceived ability of the embryo to feel pain. If this criterion was accepted, the time-limit for research on 'human' embryos would be: 'either when the first beginnings of the central nervous system can be identified, or when functional activity first occurs' (Warnock, 1985, p. 65). At the moment, it is thought that the beginnings of a central nervous system can be perceived (by embryologists) twenty-two to twenty-three days after fertilisation.

As for the use of the initial 'functional activity' of an embryo as a marking point, the Report judged that: 'in the present state of knowledge, the onset of central nervous system functional activity could not be used to define accurately the limit to research, because the timing is not known; however, it is generally thought to be considerably later in pregnancy' (Warnock, 1985, p. 65). In other words, the standards used to make judgements were based on what it was possible, at that stage, to 'know' about embryo development.[22]

Another criterion suggested for denoting a significant stage in embryo development was the point at which early neural development was perceived to begin. The Royal College of Obstetricians and Gynaecologists (RCOG) proposed this as the crucial point in the development of an embryo. The RCOG was concerned, as was the Warnock Committee, with the question: 'At what point in the development of an embryo do we attribute to it the protection of a human being?' (RCOG, 1983, p. 13), rather than 'when does life begin?' The RCOG dismissed the idea that an organism (presumably it is referring to a fertilised egg) should be inviolable. It stated: 'Knowing as we do that in the natural process [that is, the reproductive processes occurring in women's bodies] large numbers of fertilised ova are lost before implantation, it is morally unconvincing to claim absolute inviolability for an organism with which nature itself is so prodigal' (RCOG, 1983, p, 13). The RCOG proposed that judgement of a time-limit 'must relate to its growth, especially its neural development' (RCOG, 1983, p. 14). At this stage in the development of scientific knowledge, early neural development was perceived to take place around day seventeen after fertilisation.

The Medical Research Council (MRC) expressed concern that legal prescriptions regarding embryo research could hinder scientific investigations. It stated: 'Good research often depends on exploiting the chance or unexpected finding' (MRC, 1985a, p. 4). The MRC considered that difficulties may arise in the formulation of legislation 'which could encompass the precise nature of individual research projects in this rapidly expanding field' (MRC, 1985a, p. 5). It suggested that, although fourteen days is thought to mark the end of the implantation stage, 'because of variations in the rate of development of the embryo there are advantages in specifying the limit in terms of stage of development rather than days after fertilisation' (MRC, 1985a, p. 5).

The Royal Society considered embryo experimentation necessary for several reasons: to improve current IVF techniques, to increase knowledge relating both to infertility and to inherited genetic disease by a development of current IVF practices, and to develop knowledge of 'human development and its disorders' (Royal Society, 1983a, pp. 5–6).[23] It also proposed that limits to embryo research should be determined according to each particular case, and stated that 'adoption of implantation as the end point is unduly restrictive . . . Likewise, it would be restrictive to have to specify the precise research purposes for which any given specimen of human embryonic material is obtained' (Royal Society 1983a, pp. 10–11). Accordingly, it was not surprising to find that: 'Generally, a degree of flexibility is advocated in the regulation of work on human fertilisation and embryology' (Royal Society, 1983a, p. 12).

Edwards and Steptoe favoured a limit based on a stage of the neural development in the embryo, and they suggested an eighteen to thirty day limit to research (Prentice, 1984, p. 2). In general, individual scientists and medical/scientific organisations making recommendations on embryo experimentation based their criteria on an evaluation of existing knowledge about embryo development. The delineation of various perceived stages in embryo development and the meaning attached to these was articulated in terms of what it was considered physically or materially *possible* to apprehend. Conceptualisations of what it was possible to perceive were framed exclusively by current understandings and accepted interpretations within the scientific community.

The Warnock Committee had decided that embryo experimentation was necessary both for the 'treatment of infertility' and for the development of scientific knowledge. The issue for the Committee then was how to establish a time-limit for such experimentation. Mary Warnock herself felt that the time-limit set for embryo research must be unambiguous: 'The point was not . . . the exact number of days chosen, but the absolute necessity for there being a limit set . . . in terms of number of days from fertilisation' (Warnock, 1985, p. xv). She thought that criteria such as the perceived capacity of an embryo to feel pain, for example, would be ambiguous because this is open to various interpretations. She also felt that disputes may arise within the scientific community if an ambiguous indicator such as a particular 'stage' of embryo development were used. She suggested that scientists could circumvent the time-limit if it was based on criteria such as the ability to feel pain: 'I persuaded my colleagues not to use the criterion of the fetus feeling pain . . . because I was afraid that some smart surgeon would come along and say "my" [*sic*] embryo doesn't feel pain because I anaesthesitised it' (Dunn, 1984).

In the end, the Committee decided that the perceived formation of the 'primitive streak' should be the criterion by which to set a time-limit. At this stage, as with other 'early' stages, scientists may perceive differentiation of cells according to the way cells function. This perception is explained in terms of the recognition that a small percentage of cells which have already formed after fertilisation will coalesce and form tissue which contributes to the embryo. Other cells will form tissue which contributes to the placenta. The 'primitive streak' is thought to have come into existence at day fifteen after fertilisation.

According to Warnock: 'The genetic composition of the resulting child isn't determined for fourteen days. Therefore you might say that *continuity with your past* [my emphasis] begins at fourteen days. This seems to me the important point, rather than when the embryo is alive' (Dunn, 1984). One's 'past', in this instance, is viewed exclusively in terms of genetic connectedness. This again reflects the medical/scientific orientation in which one's 'past' is interpreted exclusively as 'biology'.

Establishing the 'Pre-embryo'

The Warnock Committee had received various proposals of possible criteria for judgements concerning embryo research. These included the perceived pre- and post-implantation stages, recognition of the beginnings of central nervous system activity, and the onset of central nervous system functional activity, amongst others. The Committee recommended a fourteen day limit to such research. Its judgement was contingent on the formation of the perceived 'primitive streak'.

The articulation of the significance of perceived qualitative differences in the development of a fertilised egg between day fourteen and day fifteen after fertilisation reached a point where a change in classification began to take place within the scientific community. The fertilised egg up to fourteen days after fertilisation began to be termed the 'pre-embryo'; after day fourteen, the same entity was termed an 'embryo'. The term 'pre-embryo' is not mentioned in the *Warnock*

Report. The Committee made a point of clarifying the term 'embryo': 'we have taken as our starting point the meeting of egg and sperm at fertilisation. We have regarded the embryonic stage to be the six weeks immediately following fertilisation' (Warnock, 1985, p. 5).

In 1984 the Conservative MP Enoch Powell's Unborn Children (Protection) Bill brought to public attention the issue of whether embryo research should be permitted. Hence, reclassification of perceived data relating to early embryo development (that is, the significance of the 'primitive streak') and the concurrent revision of the term 'embryo' began at a time when the issue of the legitimacy of embryo research itself was being contested. So, in the same year that the *Warnock Report* was published, a Bill came before the House of Commons which, if passed, would have prohibited embryo research altogether. Certainly, the Warnock Committee was aware of public sensibilities and made reference in their Report to decisions being partly based on the desire not to cause public anxiety (Warnock, 1985, p. 65). In putting forward the Unborn Children (Protection) Bill, Powell argued against embryo research on the grounds that a woman's fertilised egg should have the same rights to protection in law as an adult human being. He maintained that all fertilised eggs resulting from IVF procedures should, therefore, be used for the express purpose of enabling a specified woman to have a child.

In April 1985, Sir Andrew Huxley, then president of the Royal Society, attempted to justify embryo experimentation in the light of the fact that the Powell Bill was coming before Parliament (Huxley, 1985, p. 2).[24] Huxley attempted to clarify 'misunderstandings' appearing in the discussion: 'Unfortunately, the public debate . . . is taking place against a background of widespread ignorance about the earliest stages of development of the fertilised egg' (Huxley, 1985, p. 2). He stated that there was 'an unfortunate ambiguity in the word "embryo"', and drew a distinction between 'extra-embryonic tissue' and the 'embryo proper' (Huxley, 1985, p. 2). Huxley does not use the term 'pre-embryo', but the distinction he makes between 'extra-embryonic tissue' and 'embryo proper' is in accordance with the differentiation which was made significant in the recommendations proposed by the Warnock Committee – that is, the formation of the 'primitive streak'. Until this point, the term 'embryo' had been adequate as a resource for descriptive purposes in the scientific community. The conventional meaning of the term within the community had sufficient scope to accommodate its use in different contexts. In other words, the descriptive capacity of the term 'embryo' had hitherto been sufficient to cover any exigent circumstances.

The Warnock Committee chose as its criterion for judgement the formation of the 'primitive streak' as designating a time-limit for embryo research. The significance of scientific knowledge pertaining to the perceived 'primitive streak' (as opposed to scientific knowledge of any other stage, for example) was, at this point, being consolidated in a particular social context. This context included the publication of the *Warnock Report* recommending fourteen days after fertilisation as a limit for embryo research. Another element in this context was the contesting of the legitimacy of embryo research itself, particularly Enoch Powell's Bill. Hence, the concept 'embryo' and the term were increasingly found to be inadequate, as manifested by the instigation of a change in classification within the scientific community. Indeed, in the light of the imminent debate of the Powell Bill, this term came to be seen by those advocating embryo research as 'misleading' when used in public discussions.

Although Enoch Powell's Unborn Children (Protection) Bill was ultimately defeated in the House of Commons in October 1985, it was, for a time, popular with many MPs. Maxine Clarke suggests that part of the explanation for the Bill's decrease in popularity with MPs may lie in the lobbying activities of a group which eventually formally constituted an organisation called PROGRESS (Campaign for Research into Reproduction) (Clarke, 1985, p. 197). This organisation was formed in November 1985, in the aftermath of the Powell Bill. Although the Powell Bill was eventually defeated, its popularity amongst MPs was a cause for concern amongst those interested in 'research' on women's embryos. It was formed by a group including scientists, physicians and medical organisations. Dr Anne McLaren, Director of the MRC Mammalian Development Unit in London, and a member of the Warnock Committee, Professor Martin Bobrow, a geneticist, and Dr Robert Winston, from the IVF clinic at Hammersmith Hospital are prominent members (Ironside, 1985, p. 10; Cantacuzino, 1986, p. 28).

PROGRESS was formed, amongst other things, as a 'campaign for research into reproduction' (PROGRESS, 1986, p. 1). The kind of research into reproduction proposed by PROGRESS specifically involves the use of embryos for research into 'prevention of genetic disease, infertility treatment, diagnosis of infertility, miscarriage, contraception' as well as, in some circumstances, 'pre-embryo diagnosis' to replace existing pre-natal diagnosis techniques (PROGRESS, 1985, pp. 2–3). Members of PROGRESS 'are seeking to

educate MPs and encourage a more rational and humane judgement' (concerning embryo experimentation) (Clarke, 1985, p.
197). Indeed, PROGRESS states:

> people often have limited information about medical and scientific re-
> search. Exaggerated and emotive propaganda distorts the facts and causes
> confusion and anxiety . . . PROGRESS aims to increase knowledge about
> research into the earliest stages of human conception through a wider
> exchange of discussion between the public and scientists. Legislation
> should be based on full and factual understanding of the issues involved.
> (PROGRESS, 1986, p. 1)

In its literature PROGRESS uses the term 'pre-embryo': 'What has
popularly been called "embryo" research is not really that at all. It is
research using "pre-embryos"' (PROGRESS, 1986, p. 1). The em-
bryo/'pre-embryo' distinction proposed by PROGRESS is in accordance with differentiation of stages in embryo development which had
been made significant in the recommendations of the Warnock Committee.

In March 1985 members of the Medical Research Council (MRC)
and the Royal College of Obstetricians and Gynaecologists (RCOG)
established and jointly sponsored the Voluntary Licensing Authority
for Human In Vitro Fertilisation and Embryology (VLA). The MRC
and RCOG established the VLA in response to recommendations in
the *Warnock Report* that a statutory licensing authority be set up to
regulate embryo research and specific types of 'infertility services'
(that is, IVF clinics) (Warnock, 1985, p. 75).

At present, the VLA is not a legislative body. As yet, its guidelines
carry no authority outside the scientific community. It seemingly
serves as a regulator of standards and practices within its own
community. Nevertheless, it has provided a model which will be
influential when a Statutory Licensing Body is established.

In its first report the VLA introduced the term 'pre-embryo'
(VLA, 1986). It stated that the development up to fourteen days of a
fertilised egg constitutes: 'not an embryo, but a pre-embryo: a
precursor of the embryo just as the separate sperm and egg were its
precursors' (VLA, 1986, p. 39). Members of the VLA discussed
various terms which might be used to define the stages in the development of the fertilised egg before the appearance of the 'primitive
streak'. The term 'pre-embryo' was favoured by lay members of the
VLA (Turney, 1985, p. 2). As Pat Spallone explains: 'It was coined
by a lay member of the VLA in preference to other terms . . . such as

conceptus and zygote and pro-embryo' (Spallone, 1989, p. 53). Dr Anne McLaren, a member of the VLA and of the Warnock Committee, has been reported as saying that 'the problem was that scientists use the word "embryo" to mean different things in different contexts' (Turney, 1985, p. 2). McLaren's statement, made around the same time as Huxley's discussion of the 'unfortunate ambiguity in the word "embryo"'', (Huxley, 1985, p. 2) articulates what may be described as a 'tension' (Barnes, 1983, p. 45) around the word 'embryo'. The term 'tension' is used to denote the situation which occurs within the scientific community when a word no longer has the capacity to meet all exigent circumstances. Resolution of such a tension can occur when that term's meaning has slowly changed and when this has only been noticed upon reflection (Barnes, 1983, p. 45). In this particular case, the adoption of the term 'pre-embryo' represents a more explicit resolution of the tension around the term 'embryo'.

Whether the scientific community takes up this term will depend, to a considerable extent, on the achievement of consensus. The sanctioning of such a concept through communal authority involves a process of negotiation about meaning, and of co-operation in the usage of the term. The concept 'pre-embryo' is a relatively recent formulation, and there have been challenges to its use from within the scientific community. Dr David Davies,[25] a member of the Warnock Committee, has contested the use of the term 'pre-embryo'. He is 'reasonably sure that at least in our [the Warnock Committee's] discussions the word "pre-embryo" was never used' (Davies, 1986, p. 208). He claimed: 'if research on embryos were an uncontentious matter, and if scientists were genuinely of the opinion that the new terminology helped their understanding, nobody would have many qualms at the name change' (Davies, 1986, p. 208).

Davies does not challenge the articulation of a perceived qualitative difference in stages of early embryo development inherent in the term 'pre-embryo'. He contends that the legitimacy of the term should be questioned because of the *context* of its introduction. By highlighting the conditions of the introduction of the term, Davies demonstrates the social nature of the formation of scientific knowledge. In other words, Davies is withholding his co-operation in legitimating a concept within science. This refusal, together with that of other members of the scientific community, could undermine the legitimacy of this particular concept. In order for a concept to become routinely accepted as part of conventional knowledge within science, social forces which give legitimacy to the knowledge must cohere.

Dr Anne McLaren has attempted to clarify the origin of the term 'pre-embryo'. She explains that confusion has arisen because embryologists have 'adopted the sloppy practice of using the same term for the entire product of the fertilised egg' (McLaren, 1986a, p. 570). In an article outlining the stages in early embryo development, in which McLaren describes the formation of the 'primitive streak', she states: 'In recent years, we researchers have developed the bad habit of calling the whole set of cells, at each prior stage, the embryo as well' (McLaren, 1986b, p. 49). That is, although various stages in the development of a fertilised egg had previously been recognised, circumstances in the field of embryology had not given rise to the need for such an explicit articulation of differentiation.

A sense of what constitutes a routine or legitimate interpretation of observations can be viewed as a product of the relationship between the activities of individual members of the scientific community and the communal ascription of significance to that which is observed. A specific interpretation must be used by individuals in their everyday activities for it to gain credibility. The various activities of a community yield a sense of 'normality' to newly introduced (and existing) concepts.

The perception of entities as having either similarities or differences, for example, may be understood by reference to the context in which the perceived similarities or differences are articulated. The debate taking place at present within the scientific community in relation to the concept of 'pre-embryo' centres on the negotiation of the communal ascription of meaning to perceived sets of similarities or differences in the process of development of the embryo. In the United Kingdom, the notion of the 'primitive streak' as denoting qualitative differences in embryo development between day fourteen and day fifteen after fertilisation is currently being contested. Whether or not the concept of 'pre-embryo' will be incorporated as a new concept within the scientific community remains to be seen. If it is, this will come to be recognised and accepted as a routine differentiation and form part of conventional knowledge within science. Within the scientific community, the Warnock Committee's recommendation on embryo research is a crucial element in the relationship between social forces and the scientific enterprise. The acceptance of the formulation of the 'primitive streak' as denoting a legitimate limit for embryo experimentation would bring about a re-examination and reorientation of research questions, methods and possibilities. For example, subsequent formulations of procedures and methods relating to embryo research, together with 'stages' recognised, developmental processes classified and terminology employed, would be framed in relation to the formation of the 'primitive streak'. The introduction of the concept 'pre-embryo' does not simply represent an increase in scientific knowledge. Rather, its introduction will involve qualitative changes for related concepts and already constituted conventional knowledge.

In addition to involving communal activities which invoke a feeling of the 'normality' in the use of the concept, a new concept must 'make sense' in its surroundings. An understanding of the concept 'pre-embryo' relies on a shared understanding and agreement on terms such as 'fertilisation', 'embryo' and indeed 'pregnancy'. The term 'embryo' has been explicitly redefined as a result of the introduction of the term 'pre-embryo' (that is, an 'embryo' exists after day fifteen following fertilisation). Although the emphasis within the scientific community has been directed at validating the term 'pre-embryo', the 'correction' of the term 'embryo' has necessarily taken place. This is an example of a resolution of a tension whereby, as Barnes describes it, 'the community claims finally to have found out what a term has always "really" meant' (Barnes, 1983, p. 46). The connotations of the concept of fertilisation may also be altered. In outlining stages leading up to the development of the 'primitive streak', the VLA stated: 'An individual baby cannot begin *without* fertilisation but fertilisation does not start an individual baby but merely sets in motion a train of events which can lead to such a beginning' (VLA, 1986, p. 39). Indeed, the understanding of 'pregnancy' itself may also shift with the introduction of the term 'pre-embryo'. PROGRESS has stated that 'When an egg is fertilised within a woman's body and begins to divide into more cells, it does not complete implantation in her uterus until about the fourteenth day. *Only after that is she said to be pregnant*' (PROGRESS, 1986, p. 1, my emphasis).

The enunciation of scientific knowledge pertaining to the appearance of the perceived 'primitive streak', as opposed to any other potentially meaningful stages in the development of an embryo, has occurred as an outcome of the process of negotiation. This negotiation has taken place between various interest groups. The Warnock Committee with its particular terms of reference constitutes one such group. The Committee's interpretation of the issues as medical/

scientific ones which required a set of medical/scientific solutions further legitimated this conceptualisation by giving legitimacy to procedures such as IVF and embryo experimentation. In so doing, the Warnock Report was contributing to the constitution of scientific practices. A majority of the Committee viewed embryo experimentation as an exclusively medical/scientific issue in which possible future benefits may outweigh harm. This gave rise to a second element for negotiation: the setting of a time-limit for embryo experimentation. It is highly probable that the British government will adopt the time-limit recommended in the Warnock Report. The time-limit will then not only gain significance as a reference point for experimentation *within* the scientific community; its status will be further enhanced by its institutionalisation within law.

As I have illustrated, the options selected for consideration as possible indicators for the time-limit for embryo experimentation, as well as the values ascribed to these options, arose in a specific socio-political context. Considerable controversy was (and indeed, still is) taking place about the desirability of embryo experimentation. One way this controversy became evident was in Enoch Powell's Bill calling for a ban on all such research. Individuals and organisations with various interests were vying to have their particular interpretation of the issues taken as the determining one. The Warnock Committee received various submissions relating to embryo experimentation. Medical and scientific organisations submitting proposals based their recommendations on different criteria. These criteria were manifestations of their technical competency to determine various stages of cell differentiation. Thus, what was considered feasible in their research objectives was articulated in terms of their technical competency to perceive differentiation in early embryo development. As Barnes states: 'It is not that agents operate by reference to goals and interests *instead* of considerations of technical and empirical adequacy; rather it is their sense of technical and empirical adequacy which is itself intelligible only in terms of contingent goals and interests' (Barnes, 1983, p. 44, my emphasis).

The decisions by organisations representing scientists, physicians and medical groups about adopting the term 'pre-embryo' and about emphasising the difference between cells at one given point, indicate the emergence of a scientific consensus from a particular social and political context where strategic classification was required.

Conclusion

In this chapter I have examined the introduction of the term 'pre-embryo' and shown the social processes which constructed this scientific knowledge. These processes include a specific set of practices within science which have legitimated the methods employed in the initial experimentation on women and the use of women's bodily parts in the development of the IVF procedure. The current practice of IVF demonstrates the continuation of these methods and procedures developed during its innovation. Women's bodies are employed as a resource for extraordinary egg maturation; these eggs, which are parts of women's bodies, become, in turn, the discrete objects of scientific experimentation. In the development of IVF, those practices taken as 'routine', such as gathering pieces of women's reproductive organs for experimentation, using parts of women's bodies as sites for sperm maturation, or using women as locations for egg maturation, create the foundations for scientific knowledge relating to embryo development.

The discussion of a time-limit for 'embryo research' in the *Warnock Report* is one which supports the medical/scientific perception of IVF. In this version of the issue, focus has centred on 'the embryo' as an entity separate unto itself. The Warnock Committee's discussion of 'research' on embryos did not acknowledge that such 'research' constitutes experimentation *on* women's bodies, both in terms of the way 'material' for experimentation is gathered, and in the nature of the appropriation of these bodily parts as resource material.

The only opposition to embryo research cited in the *Warnock Report* (by groups which advocated the 'rights of the unborn child') was articulated in terms of the embryo as constituting an entity which is separate from a woman. Indeed, in the report, there was no recognition of any representation on behalf of women or of the contribution of women's groups to the debating of IVF and embryo experimentation. In effect, in its decision about the formulation of the question to be addressed, the Warnock Committee chose one embryo-centred interpretation (the medical/scientific view) over another (the 'right to life' of an 'unborn child') embryo-centred position.

The terms with which the issues are discussed in the *Warnock Report* give credence to the medical/scientific interpretation in which

IVF and 'embryo research' are comprehended exclusively as medical/scientific solutions to medical/scientific problems. At the same time, the decision to establish the time-limit for embryo experimentation lends legitimacy to the experimentation itself. Such a decision about standards of operation within science, made by an ostensibly 'non-scientific' committee, imparts a sense of 'normality' and validity to those practices. As such, the Warnock Committee's recommendations exemplify the way a specific form of scientific inquiry gains authorisation from 'outside' the scientific community. The perceived formation of the 'primitive streak' was accorded significance in the context of negotiation between a committee representing the state and various medical/scientific organisations advocating embryo experimentation. The implicit objective of those participating in the process of negotiation for a time-limit was the establishment of 'embryo research' as both an orthodox and an essential area of 'research' in science.

The Warnock Committee's decision on a time-limit for embryo research was expressed in terms of the medical/scientific interpretation of perceived phenomena related to early embryo development – the formation of the 'primitive streak'. Through this interpretation, various groupings of cells are attributed significance in terms of arrangements of similarities and differences. Several 'stages' which denoted similarities and/or differences were proposed by advocates of embryo experimentation as criteria for making judgements concerning the time-limit for 'research'. The stages were presented as being a *description* of events which occur 'in nature'. Hence, what an observer can 'see' depends upon the technical skills and techniques employed to investigate the phenomenon. The foundations for this understanding came from the epistemological assumptions that science can apprehend phenomena from the 'natural world' and mimic those processes as part of its practices. Thus, it is presumed that the associated development of technical capabilities will allow one to 'see' phenomena and will, in this case, reveal further stages in embryo development.

In the examination of the development of IVF procedures and the concomitant development of techniques for embryo experimentation, I have tried to demonstrate that it is the interests and objectives of participants that form the *context* in which developments are made intelligible. In other words, goals and interests of researchers form part of the constitution of knowledge within science as they endow that which is perceived with meaning.

Notes

I wish to thank Jalna Hanmer for the original suggestion that I contribute to the BSA conference. Sarah Franklin and Annette Burfoot provided inspiration and support in the formation of my paper. In particular, I would like to thank Patricia Spallone for helping me locate much of the information necessary for this project. Debbie Steinberg's invaluable support and assistance have helped me develop my argument. Maureen McNeil has greatly helped me bind together and make coherent in this chapter some of the themes I have been developing in a larger project.

1. Whether to use the term women's 'eggs' or women's 'ova' when referring to those cells of a woman's body which have the potential to begin her pregnancy is a choice where the options are limited. 'Eggs' contains connotations that these cells are commodities and therefore can be perceived in terms of market relations. 'Ova' (meaning 'eggs') is a term which clearly derives from the medical/scientific framework. I have used the term 'eggs' because it is more accessible. The language employed reveals secrets of the culture. The paucity of options with which to refer to the particular cells in a woman's body which have potential in reproduction reflect dominant patterns of perceiving women as divisible from their bodily parts. I appreciate a conversation with Sarah Franklin which enabled me to clarify some of my ideas on this subject.
2. For the purposes of this chapter, I use the term 'embryo' to denote the result of fertilisation before and after the proposed fourteen/fifteen day demarcation being discussed. I use the term 'embryo experimentation' rather than 'research' as the term 'research' itself implies the social sanctioning of such activity. The issue of experimentation on embryos derived from women's eggs is by no means resolved. I use the term 'experimentation' as the connotations suggest the possibility that the practices may be contested.
3. A description of the technical aspects of an IVF procedure can only give some idea of the demands placed upon women who enter such a programme. Women's experiences of IVF have been documented by Crowe, 1987; Klein, 1989.
4. Clomiphene citrate diminishes the effect of oestrogens which are already present in a woman's body. Since eggs develop as an oestrogenic effect, a woman's body is led to act as though no eggs have been developed. Her pituitary gland then releases more hormones such as follicle stimulating hormone (FSH) and luteinizing hormone (LH) for the ripening and releasing of eggs from her ovary.
5. Human menopausal gonadotrophin (HMG) is a purified extract of FSH and LH (see note 4 above) obtained from the urine of women who have reached menopause. HMG is injected intramuscularly, and bypasses the pituitary gland as a source of ovarian stimulation. Human chorionic gonadotrophin (HCG) is a placental hormone obtained from the urine of pregnant women. HCG mimics the action of LH; it stimulates ovulation in a follicle.
6. Klein and Rowland have examined the gross inconsistencies regarding

'recommended' dosages. They also describe women's experiences of taking the drug. See Klein and Rowland, 1988.

7. These include luteinizing hormone. This hormone is produced by the pituitary gland and released into the bloodstream.

8. Indeed, as Klein and Rowland put it, the *failure* rate of 92.6 per cent in Australia and 91.4 per cent in the United Kingdom is a more significant interpretation of 'success rates' (Klein and Rowland, 1988).

9. Haploid embryos develop when only half the number of chromosomes contribute to its formation.

10. I wish to draw attention to the point that women's specific agency in reproduction is negated by the use of terms such as 'human'. Eggs used in IVF-related experiments are eggs derived from women's bodies. To refer to 'human' eggs obscures the fact that IVF is oriented around gaining *women*'s eggs for experimentation.

11. Here it was evident that Edwards's interests were oriented towards experimentation in general rather than a particular orientation towards helping women 'overcome' an 'infertility problem'.

12. The drugs which caused superovulation also caused a speeding up of the woman's reproductive cycle. By the time any fertilised egg was transferred to her uterus, the uterus was preparing to shed its lining, thus making implantation of the fertilised egg highly unlikely.

13. Women are usually 'invisible' in medical/scientific discussions of the IVF procedure (see Steinberg, this volume). It is significant that, if and when any allusions are made to 'patients' as women, they are couched in terms of women as 'mothers', highlighting the fact that women as women are not recognised in the medical/scientific framework.

14. Moreover, the incidence of multiple births would be reduced if only a single egg were used.

15. Klein and Rowland have discussed the possible effects of the use of superovulatory drugs (Klein and Rowland, 1988).

16. Of course, if 'egg freezing', or 'egg cryopreservation', is developed, the eggs may not all be fertilised at the same time.

17. 'Childlessness' and 'infertility' can, of course, only be perceived as 'problems' where the childlessness is involuntary.

18. For a discussion of the assumptions underlying recommendations, and the implications of the Committee's recommendations and omissions in the *Warnock Report*, see Spallone, 1987.

19. The first part of the Report 'concerned processes designed to benefit the individual within society who faced a particular problem, namely infertility; the second concerned the pursuit of knowledge, much of it designed to benefit society at large rather than the individual' (Warnock, 1985, p. 5).

20. For a list of individuals and organisations submitting proposals to the Warnock Committee, see Warnock, 1985, pp. 100–5.

21. For a list of members expressing dissent on the issue of embryo research, see Warnock, 1985, pp. 90–4.

22. It is clear that Warnock required that the time-limit be empirically defined. Proponents of various stages of central nervous system functional activity as a time-limit did not require such precision. For example,

proponents advocating either the identification of the 'first beginnings of [the] central nervous system' or the occurrence of 'functional activity' suggested 'subtracting a few days in order that there would be no possibility of the embryo feeling pain' (Warnock, 1985, p. 65).

23. The Royal Society was constituted in Britain in 1660, and is the oldest scientific society known. Its general purpose is the 'advancement of science'.

24. Huxley's justification of embryo experimentation was in terms of the medical/scientific perspective: potential 'benefits in the treatment of infertility' and the 'reduction of inherited disease' (Huxley, 1985, p. 2).

25. Davies was also editor of the British science journal *Nature* from 1973 to 1980.

3 The Normalisation of a New Reproductive Technology
Annette Burfoot

Introduction

To counter the prevalent and misleading assumption that technology is a self-determining enterprise abstracted from competing human interests, it is necessary to state simply and repeatedly that technology is social in its formation and its application. Since the early work in the relatively new field of sociology of technology (Mumford, 1967; Kuhn, 1970; Sklair, 1973) we have learned more about various socio-technical relations and about the way power structures and guides the development of technology as shared but restricted knowledge, as recognised techniques and caches of characteristic tools to be used by experts only. There is a gender dimension to this as Cynthia Cockburn (1985) explains in sketching the features of men's appropriation of technology and with it technological domination in our post-agrarian, centralised and industrial society. With the advent of new reproductive technologies, particularly *in vitro* fertilisation (IVF), gamete intra-fallopian transfer (GIFT) and embryo freezing, other feminists have given warning about the specific physical, psychological and social implications these technologies have for women's well-being (Arditti *et al.*, 1984b; Corea, 1985). Meanwhile, the medical and scientific interests involved with emergent reproductive technologies continue to organise themselves into new practices of reproductive medicine, supported by a pharmaceutical industry drawing on a burgeoning market in hormones and infertility services.

A citation analysis of scientific research into IVF[1] and a description of the professional organisation of European IVF, along with the documentation of international commercial market behaviour of companies with interests in the new reproductive technologies, are the components of this chapter. These are used to indicate the normalisation of increased, high-technology intervention in female procreation and are interpreted as part of the tradition of male control of technology and technology as social control.

The term 'normalisation' refers in this chapter to the establishment of an innovative technique as routine procedure. As mentioned above, this process never occurs outside structures of power and becomes one itself as the naturalisation of a new technique involves conformity and ideology. Lewis Mumford pointed out how technological ideology is formed, beginning with the elitism of technological expertise first witnessed in ancient Egyptian cultures (Mumford, 1967). By making knowledge and technology a secret and 'wonder'-full thing (the high priests were the keepers of technical information) these early civilisations were able to create a hegemonic 'mega-machine' or a socio-technical system based on domination.

Cynthia Cockburn agrees with Mumford that, with the beginning of centralised government (with its restricted information and access to technology) and an agrarian base in prehistorical society, came technological domination (Cockburn, 1985). Unlike Mumford, Cockburn explains how this domination was gendered and that the practice remains with us today as 'men's appropriation of technology'. It is remarkable that women cannot be found in any substantial numbers in engineering and most other science and technological fields (except, of course as cheap, unskilled labour). In Britain, this fact contributed to the establishment of the Women into Science and Engineering (WISE) programme in 1984. This event was one of the factors which prompted feminists worldwide to examine the meaning of science and its masculine epistemological bias (Fox-Keller, 1985; Harding, 1986; Birke, 1986). Women are largely absent as producers in socio-technical systems; but as reproducers they are not. They are the main consumers in a growing market of reproductive technologies. It is argued in this chapter that men's appropriation of technology continues in the realm of reproduction and that the development and dissemination of new reproductive technologies as normalised procedures and techniques reflect and protect male interests.

In 1969 Robert Edwards reported from his Cambridge laboratory on the first human embryo to be conceived *in vitro* (Edwards *et al.*, 1969). The scientific community responded to this development with obvious interest: over the next eighteen years awareness of IVF within the scientific community spread and the field gained credibility. With the much-publicised birth in 1978 of the first successful IVF-conceived child, Louise Brown, this field was brought to the public eye as yet another miracle of modern science with the power to harness nature and save the infertile. A new area of research was established and the European Society of Human Reproduction and Embryology (ESHRE) was founded.[2] Now strong as a new scientific field, organised into a professional society and gaining public acceptance, IVF is well on its way to becoming medical convention.

The process of IVF is, literally, the conception of an embryo in glass. The newly formed embryo is kept there from several hours up to three days. It is then placed in the uterus of either the genetic or surrogate mother in the hope of its successful implantation and development to term. The process of gathering the eggs for this procedure is complex and involves an operation to pick them up from an ovary hyperstimulated with hormones to produce more than the usual, single egg. Most IVF programmes pick up at least six eggs, some as many as fifteen, at one time. Almost all programmes implant at least three embryos shortly after their retrieval to cope with the high rate of embryo rejection and loss. The left over or 'spare' embryos are most often used in experimentation (which is not always related to the development of IVF) and, to a lesser degree, in donor programmes where they are brought to term in women with no genetic relation to the embryo.

It has taken eighteen years to develop IVF from initial scientific discovery to routine infertility service. The most obvious obstacle to the normalisation of IVF came from a public disturbed by the prospect of research on human embryos. Objections to IVF development focused on embryos' right to life and challenged the right of scientists to conduct research on disposable human embryos. Besides much publicised concern about embryo research in local and national papers and magazines in Britain, the Powell Bill, a private member's bill, was introduced in Parliament in 1985. The Bill called for a ban on embryo research because such research was seen to interfere with the embryo's right to life. PROGRESS, a professional lobby of scientists and physicians, was established to fight the Powell Bill, since such a research ban would severely hamper IVF practice and development (see Crowe, this volume). Such a ban would mean that all eggs taken from a superovulated woman would have to be fertilised and implanted (which is the procedure used in the Republic of Ireland). This is particularly difficult since the number of eggs produced by superovulation drugs cannot be controlled. It would also mean that embryo research designed to improve IVF success rates could not be undertaken.

Despite such objections, the establishment of IVF and its accompanying technologies as parts of routine infertility service has progressed by appeasing or bypassing moral reservations. For example, the term 'pre-embryo' was coined in official reports (the *Warnock Report*, 1984; the VLA Report, 1986; Crowe in this volume) mainly to deflect public concern from embryo research. It seems to be more acceptable to say you are using 'pre-embryos' in research than to use the term 'embryos'.

Commercial interest has encouraged and supported the normalisation of this reproductive intervention. Commercial commitment to IVF is obvious. At least two major pharmaceutical firms (Organon and Serono) are interested in the profit to be gained in providing the hormones required for hyperovulation and control of ovulation in IVF. There is also the potential use of human embryos (the 'spare' embryos that are by-products of IVF) as new natural resources in genetic and other types of scientific experimentation. Financial interest extends beyond the expected sources (such as pharmaceutical firms) to venture-gain companies which regard IVF as a sound financial investment with the prospect of high financial return.

The growth of scientific interest in IVF, the establishment of a new medical/scientific field in reproduction and their support from professional and capital interests are key features of the normalisation of a new reproductive technology. Such growth and support can be measured and observed. A citation analysis complemented by indications of the new, professional organisation surrounding IVF and the rate and intent of commercial support can all be taken as indices of the normalisation of this technology. It is these developments which this chapter will trace.

Citation Analysis of Robert G. Edwards: The Emergence of a New Medical/Scientific Field

Introduction to Citation Analysis
Citation analysis is a method of investigation of scientific research and an index of relative success within various scientific fields. Such analysis indicates the rates of citation of scientific papers. This information is conveniently stored in the Scientific Citation Institute's (SCI) annual volumes listing citation and related statistics for the international scientific community (for English publications only). The SCI's *Journal of Citation Reports* complements the SCI's

Citation, Source and Corporation indices with information on the impact of scientific journals (in terms of the rate of citation of the averagely cited article for each journal in a given year).

Patent analysis is another useful indicator of scientific and technological innovation. Using the information available in national and international patent libraries, such analyses map what is being patented, by whom and to what degree. It is a research method best used in fields which exhibit high patent activity, such as manufacturing. Biomedical innovations are more difficult to patent as procedures. Also, discoveries in these areas are more likely to be shared than in the industrial sectors, since competition between innovating groups is not so stiff. As a result, there are not so many patents in biomedicine as there are in other technological sectors, which restricts the use of patent analysis in examining biomedical innovation, such as IVF.

A citation analysis helps in mapping trends in scientific enterprise, in defining borders to discoveries and developments and in indicating a particular type of success of the actors in the scientific arena where rank and influence are linked to high rates of publication in prestigious journals. Robert Edwards has been chosen as the subject of this citation analysis because he, along with the late Patrick Steptoe, was the first to bring to term a foetus conceived in a Petri dish and then replanted in the genetic mother's uterus (Louise Brown, 1978). Also, Edwards has become something of a spokesman for IVF technology and was instrumental in the formation of the European Society of Human Reproduction and Embryology (ESHRE) in 1985. His career, to date, is long (over thirty years) and substantial in terms of articles published. A citation analysis of his work also reveals the great extent to which he has led developments in IVF technology over the past twenty years. Although Edwards is not the only researcher of importance in the field of IVF, he is highly notable as the field's leading spokesman.

Rate of Citation

An eleven year period of citations of Edwards's work (between 1975 and 1986 inclusively) is examined from the SCI *Citation and Source Indices* and in the SCI *Journal of Citation Reports* (1975 is the first year of publication of the indices). All articles written by Edwards throughout his career that were cited three or more times during the study period are included in the analysis. Except for his very early work on muscle fatigue, all articles cited relate to IVF. The citations

Figure 3.1   Citation analysis: Robert G. Edwards, 1975–86, rate of citation (total per year and by article)

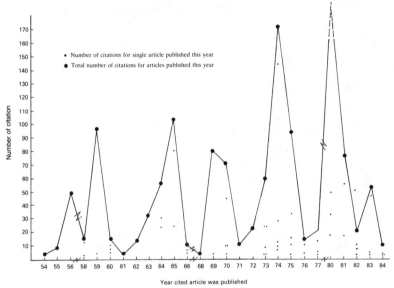

Source: SCI Citation Index (1975–86).

are categorised by year and by 'impact factor'. Impact factor is a statistical procedure used by the SCI in measuring the impact of scientific journals. It is 'a measure of the frequency with which the average article in a journal has been cited in a particular year' (SCI, Reports, 1986) where the 'average' is taken from all the journal's articles for a specified year. Impact factors in this analysis are taken from the latest report, 1985, and are applied to articles published from 1954 to 1985.[3] The database of the Institute for Scientific Information is searched when determining the impact factor.

Figure 3.1 displays the number of citations per article and the total citations per year throughout Edwards's career. Peer interest in Edwards's work reached a peak most noticeably in 1974 (owing chiefly to the article 'Follicular Fluid' in the *Journal of Reproduction and Fertility*) and again in 1980 (as a result of the article 'Establishing Full-term Human Pregnancies Using Cleaving Embryos Grown *In Vitro*' in the *British Journal of Obstetrics and Gynaecology*). Edwards's (1974) article was cited 144 times, while the 1980 article was cited 166 times. Other articles that are highly cited are:

(a) 92 citations (1959) 'Timing of the Stages of the Maturation Divisions, Ovulation, Fertilisation and the First Cleavage of Eggs of Adult Mice Treated with Gonadotrophins', *Journal of Endocrinology.*

(b) 80 citations (1965) 'Maturation *In Vitro* of Mouse, Cow, Pig, Rhesus Monkey and Human Ovarian Oocytes, *Nature.*

(c) 77 citations (1969) 'Early Stages of Fertilisation *In Vitro* of Human Oocytes Matured *In Vitro*', *Nature.*

(d) 55 citations (1981) 'Test-tube Babies', *Nature.*

(e) 46 citations (1983) 'Current Status of IVF and Implantation of Human Embryos', *Lancet.*

(f) 44 citations (1970) 'Fertilisation and Cleavage *In Vitro* of Pre-ovulatory Human Oocytes', *Nature.*

(g) 30 citations (1964) 'Immunological Control of Fertility in Female Mice', *Nature.*

The years indicated in this list refer to the date of the published article; the number of citations are total citations per article between 1975 and 1986.

Impact Factor of Journals

Besides rates of citation, it is important to consider where Edwards's work is published and the rank of journals that publish his research. Of these journals, clearly the most prestigious (assessed both in terms of SCI impact factor and in terms of popular attitudes) are *Nature* and *Lancet*. Figure 3.2 shows the 1985 impact factor of all the journals in which Edwards has published throughout his career. The SCI impact factor (IF) ranges from 0 to 39.723 with a considerable leap from 15 to 39.723; only ten journals have an IF of fifteen or more, out of approximately 7000 ranked journals. Most journals are ranked below a factor of four. In Edwards's case, *Nature* and *Lancet* are the highest ranked at 12.863 and 12.165 respectively.

Edwards's articles in these two high-status journals are cited extensively: the 1965 and 1969 articles are cited eighty and seventy-seven times respectively. The 1981 and 1970 articles in *Nature* are cited fifty-five and forty-four times respectively. A 1983 article in *Lancet* is cited forty-six times; a 1965 article in *Nature* is cited twenty-four times.

A cross-tabulation of journals of high IF with Edwards's most highly-cited articles results in the list below (in order of IF). The purpose of the cross-tabulation is to reveal Edwards's most popular

Figure 3.2   Citation analysis: Robert G. Edwards 1975–86, impact factor of journals

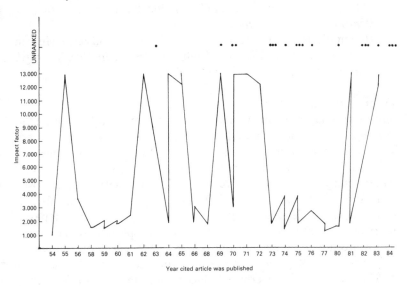

Source: SCI journal reports (1985)

articles (in terms of citations) which are also in the most highly respected journals (in terms of IF). This would indicate his level of popularity combined with prestige:[4]

(a) 80 citations – 12.863 IF (1965) 'Maturation *In Vitro* of Mouse, Sheep, Cow, Pig, Rhesus Monkey and Human Ovarian Oocytes', *Nature*.

(b) 77 citations – 12.863 IF (1969) 'Early Stages of Fertilisation *In Vitro* of Human Oocytes Matured *In Vitro*', *Nature*.

(c) 55 citations – 12.863 IF (1981) 'Test-tube Babies', *Nature*.

(d) 44 citations – 12.863 IF (1970) 'Fertilisation and Cleavage *In Vitro* of Pre-ovulatory Human Oocytes', *Nature*.

(e) 30 citations – 12.863 IF (1964) 'Immunological Control of Fertility in Female Mice', *Nature*.

(f) 46 citations – 12.165 IF (1983) 'Current Status of IVF and Implantation of Human Embryos', *Lancet*.

(g) 92 citations – 1.943 IF (1959) 'Timing of the Stages of the Maturation Divisions, Ovulation, Fertilisation and the First

Cleavage of Eggs of Adult Mice Treated with Gonadotrophins',
Journal of Endocrinology.
(h) 144 citations – 1.834 IF (1974) 'Follicular Fluid', *Journal of Reproduction and Fertility*.
(i) 166 citations – 1.542 IF (1980) 'Establishing Full-term Human Pregnancies Using Cleaving Embryos Grown *In Vitro*', *British Journal of Obstetrics and Gynaecology*.

Types of Journals
More information about the direction of research and development in IVF can be gained from a look at where Edwards has published. There are three levels of specialisation and two types in the range of journals listed above: the levels of specialisation vary from general (where many scientific fields are involved, that is, IVF) to specialised and then to highly specialised (where only one scientific field is involved, that is, endocrine or hormone function). The two types of journals are those directly related to human reproduction and those which are not. Examples of the ranges in specialisation are *Nature* (covering all biological sciences) as a general journal, *Lancet* as a specialised journal (covering medicine), and the *British Journal of Obstetrics and Gynaecology* (covering a specific field of medicine). Examples of types include the *Journal of Reproduction and Fertility* as a directly-related type and *Nature* as one that is not.

The following list is generated by comparing the list above (of prestigious journals in which Edwards is also highly cited) with degrees of journal-specification and the relationship of the field to human reproduction. Each line contains the year the article was published; whether the journal in which it was published is of very high IF (above 5.500), medium high IF (between 2.485 and 5.499) or of relatively low IF (below 2.485); the total number of times the article has been cited between 1975 and 1986; the journal's specificity; and its relation to human reproduction. The point of this comparison is to determine where Edwards is popular (in terms of specificity of field), how much status is attached to that popularity and to see whether there is any indication of how IVF crossed scientific fields.

Year	IF	Citations	Specificity	Reproduction-related
1983	very high	46	specific	no
1981	very high	55	general	no
1980	low	166	very specific	yes

1974	low	144	very specific	yes
1970	low	44	general	no
1969	very high	77	general	no
1965	very high	80	general	no
1964	very high	30	general	no
1959	low	92	very specific	yes

Conclusions from the Citation Analysis

Robert Edwards has enjoyed a remarkable success since his career began in 1954. Clearly the most successful article in terms of the number of citations it has received is the one written with Patrick Steptoe and J. M. Purdy, 'Establishing Full-term Human Pregnancies Using Cleaving Embryos', in the *British Journal of Obstetrics and Gynaecology*, with 166 citations. This is a remarkable number even allowing for the fact that biological articles are more cited than any other in science (SCI *Journal Citation Reports*, 1985). As with his 1974 article in the *Journal of Reproduction and Fertility* which was also extensively cited (144 citations), the journal does not enjoy a high impact factor in the scientific community. In relation to all other articles with high citation rates, these two are in the lowest IF category.

The articles in journals with higher IF ranks have lower citation rates than those above, but still have high citation rates in comparison to other authors in the same field. Of those journals ranked for IF, the most influential and those for which Edwards receives the most citations are *Nature* (1965, 1969, 1981 and 1970) and *Lancet* (1983). *Nature* is considered a general publication; *Lancet* is more specific. Neither journal is directly related to the field of human reproduction. The conjunction of such prestigious exposure and the general audience of the journal are evidence of the cross-disciplinary interest IVF technology has generated, particularly after 1969 when IVF was first used in humans; Edwards's article in *Nature* of that year is frequently cited.[5]

The titles of the articles with high citation rates in journals with high IF also indicate Edwards's rise from being a leading-edge scientist to becoming a spokesperson for the new field, IVF. Early papers (some highly cited) tend to have titles that are in the spirit of pure scientific research (for example, 'Immunological Control of Fertility in Female Mice'). Later, article titles become more generalised and indicate an enhanced position in the newly formed field. For example, they report on the state of research to date ('Current Status of IVF . . .') and they obviously speak to a wide audience ('Test-tube Babies'). There is a great deal of confidence expressed in the articles that appear after 1979 (shortly after the birth of Louise Brown in 1978 and the popularisation of IVF that followed).

In the list above (pp. 66–7) which delineates Edwards's popularity, status and the specificity of the field in which he was publishing, three distinct stages can be seen in the development of IVF: it clearly moves from being of general, scientific interest to becoming highly specific, and then finally reverts to a position of general scientific appeal. Also it can be seen how IVF began as a pure research problem and evolved into a specific human application (around the time of the first success with humans) and then returned as a human application with appeal to scientists in general. However, it returned transformed into accepted practice as a newly established procedure in gynaecology and obstetrics. This is how IVF was normalised as a reproductive intervention in published scientific and medical research. Once established as a new field in science and technology, the next step for those now in the field of IVF was one designed to protect professional interest and to secure the emergent field's future.

The Protection of a New Medical/Scientific Field and Commercial Interest in IVF

The Rise of ESHRE
Late in June 1986, over 650 scientists and doctors met in Brussels in a well organised and very well funded conference on human reproduction. They met as members and guests of the ESHRE, a recently formed society (1985) of scientists and medical practitioners interested and involved in the science of human reproduction. According to Edwards (one of the society's chief founding fathers) there are three objectives of ESHRE: 'One, to join scientists, doctors, philosophers and ethicists in this area of research and practice; two, to encourage young people into the area; and three, to unite Europe in this endeavour.'[6] Not referred to in the formal objectives of the Society was Edwards's fear that he and his European colleagues would be overtaken in advancing IVF research by their American and Australian counterparts. Edwards complained during the press conference in Brussels (the Second Annual Meeting of ESHRE) that the British code of practice forbidding the experimentation on embryos beyond fourteen days was to blame.[7]

According to Edwards, 750 people registered for the conference, more than fifty companies participated in the commercial exhibition, and 305 abstracts were submitted to the conference organisers. Participants came from all over the world and included general practitioners and medical specialists, as well as a variety of scientists. The international drug companies, Organon and Serono were the prime sponsors of the conference. Both companies provide the drugs necessary for hyperstimulation of the ovaries in the IVF procedure. Organon offered free video tapes on how to perform IVF to the medical practitioner participants.

Besides providing financial backing, the conference entertained professionals from many scientific and health-service areas. Gynaecologists, general practitioners, medical and laboratory assistants, nurses, endocrinologists, embryologists and comparative physiologists were present. Rarely do doctors, scientists and paramedics mingle in this way. This is therefore further evidence of a new area of specialisation in reproductive intervention, one that requires a team of basic scientists, medical specialists and general practitioners.

Commercial Interest in IVF and its Commercialisation
As the newly formed area of IVF research and practice gains momentum through professional organisation, so commercial interest in its research and development has blossomed. Organon and Serono are two pharmaceutical companies which have substantial financial interest in the promotion of IVF technology. 'Ares-Serono's sale of products for treating infertility rose by 33% as the result of sales of Perganol [hypopituitary gonadotrophin] and of the launch of Metrodin [Follicle Stimulating Hormone, FSH] in European markets' (Ares-Serono Pharma Sales, 4 April 1986). Both these products are used in IVF procedures. Another financial report announced that Serono is to spend 100 billion Italian lire (£40–45 million) on research into genetic engineering, which directly profits from IVF as a production system of embryos and embryonic material for genetic research.[8]

Organon, a subsidiary of the Dutch multinational, AKZO, N.V., is part of a worldwide system of companies with forty-six branches in twenty-eight countries including most Western European countries, America, Australia, countries in South America, the Pacific Rim, and the Far East (*Who Owns Whom*, 1986). AKZO was formed in 1969 by the merger of two large Dutch chemical companies. Its numerous subsidiaries produce man-made fibres, chemicals, coatings, pharmaceuticals (including veterinarian products), consumer products and some machinery. In 1981, 10 per cent of AKZO's net sales were from the sale of pharmaceuticals: approximately 1466 million Dutch florins (£419 million) (Stopford, 1982). Both Organon and Serono continue to finance ESHRE and were well represented as prime sponsors at the July 1987 Annual Meeting in Cambridge.

Besides multinational, pharmaceutical interest, there has been a more direct form of commercialisation of IVF. In 1985 Monash University (Melbourne, Australia) agreed to market its IVF techniques in the United States. The company IVF Australia Ltd was created to handle the transaction. The company began with five million Australian dollars (£2 million) capital and immediately opened an IVF clinic in New York State. IVF also draws commercial interest from unexpected areas in capital investment: 'Licensed management investment company, CP Ventures Ltd, has chosen the two highest profile areas of high technology for its first investments, satellite communications and *in vitro* fertilisation'(CP Ventures).

The Face of Commercialised IVF
Organon produced a video to be shown to prospective IVF clients which was distributed free of charge during the 1985 ESHRE conference. The title of the video is 'When Nature Fails' and it features a happily married, but tragically infertile couple. The video begins with the scene of a lonely couple, visibly unhappy while watching another couple playing with their child on a beach. A voice begins to tell us the statistics concerning infertility and what an unhappy situation it is inasmuch as 'most couples have a natural desire to fulfil their relationship with one or more children . . .' and 'fifteen per cent of couples do not succeed because infertility stands between them and their desire to have children'. Infertility is later referred to as a 'failure' and a 'shortcoming'.

The video speaks briefly of male infertility (50 per cent of all infertility occurs in men) and describes how simply and quickly it is tested (all that is required is an external examination and the provision of a sperm sample). On the other hand, the infertile woman is presented as a more complex problem worthy of a variety of investigations, including internal examinations of the cervix, the uterus, the fallopian tubes, the ovaries and analysis of thalamic and pituitary functions. The various forms of female infertility investigation are explained: internal examination, visual inspection, laparoscopy, hysteroscopy, hormone testing and ultrasound scanning.

The video then explains how, once the extensive series of tests has been performed, IVF treatment is recommended. After many shots of women's abdomens pierced by laparoscopes and women in the prone position typical for internal examination, the IVF procedure begins. The viewer is then told about 'eggs *resting* in incubators (my emphasis)' and is shown more shots of women in prone positions as their ovaries are penetrated during egg collection through trans vaginal/trans urethral pick-up' which is described as 'less invasive' than trans-abdominal pick-up (the former requires no general anaesthetic nor any incision through the abdominal wall as does trans-abdominal pick-up). The video concludes with a review of the possibilities IVF opens up for reproduction with the variety of combinations of genetic and non-genetic parents possible. It notes how women can carry an embryo genetically unrelated to them (egg donation) or to their partner (sperm donation) or to either social parent (embryo donation).

Organon has an obvious financial interest in the promotion of IVF. The production and free distribution of this video not only emphasises this interest but its content also provides an example of how infertility is conceptualised. Childlessness is depicted as a tragedy and infertility as failure. Owing to the video's focus on female infertility, it is women who emerge as unsuccessful in satisfying that 'natural desire to fulfil their relationship with one or more children'. At the same time as they are made visible in the light of this failure, women's experiences of IVF treatment are trivialised. Therefore, as whole bodies that experience pain and as people who are tired and tested from continuous medical evaluation, they are rendered invisible.[9]

The video's positive image of new genetic familial ties ignores the potential exploitation of women in surrogate arrangements and misleadingly equates sperm donation with egg donation and embryo donation. We are left with the idea that IVF is a completely safe and routine practice in reproductive medicine and a salvation to the tragically infertile and fundamentally unfulfilled *couple*.

Conclusion

In its eighteen year history, IVF technology for humans has evolved from a minor scientific interest to a major field that spans scientific and medical disciplines and relies heavily on commercial markets for support and distribution. This professional and economic organisation of reproductive technology represents the emergence of IVF as a routine practice with specific implications for women and their relationship to procreation.

This chapter has documented some of the signs of the 'normalisation' of IVF as a field of technological medical practice. In the case of Robert Edwards's research career, I have shown his rise to the position of a highly influential spokesperson for the new field. Citation indices were used to trace the simultaneous emergence of interest in his work and a new field in reproductive medicine. In the citation analysis, it is remarkable that there is virtually no regard given to the health risks for women involved in IVF. In the second section of the chapter it is made clear how the consolidation of IVF within professional practice (particularly in the ESHRE) has been sponsored by commercial interests. The Organon video distributed to those medical practitioners attending the ESHRE conference indicates some of the qualities of this professional–commercial link, in particular how IVF is promoted as a routine and virtually trouble-free procedure.

Absent from the IVF research agenda and the commercial enthusiasm surrounding its development and dissemination is any consideration of the new forms of procreation that its routine procedure represent. The misleading language (indicated in the Organon video) of the new high-technology, reproductive medicine speaks of treating the tragically infertile couple without reference to potential health risks for women or to the pressures it reinforces to perform and produce a baby within the traditional family unit. As such, reproduction is sanctioned within prescribed social arrangements and paternity is ensured at the expense of increased medicalisation of women's procreation. Women need to be aware of the extent to which IVF has become normalised as a field in reproductive medicine and to realise that the high commercial gains at stake in IVF's development and dissemination are likely to prevail against a women-centred approach to infertility and reproduction. It is important that notions of 'normal' and 'routine' in IVF be challenged despite the scientific approval, the technological expertise and the commercial investment behind them.

Notes

1. IVF is central to a variety of new reproductive technologies including embryo freezing, embryo flushing and pre-implantation diagnosis. IVF preceded these related developments and remains central to their continuation. As such, IVF is the focus of this chapter.
2. ESHRE was officially established in June 1985. Robert Edwards was one of the founding members.
3. Although journals' impact factors may have changed over the time Edwards's career spans (that is, a 1985 ranking may not apply to the journal in 1954 when the article was published), the highly prestigious journals in this study (such as *Nature* and *Lancet*) have been ranked as such longer than Edwards has published.
4. Because seventeen of the thirty-five journals selected for this analysis according to the high rates of citation of Edwards's articles have no ranked IF, the IF should not be the only guide in indicating influential research. The *Journal of Reproduction and Fertility Supplement* is not ranked. Nevertheless, Edwards's three articles published there received a total of sixty-one citations during the period studied. Edwards's 1963 article in the unranked journal, *Genetic Research, Cambridge*, received thirty-two citations.
5. A further support for the argument that IVF has become a cross-disciplinary field is that Edwards has published in genetic journals (for example, *Genetic Research, Cambridge*), in journals on world population (for example, *Human Population*), and in animal research journals (for example, *Journal of Experimental Zoology*).
6. Press conference, at the ESHRE's Second Annual Conference, Brussels, 27 June to 1 July 1986.
7. Transferring research to nearby European countries would be an easy solution to this inconvenience and may advance British research teams in the international race towards increased control of reproductive processes.
8. 'Ares-Serono has Announced it is to Spend 100 Billion Lire on Research into Genetic Engineering', *Sole Venti Quattro Ore* (7 October 1984).
9. The potential long-term health hazards created by the massive doses of hormones used to hyperovulate women's ovaries are also left unexplored. For more information on these hazards see Direcks and Holmes, 1986.

4 The Depersonalisation of Women through the Administration of '*In Vitro* Fertilisation'
Deborah Lynn Steinberg

Introduction

'*In vitro* fertilisation' is a series of technological procedures designed by medical scientists to intervene in, alter and extract parts of the bodies and to interfere with the reproductive processes of women. It has been offered, received and lauded by medical scientists, the press and various government committees as 'progress', as caring, and as a response to the needs and demands of infertile couples. Representations of, descriptions of and public debates about '*in vitro* fertilisation' have been dominated by a rhetoric of benevolence and remarkably lacking in critical assessment, particularly regarding its impact on women's health and autonomy. Feminist challenges and resistance to this *a priori* assumption of medical scientific beneficence and particularly our attempts to re-orient analysis of '*in vitro* fertilisation' in terms of women's reproductive rights and women's liberation, generally have not been given recognition or serious consideration in so-called 'public' forums of discussion about the implications of this technological innovation. My intention in this chapter is critically to examine '*in vitro* fertilisation', specifically in terms of how it effects women's health and social status. In so doing I will challenge the image of benevolence that has so far dominated its representations. I will argue that it is an image which has depended on, and is only possible through, exclusion of attention to the meaning of '*in vitro* fertilisation' for women.

This chapter rests upon four central premises. The first is that the tools and processes of Western medical scientific technologies, of which '*in vitro* fertilisation' is one example, do not exist or function autonomously. They are designed, developed, named and utilised by exclusive communities of medical and scientific professionals who are nearly always men (Zimmerman, 1986; Rosser, 1988).

The second premise is that medical scientific technologies are never value-free or neutral, devoid of historical specificity, context or the values of those who, in the first place, developed them and, in the second place, use them. Technological apparatuses and procedures are at once a concrete manifestation and practice of the particular values and ideas of their originators. Technologies are, in this sense, a language or discourse of values, a structural (materially structured) encoding and expression of the priorities and consciousness of those who invent and then utilise them. The design of the machine, as it were, reveals much about the mentality and objectives of its makers as well as the parameters or limitations of its uses.

The third premise is that the medical scientific community is a white, patriarchal (male dominated) and powerful community – that is, a community which exercises white male power (Daly, 1979, pp. 223–92). Historically, the members of this powerful community have been remarkably free from accountability to anyone but themselves for the power they exercise and for the tools and procedures they develop for their own use in projects they initiate. The individual members of this community, their technologies and projects are necessarily invested in some way with the power and self-interests of the community. Thus, medical scientific technologies also constitute a structural language through which power is expressed in both material and social practices.

The fourth premise of this chapter is that women are globally and differentially subordinated to men, male power and men in power. Women are discriminated against and disempowered materially, civilly, sexually and reproductively. The social oppression and subordination of women is constituted within an overarching, rigid and systematic and yet, at the same time, differential, arbitrary and impersonal regime of sexism, racism and classism (among other bases). At the same time, violence towards women in any sphere is rarely considered noteworthy by either the patriarchal media or institutions of patriarchal 'justice', most notably the law and the police (Hanmer and Saunders, 1984). Consequently, the agents (particularly institutions) of violence against women are rarely acknowledged as such. The medical scientific community has historically counted among the institutions of patriarchal power which do particularly extensive violence to women and yet at the same time maintain the reputation of a benevolent and caring profession.

Feminists have always recognised that violence against women *exists* and that it is a central and necessary tenet of male dominance (Dworkin, 1974; Frye, 1983; French, 1986). Any artifact, process, law and so on that emerges from patriarchal institutions is, in relation to the status of women, suspect. That is, it is presumptively consistent with the central feature of patriarchal power – it discriminates against women. Feminists have also long recognised that the history of medical science, particularly obstetrics and gynaecology, has been, on the one hand, the history of abuse and injury for women. It is, at the same time, a history of feminist resistance to ideologies and acts which jeopardise women's health and well-being and deprive women of rights (civil or otherwise) and of a concomitant struggle for women's reproductive autonomy (Daly, 1979, pp. 223–92; Corea, 1979; Rothman, 1982). In the light of this history, feminists have understood that any medical scientific innovation, particularly in obstetrics and gynaecology, should be considered suspect and pre-sumptively (likely to be) injurious to women. Any new development in this field should be viewed with suspicion by women and scruti-nised for its effects on women's health, well-being and social status.

This chapter is about the impact of '*in vitro* fertilisation' on three aspects of women's personhood: women's health, women's repro-ductive autonomy, and women's civil status. In the first section of this chapter, I shall examine the procedures and nomenclature of '*in vitro* fertilisation' at four levels. First, I shall decode the meaning and structure of '*in vitro* fertilisation' treatment and language in terms of how they represent the consciousness and priorities of the medical scientific community regarding their construction of the status of women, their perception of their own legitimate power, and the status of their '*in vitro* fertilisation' project. I shall examine how '*in vitro* fertilisation' procedures delineate and structure a particular position for women within the context of treatment. In the next part of this section, I shall discuss the ontological implications of '*in vitro* fertilisation' for women's lives and status, particularly in relation to women's reproductive autonomy. I shall then contextualise '*in vitro* fertilisation' within the medical framework of 'infertility' and discuss the centrality of the meaning of 'infertility' to the treatment of women with '*in vitro* fertilisation'. I shall also discuss the conceptual interrela-tionship of '*in vitro* fertilisation' and the medical model of 'infertility' as it impacts upon the personhood of women. I shall conclude this section by distinguishing '*in vitro* fertilisation' from other medical treatments.

The focus of my discussion will be, in particular, on the research potential of '*in vitro* fertilisation' (as defined by practitioners) and the position of women as subjects of a research project.

In the second section of this paper I shall discuss the impact of the current British medical scientific framework for self-regulation of '*in vitro* fertilisation' (the Voluntary Licensing Authority's code of practice) on the civil status of women. Using this framework as a case study, I shall discuss how the implicit medical scientific objectives and priorities within the procedures and language of '*in vitro* fertilisation' are explicitly codified and consolidated within the overall power structure of medical science.

I Erasure and Recombination: 'IVF' Language and Procedures and the Status of Women

To understand the status of women within the context of '*in vitro* fertilisation' treatment, it is necessary to examine both the procedures and terminology of 'IVF': how they physiologically and materially affect and metaphysically represent women. The procedures incorporated under the heading of '*in vitro* fertilisation' and the language used to denote them have direct and detrimental bearing on the status of women, both within the specific 'IVF' context and more generally.

The status of women in the context of 'IVF' is constructed and reflected by means of two fundamental processes which I call *erasure* and *recombination* of women. The former refers to those processes which obscure or remove women from recognition within the 'IVF' context. This erasure occurs at two levels, those of *representation* and *ontology*.[1] Recombination refers to the effects of 'IVF' procedures on women: the alteration, removal and reconstitution of parts of or affecting women's whole bodies. I shall argue that both these processes of erasure and recombination of women within the context of 'IVF' operate to depersonalise, that is to fragment, alienate and injure, women.

'*In Vitro Fertilisation*'
'*In vitro* fertilisation' means literally *fertilisation in glass*. It identifies only one part of an extensive series of procedures performed on women. While the process as a whole constitutes a recombination of women's bodies and reproductive processes, principally to extract women's body tissues (their eggs), the label '*in vitro* fertilisation'

names only the act of fertilisation and the place, Petri dish (glass), where it occurs. In naming only this one part, the phrase '*in vitro* fertilisation' obscures the rest of the procedures which make such fertilisation in glass at all possible. The term conceals: (1) procedures, all of which, including surgeries and hormone treatments, are and can only be performed on women; and (2) that fertilisation in glass is *predicated* on, (not possible without) prior, protracted and intensive intervention, manipulation and scrutiny of women. In fact, '*in vitro* fertilisation' names the one part of the process from which women are physically absent.

The more popular term 'test-tube babies' replicates this erasure of women and the procedures performed on them. It also compounds this erasure in several ways. It misnames even the site of fertilisation which does not, in fact, occur in a test-tube. Moreover, the term 'baby' modified by 'test-tube' suggests that the act of fertilisation, and even the entire process of conception and 'pregnancy' is not only unrelated to women, but entirely extra-corporeal, outside a woman's body. Furthermore, this term names only the product of the (misnamed) process – the 'baby', instead of the persons (women) who undergo the process.

Both of these terms, '*in vitro* fertilisation' and 'test-tube babies' with the Latin (technical jargon) words of the former and the reference to laboratory paraphernalia in the latter, implicitly recognise medical science as the central (if not the only) domain of reproductive practice. By extension, these terms implicitly recognise medical and scientific practitioners – the 'IVF' team, the 'test-tube baby' doctors. They are not only implicitly identified as present, as *constituents*, but as *agents* of 'IVF' and most importantly as *agents of (women's) reproduction*; the ones who make it happen. Women, who *undergo* 'IVF' on the other hand, are not only *not* identified as agents of their reproduction, but they are not identified in any capacity; neither as participants nor, more specifically, as patients.

This erasure of women in the context of 'IVF' is further portrayed, perhaps most overtly, through consistent references to 'IVF' patients as 'IVF couples', (by which is meant heterosexual couples). The phrase 'IVF couples' linguistically denies the autonomous individuality of women, conflating them with their male partners (or husbands) under the heading 'couple'. It also implicitly suggests that being part of a heterosexual couple is a fundamental standard for women's eligibility for 'IVF' treatment. Moreover this *gender-blurred* nomenclature connotes a false equivalence of women's and men's positions in relation to 'IVF' treatment. It suggests that both receive it, and that they do so equally. This is despite the fact that 'IVF' procedures, by design and structure, *can only be performed on women*.

The procedures which constitute the 'IVF' process and which are obscured by the term '*in vitro* fertilisation' comprise an ever-growing, extensive array of physiological interventions practised on women. These include: (1) continuous and varied chemical alteration and reconstitution of women's reproductive functions; (2) removal and transfer of women's body tissues to medical scientific custody and treatment; and (3) replacement of women's altered and fertilised tissue into their bodies. These procedures women undergo, and the names identifying them have profound bearing on their position, status and personhood, not to mention their health and safety.

The components of the misleadingly termed '*in vitro* fertilisation' process can vary widely, although they all depend on similarly extensive intervention into women. The basic or routine 'IVF' protocol includes four stages of treatment: 'superovulation', 'egg recovery', fertilisation and 'embryo replacement/transfer'.

'Superovulation'

'Superovulation' entails the administration of large doses of various synthetic hormones. These include, but are not limited to: clomiphene citrate (Clomid), human pituitary gonadotrophins HCG and HMG[2] (Pergonal) and progesterone (Walters and Singer, 1984, pp. 5–6). The designated function of these drugs is to induce women to ovulate more than one egg, in fact, as many eggs as possible. The greater the number of women's eggs ovulated, the more likely it is that practitioners will extract one or more viable (sufficiently mature) eggs for fertilisation and the greater is the potential number of women's eggs which can be fertilised in glass. Equally important, hormonal induction of women's ovulation makes it possible for 'IVF' practitioners to time the next phase of the procedure – the removal of women's eggs. According to Carl Wood and Ann Westmore:

> the use of fertility drugs also makes organisation of the procedure considerably easier. Operating theatres can be pre-booked for egg pick-ups at times compatible with the staffing situation and other requirements of the hospital. (Wood and Westmore, 1984, p. 60)[3]

The overall effects of these hormones on women's health have not been extensively documented, or explored in any depth by that sector of the scientific community particularly concerned with the development of 'IVF'. Nowhere, for example, in the abstracts of the 1986 conference of the European Society of Human Reproduction and Embryology (ESHRE) was there any expressed concern for, let alone discussion of, the effects of superovulation on women's health.[4]

Most research and documentation on the long-term effects of Clomid (like those of Diethylstilbestrol (DES) and Thalidomide) are limited to its effects on foetuses and offspring rather than on the women who take it. These include teratogenic (producing congenital abnormalities) malformations such as hydatidiform moles,[5] anencephalics (absence of brain), ovarian dysplasia (abnormal ovarian cell) growth in female foetuses, congenital retinopathy, and bilateral breast cancer (in two daughters of women who took these drugs) (Crook, 1986; Cunha *et al.*, 1987).

Detrimental effects of Clomid on women noted briefly by Mary Anderson include 'hot flushes, palpitations, visual blurring and abdominal discomfort'. Anderson reports, moreover, that one risk of gonadotrophin therapy is excessive stimulation of the ovaries with cyst formation and in the worst cases 'blowing up' of the ovaries, producing acute abdominal pain (Anderson, 1987, p. 68).[6]

Practitioners name and describe the administration of 'IVF' hormones to women strictly in terms of their *desired effect*, that is, the effect desired by practitioners. Thus, hormone administration is called 'superovulation', and described only in terms of stimulation to 'the' ovaries. This misleadingly suggests that these hormones affect *only* the organ or tissue to which they are directed and act on women *only* in the way practitioners purposefully administer them. Hormones, however, are administered in tablets (orally) or by injection (intravenously) and therefore circulate through a woman's whole body, systematically affecting not only the balance of her entire endocrine (hormone) system, but *all* organs and tissues that constitute her body. By definition, they cannot affect just her ovaries.

It is clear, despite the scarcity of research and documentation on the subject, that 'superovulation' entails barely estimated and perhaps even immeasurable risks to women's health and that of their offspring (Crook, 1986). Moreover, practitioners' representations of 'superovulation' procedures reveal a singular lack of concern for the risks 'IVF' hormone administration pose for women. Practitioners narrowly focus on their intention to control women's ovulation and induce them to produce many eggs, and on the disembodied objects of their intention, 'the' (women's) eggs, ovaries and ovulation. They omit reference to women as persons and to women's whole bodies.

Finally, the 'superovulation' phase of 'IVF' treatment necessitates that women are monitored throughout the period of the adminis-tration of fertility drugs, with procedures that include blood tests and ultrasound scans. This continuous scrutiny is requisite as prac-titioners attempt to time the actual moment when women are ready, through hormonal induction, to 'release' their eggs (their point of ovulation). This point, where women are ready (made ready) to ovulate, is the point of transition to the next phase of 'IVF' – 'egg recovery'.

'Egg Recovery'

'Egg recovery' is the most common of the names given by 'IVF' practitioners to the second phase of the 'IVF' process. The *Oxford English Dictionary* defines the term 'recover' as 'to regain possession of or use or control of'. The term 'egg recovery' implies that 'IVF' practitioners are *regaining* possession of something that is theirs, when, in fact, they are *dispossessing* women of what is ours. Other terms for this procedure, including 'egg pick-up', used by Carl Wood and Ann Westmore, share with 'egg recovery' a focus on the tissue removed and the medical/scientific process of removal without refer-ence to the person (a woman) from whom it is removed (Wood and Westmore, 1984, p. 66). The term used by Mary Anderson, egg 'harvest' (Anderson, 1987, p. 71), an agricultural term, connotes the gathering of a (disembodied) 'crop' from a genderless 'field' rather than a surgical removal of (women's) body tissue. 'Harvesting', a term denoting the picking of ripe produce, implies that the maturity of women's eggs, their very 'ripeness' is functionally a *ripeness for removal*. Do we speak of a hysterectomy or appendectomy as 'harvesting' uteri or appendixes, or in the case of transplant surgery of 'harvesting' kidneys or corneas or hearts and lungs?[7] This term, moreover, describes a process of *separating* what is reaped (in this case, women's body parts) from its source (women's bodies) and then *transferring* it (or them) for *consumption* by those who did the reaping ('IVF' practitioners).

In the 'egg recovery' phase of 'IVF', women undergo one of two surgical procedures, *laparoscopic egg retrieval* or one of at least three methods of *ultrasound directed 'egg recovery'*, that enable prac-titioners to extract women's eggs from women's ovaries. *Laparos-copic 'egg retrieval'*, the original procedure for 'egg pick-up' is a surgical procedure women undergo under general anaesthetic. Three incisions are made through a woman's abdomen so that practitioners can insert a laparoscope (a fibre-optic viewing tube), forceps and a teflon-coated needle. Practitioners hold her ovaries with forceps while inserting the needle into each of her stimulated follicles and, using a vacuum pressure device, extract her eggs. This procedure can damage women's ovaries and poses additional risks that are attendant upon general anaesthesia (Wood and Westmore, 1984, pp. 66–8).

Ultrasound directed 'oocyte recovery' is the more recently developed procedure for 'egg pick-up'. In this type of procedure, women are awake. Practitioners may first 'overfill' women's bladders with a saline solution. They then distend women's abdominal cavities with a carbon dioxide gas mixture. Under continuous ultrasound monitoring, they guide a hand-held instrument with a needle at one end through women's bladders and into each of their mature (stimulated) follicles to suck out their eggs. According to Bruel and Kjaer, who manufacture ultrasound 'oocyte pick-up' equipment: 'The puncture procedure can be performed by three different routes for needle insertion: A) Transvesical [through the bladder with an abdominal transducer]; B) Perurethral [through the urethra with an abdominal transducer]; C) Transvaginal with an abdominal transducer or *a vaginal transducer*' (Bruel and Kjaer (UK) Ltd., pp. 4–5, their emphasis).[8] As documented on film, this method of 'egg recovery' is painful for the women and poses the risk of infection from the incision through their bladders (Panorama, 1988).[9]

As a sales pitch in another of their brochures, Bruel and Kjaer report their 'high recovery [of women's eggs] rate':

On average five eggs are obtained per patient; the largest number of eggs retrieved from one patient so far is twenty-two. (Bruel and Kjaer (UK) Ltd., 1986, p. 2)

They do not mention or assess how this 'high recovery rate' affects women's health.

Fertilisation
Assuming that women's eggs have been 'successfully' removed from their bodies, alive and sufficiently mature, the phase for which the process is named 'IVF' – fertilisation in glass, follows. Women's extracted eggs are placed in a Petri dish with (usually their husbands') sperm with the objective that some or all will fertilise. Any resultant embryos are maintained *in vitro* for at least twenty-four hours.

During this time a woman is continuously administered hormones to prepare her for the final phase of the 'IVF' process, 'embryo transfer/replacement'.

'Embryo Transfer/Replacement'
This procedure, as described by Mary Anderson, entails the

> transfer [of] *the* now growing *egg* and implant[ation of] it into *the* uterus previously primed with hormones so that its lining endometrium is in a receptive state. (Anderson, 1987, p. 71, my emphasis)

Typically, the language practitioners use to describe 'IVF' procedures does not refer to women as persons. Instead, women's organs and tissues are described in a disembodied way – as 'it' or 'the uterus'.[10] This language, besides being depersonalising, can be both subtly and overtly misleading. For example, the phrase 'the uterus previously primed with hormones' implies that only this (disembodied) organ was administered hormones when, in fact, women's whole bodies are affected by them. Furthermore, Anderson writes of 'it' or 'the egg' – as singular and independent entities. Eggs, like uteri, are women's body tissues and organs. Moreover, there is rarely only one fertilised egg reimplanted in women. The whole point of 'superovulation' is to induce women to produce more than one. To write of one egg is to obscure the function and nature of 'IVF' procedures and to erase the risk to women of multiple pregnancy which is necessarily posed with a routine reimplantation of more than one of their fertilised eggs. In Britain the recommended and most common number of women's extracted, fertilised and then reimplanted eggs is three or four (VLA, 1986, p. 16). In some countries, such as Ireland, all women's extracted and fertilised eggs must by law be reimplanted in them. In both cases, particularly the latter, women face the many risks attendant on a multiple pregnancy.

Despite claims by some 'IVF' clinics of success rates of upwards of 20 per cent, Gena Corea and Susan Ince found, in a survey they conducted on clinics in the United States, that success rates for 'IVF' treatment are routinely manipulated by clinicians in various ways. These methods of 'success enhancement' include: (1) careful selection of 'IVF' patients; counting so-called 'clinical pregnancies' (a label which refers to a rise in a woman's HCG hormone level; 'clinical pregnancies' are not ongoing pregnancies and cannot lead to a live birth) and ectopic (tubal) pregnancies (which are also not ongoing pregnancies and usually lead to irreparable damage to, or loss of, a woman's fallopian tube) and; (2) removing certain (unsuccessful) patients from their accounting. Actual success rates of 'IVF', measured in terms of likelihood of a woman ending up with a live birth, are extremely low. Corea and Ince found in the United States no rates of live birth higher than 10 per cent, and even those occurred only at the best clinics. (This figure does not reflect the total number of 'IVF' attempts these women underwent.) By and large the success rate at most clinics they surveyed approached or was at 0 per cent (Corea and Ince, 1987, pp. 133–9).

In Britain, medical scientists reported a 1986 pregnancy rate of 9.9 per cent, of which 24 per cent were multiple pregnancies. They reported a live birth success rate of only 8.6 per cent. They did not, however, specify the percentage of these which were the result of multiple pregnancy. Thus, the 8.6 per cent does not represent the *number of women* who gave birth after 'IVF' treatment, but rather, the number of babies born. The success rate of live births *per woman* would therefore be lower than 8.6 per cent (VLA, 1988, pp. 21–22).

Any or all of the 'IVF' procedures can fail. These so-called 'drop cycles' (cycles which fail) 'most commonly occur because hormonal therapy has not induced an adequate number of follicles to mature, rang[ing] from less than 10 per cent to around a third of all cycles at some clinics' (Corea and Ince, 1987, p. 136). Cycles can also be 'dropped' at the 'egg recovery' stage because no women's eggs, or eggs too immature for fertilisation are 'recovered'; at the fertilisation stage where no fertilisation takes place, or fertilised eggs are too damaged to be viable; or, most commonly, at the 'embryo transfer' stage, where none of the woman's fertilised eggs implant in her uterus. Renate Klein and Robyn Rowland report a failure rate of approximately 95 per cent for embryo transfer (Klein and Rowland, 1988, p. 255). Even when (rarely) an ongoing pregnancy occurs, women frequently miscarry. As one clinician reported in the Corea and Ince study, miscarriage (so-called 'pre-clinical abortion') rates, were 25 per cent at his clinic and up to 50 per cent at others (Corea and Ince, 1987, p. 138).

Thus, owing to the high likelihood of failure at every stage of treatment, women may undergo any or all 'IVF' procedures more than once, even several or more times. This repetition of 'IVF' procedures, associated with, and perhaps necessitated by, their high failure rate, extends, by that very repetition, what is already deeply invasive intervention practised upon women. It also compounds the considerable risks to women's health already posed by a single cycle of 'IVF' treatment.

'IVF' Language and Procedures and the Status of Women
As I have shown so far, even a cursory glance at both the terminology and procedures of *'in vitro* fertilisation' reveals a complex interplay of recombination of women's bodies and a simultaneous erasure of that fact. On the one hand, because of the design and intrinsic function of 'IVF' treatment, women are administered hormones that affect their whole bodies in ways that are so far unmeasured and which may even be immeasurable. These hormones also affect particular organs of their bodies in ways which have been documented as detrimental. Women undergoing such treatment are, furthermore, subjected to surgeries and scrutiny on a continuous and usually repetitive basis, all at the risk of their health. At the same time, descriptions by 'IVF' practitioners and advocates and the language representing 'IVF' procedures focus almost exclusively on procedures and practitioners. This focus is buttressed by a simultaneous and multifaceted omission of reference to women and misrepresentation of the procedures women undergo. Women are erased both as autonomous persons and as persons central to 'IVF' treatment. Additionally, women's body parts are represented (and treated) as disembodied fragments or entities rather than as parts of their whole bodies. The fact that 'IVF' is (and can only be) performed on women is consistently obscured, as is the fact that 'IVF' recombines, that is, manipulates and reconstitutes women's bodies both in parts and as a whole.

Ontological Implications of 'IVF' for Women

The particular ways women are *procedurally positioned* and *linguistically represented* within 'IVF' treatment pose, at a broader level, profound *ontological* implications for women. The recombination of women's bodies through 'IVF' procedures and the concurrent representational erasure of women in 'IVF' terminology and descriptions constitute an unprecedented assault on the *privacy*, *integrity* and *autonomy* of women. It is this assault that characterises 'IVF' and which, in turn, makes 'IVF' possible to carry out.

Assault on Women's Privacy
Implicitly, 'IVF' procedures involve an erosion of women's bodily and metaphysical privacy. Physiologically, women's bodies must be opened, scrutinised, manipulated, parts extracted and then reintroduced. Practitioners speak, for example, of the need for women's organs (ovaries) to be 'accessible' so that 'IVF' can be carried out:

> It is important that the *ovaries are accessible* so that ripe eggs can be picked up during laparoscopy. A preliminary laparoscopy is carried out to ensure that this is so. (Wood and Westmore, 1984, p. 58, my emphasis)

'IVF' erosion of women's bodily privacy expands sequentially as each phase of intervention is strictly *predicated* on prior intervention. Thus, for example, 'fertilisation in glass' is impossible without prior 'egg recovery' from women. In turn, each successive phase of 'IVF' treatment compounds the previous level of intervention imposed on women by prior stages of treatment. Every stage of 'IVF' treatment necessitates that women are made increasingly *visible*, turned, as it were, inside out, to practitioners and then transferred to practitioners' jurisdiction. This 'imposed visibility' of women's bodies is both pre-conditional to, and for the express purpose of, effecting literal and conceptual transfer of women's private domain (their bodies) into public commodities, the disembodied 'property' of medical science. Thus, practitioners can unselfconsciously *speak* of disembodied parts of women – 'the ovaries;', 'ripe eggs', and of 'recovering' these parts even as they *materially* scrutinise, alter or remove these parts of women's bodies.

There is a concomitant expansion of women's visibility and an erosion of their privacy at a metaphysical level. In order to carry out 'IVF' treatment, procedural requirements for physiological visibility of women are matched by procedural requirements and those of practitioners that women reveal themselves and are personally accessible and accountable in various ways throughout treatment. Women are required to reveal the details of their personal lives, their sexual and reproductive practices and histories, their domestic arrangements, their relationships with (male) partners, their attitudes towards mothering, and their attitudes towards (or willingness to co-operate with) 'IVF' (Crowe, 1987, pp. 84–93). Moreover, as 'IVF' treatment entails an extensive amount of monitoring and scrutiny of women, including continuous measurement of their hormone levels, the (induced) maturation of their follicles, the 'accessibility' of their ovaries, women must be continuously *available* to the schedules, scrutiny and management of practitioners and to hospital and clinical routines. Sometimes this requires an exhausting amount of travel for women who do not live near the clinic, or that they take temporary accommodation (at their own expense) near the clinic. Moreover, the necessity that women be constantly available in 'IVF' treatment imposes considerable constraint and pressure on women's work lives, possibly jeopardising their paid employment and making it difficult, if not impossible, for them to do anything else *but* 'IVF'.

The expansion of practitioners' 'control' over 'human' reproduction effected through 'IVF' treatment is predicated on the expansion of their control over women, the extent to which they render women visible, render women's private selves public, and appropriate the rendered parts for the direction and discretion of practitioners and the domain of medical science. 'IVF' is intrinsically designed to maximise the bodily and personal visibility of women. As such, it reflects the ethical low premium, or lack of value 'IVF' innovators and practitioners place on acknowledging or respecting *boundaries* to women's bodies and selves. Perception of women as boundaried beings is fundamental to any substantive concept of personhood. I refer here to a philosophically defensive concept of women's personhood and personal liberty, that is of physical and metaphysical boundaries to women's selves whereby trespass of these boundaries oppresses, subordinates or otherwise injures women. Perception of these boundaries is implicit in the concept of violence against women; it is what makes the concept meaningful, conveying the essence of violation, of injury and of unjustified entry into a woman. Thus, a lack of recognition of these physical and metaphysical parameters of women's selves necessarily compromises and erodes women's personhood.

Assault on Women's Integrity
Intrinsic to 'IVF' at another level is the dis-integration of women's bodies and the consequent erosion of women's ontological integrity. This assault on women's integrity through 'IVF' treatment is effected through a conceptual and procedural fragmentation of women's bodies and through increasing and rarely acknowledged levels of risk to women's health.

'IVF' treatment entails an ever expanding series of concrete, repetitive hormonal and surgical interventions which disrupt and reorganise women's physiological processes and extract, manipulate, alter and finally, reintroduce parts (their eggs) of their bodies. Even as women are treated at best through 'IVF' as a compilation of discrete autonomous organs, tissues and systems, the language of 'IVF' similarly refers to disembodied parts, 'the eggs', 'the uterus', or even, in the case of embryos ('unborn children') as independent entities. Even as 'IVF' treatment by design maximises the erosion of women's privacy, so does it similarly maximise the procedural fragmentation of women's bodies. Likewise, 'IVF' language compounds this fragmentation of women even as it represents women's parts and excludes reference to women as whole persons. Thus, 'IVF' treatment intertwines both a conceptual construction of women as (already) fragmented and a series of procedures which literally fragment women's bodies.

Contiguous with this expanding level of intervention and manipulation of women's bodies is a profound and similarly expanding level of risk to women's health. However, given the fragmentary view of women articulated in 'IVF' language and procedures, and the simultaneous design and function of 'IVF' to maximise intervention, it is not surprising that these risks to women's health are seldom acknowledged or considered, let alone deeply investigated, by practitioners. The very tendency of 'IVF' treatment to maximise intervention structurally precludes (and reflects a prior conceptual preclusion of) the giving of priority to women's health and integrity.

Assault on Women's Autonomy
Also implicit in 'IVF' treatment is what may well be an unprecedented erosion of women's personal autonomy and reproductive agency. At the level of representation, women are rarely if ever acknowledged as autonomous persons in the 'IVF' context. 'IVF' patients are consistently (mis)referred to as (infertile or childless) 'couples' when it is *women* who undergo 'IVF'. This subsumption of women under the heading 'couple' linguistically denies women's autonomous personhood. It conceptually constructs women not only as *not* individuals, but categorises women, thereby obscuring them, solely in terms of their association with men (male partners). This erasure of women is compounded by the subsequent disembodied references to women's body parts.

Moreover, 'IVF' procedural requirements that women be maximally visible and subject to practitioners' and clinics' schedules, direction and discretion, impose profound constraints on women's personal liberty. Equally threatening to women's autonomy is the necessarily subordinate relationship they must have with 'IVF' practitioners. The extent to which 'IVF' treatment fragments women's reproduction and transfers their bodies whole and in parts to medical scientific jurisdiction and control is the extent to which: (1) women are alienated from their own bodies, reproductive processes and general health and well-being; (2) women are subordinated to practitioners' control and dependent on practitioners' priorities and schedules; and (3) women's reproductive agency is constrained, compromised or precluded altogether.

The Conceptual System and Structure of 'IVF'
The processes of erasure and recombination of women articulated in 'IVF' treatment and language reflect a prior depersonalised conception of women, that is, a prior understanding of women as depersonalised entities. At the same time, 'IVF' treatment and language concretely (re)construct this depersonalisation of women. The way women are represented and, in turn, positioned and (re)constructed in the context of 'IVF' treatment reveals an entire conceptual framework implicitly concerned with the social meaning of women and the relationship of medical science to women, particularly to women's reproduction. This conceptual framework is not separate from the 'machinery' of 'IVF' but is implicitly encoded into its very procedures and tools.

Linguistically and procedurally, 'IVF' treatment subordinates women. Women are endangered through procedures that haphazardly manipulate and recombine their bodies, reorganise their lives and transfer their bodies and lives to the domain of medical science. Moreover, women are linguistically erased through language which represents women as a series of fragmented parts or falsely implies their absence.

The conceptual framework of 'IVF' is reflected and constituted within and through the *structure* of 'IVF' procedures. The ways women are viewed, treated and positioned within the context of 'IVF' are inextricably confined by parameters *built into* its processes and tools. That is, not only do 'IVF' procedures *function* to depersonalise women through the processes of erasure and recombination and through the contiguous erosion of women's privacy, integrity and ever-shrinking parameters of women's personhood, status and agency are *constituted within* and *limited by*, the very design and structure of 'IVF' treatment. Therefore, the meaning of 'IVF' treatment for women is not simply determined by its (good or bad) use, or by the (good or bad) will or skill of 'IVF' practitioners. More fundamentally, the depersonalised meaning of 'IVF' to women is *in-built, encoded into its design*.

'Infertility': A Suspect Classification[11]

'IVF' is classified medically, legally and popularly as an 'infertility treatment', and more recently, as a method for diagnosing 'infertility'. Not only does 'IVF' have a bearing on the meaning and 'management' of 'infertility', but conversely, the meaning of 'infertility' itself has a *necessary relationship* to the *structure* and *implementation* of 'IVF' and therefore to the complex web of the depersonalisation of women implicit in 'IVF' treatment. To further decode the meaning of 'IVF' treatment for women's status, it is necessary to decipher the meaning of 'infertility' as a system of classification, and to examine specifically how the definition of 'infertility' facilitates the treatment of women with 'IVF'.

'Infertility' is a fundamentally *contradictory* system of classification. It displays the principle that Simone de Beauvoir defined as 'an embarrassing flexibility on a basis of rigid concepts' (de Beauvoir, 1952, p. 65). On the one hand, 'infertility' is a category which, in a general or broad sense, offers a strict conceptual framework while, on the other hand, at a specific level, it is vague, inconsistent and over broad.[12]

The Rigid Conceptual Parameters of 'Infertility'
'Infertility' is constituted as a *pathological* medical category. As a conceptual framework, it is intrinsically a 'disease' model for understanding 'childlessness'. Within the framework of 'infertility', the concept of 'childlessness' has only biological significance. It is constructed as a condition which is *physiological* in its origin and process and, most significantly, a *dysfunction* (failure). Additionally, the medical model, 'infertility', problematises 'childlessness' *individualistically*, locating 'dysfunction' or 'what can go wrong' strictly within the body of the 'infertile person' (Anderson, 1977, pp. 27–41). Likewise, the phrase 'infertile woman/man' establishes a pathological identity, orienting an individual's personhood around 'dysfunction' or 'disease'.

'Infertility' is also a rigidly *diagnostic* category. It is a system of classification which rationalises, justifies and calls for medical intervention. The way in which 'childlessness' is seen as a physiological 'dysfunction' locates it firmly (and only) within the domain of medical science. It posits not only the state of 'childlessness', but those individuals who are childless (defined as 'infertile') as appropriately, even necessarily, medical territory. In so doing, the classification 'infertility' sets up a *categorical imperative* for medical intervention. 'Infertility' is set up as a medical problem which, therefore, necessitates a medical 'solution'.

The category 'infertility' is also *covertly gendered* despite carefully worded explanations of 'infertility' as physiologically originating in either or both men and women. Underlying these 'enlightened' descriptions of 'infertility' is a bias which situates responsibility for 'barrenness' where it has historically been located, with women. Qualifying her acknowledgment that 'infertility' can be located in men as well as women, Mary Anderson writes:

> . . . some men cannot accept the possibility that they may have a problem and so refuse [infertility] investigation. There are ways of overcoming this as we shall see and the writer feels that *no criticism should be levelled at the man by the doctor, especially to the woman*. This can only increase tension, which is hardly the background for successful conception. (Anderson, 1987, pp. 2–3, my emphasis)

Anderson does not include a similar proviso for protecting the sensibilities of women. Nor does she question men's sensitivity on the subject, but she simply accepts it as given. She also expects that women will feel similarly distressed at the idea that their male partners are 'infertile' (but will apparently be able to accept the idea that they, themselves are).

The fundamental gender bias of the category 'infertility' is further revealed in the structure of 'infertility' investigations. Women bear the brunt of these diagnostic investigations, experiencing a level of intervention that is in no way comparable with the markedly less invasive investigations of male 'infertility':

> In outline, investigations for the male partner will be on his semen, and for the female partner on her ovaries and whether they are producing eggs satisfactorily, on her tubes and whether they are functioning normally, on her uterus and cervix and their capabilities and of course on the ability of her partner's sperm to enter her genital tract and reach an egg successfully. (Anderson, 1987, p.3)

Routine 'infertility' investigations of women, are primarily *internal*, entailing, at the least, post-coital internal examinations (to check the 'ability of her partner's sperm to enter her genital tract and reach an egg successfully') and, at much greater risk to her health, laparoscopic (surgical, and under general anaesthetic) examination of her reproductive organs. Investigations of men on the other hand, are primarily *external* (analysis of their sperm), obviously posing minimal (if any) risk to their health.

Finally, the gender bias of the category 'infertility' is compounded linguistically by the designation of patients undergoing 'infertility' investigations as 'infertile couples' with similar implications to those inherent in the phrase, 'IVF couple'. Moreover, the 'gender neutrality' of the phrase 'infertile couple' may appear to avoid apportioning 'blame', allocating each partner equal weight and significance in the process of reproduction, regardless of who is 'unable' to contribute to that process. But, in fact, this terminology does not equalise the position of women in relation to men. Rather, it *subsumes* and therefore *trivialises* women's unequal burden and risk in undergoing 'infertility' investigation under a rhetoric of equivalence. This erasure of women, and the procedures women undergo, is particularly manifest in the context of 'IVF' treatment where (not unlike most 'infertility' treatments) they not only bear the burden and risk of 'infertility' investigation, but also of 'infertility' treatment.

Thus, the category 'infertility' intrinsically constitutes a rigid pathological and diagnostic model for understanding 'childlessness'. Within the parameters of this framework, 'childlessness' is constructed both as a biological phenomenon and as a physiological 'problem' located in the bodies of individuals. This construction places both the 'problem' and the individuals who are diagnosed 'infertile' squarely under the jurisdiction of medical science, thereby establishing a necessity for medical management (of the 'problem'/ 'problem persons'). That women bear the primary burden and risk of 'infertility' investigations, reveals the further rigid presumption on the part of practitioners that 'infertility' itself is fundamentally located in women (whether or not the 'problem' eventually diagnosed is theirs).

The medical model of 'infertility' has further implications for women's *experiences* of 'childlessness'. Within this framework, women's feelings and experiences, their possible despair and desperation, and even guilt, are construed as part of the general 'pathology' of 'infertility'. Women's feelings and experiences are significant here, not for their own sake but only in so far as they can be used by

Deborah Lynn Steinberg

Deborah Lynn Steinberg

practitioners as indications for medical treatment. That is, they have a strictly *diagnostic* significance, and thus are taken only as further justification for medical intervention. This medicalised framework eclipses and precludes social, political and psychological analysis of the meaning of both biological childlessnes and women's feelings and experiences of biological childlessness. Thus, this framework precludes any analysis that is *divorced* from an imperative for medical intervention.[13]

Vagueness and Inconsistency of the 'Infertility' Framework in the Context of 'IVF' Treatment

While the category 'infertility' is conceptually rigid on the one hand, the specific conditions which are classified under this heading betray, on the other hand, a disquieting lack of consistency and clarity. The categorical 'flexibility' of the meaning of 'infertility' is particularly apparent in the variable ways it articulates with 'IVF' treatment. In the context of 'IVF' treatment, 'infertility' can refer to a wide range of conditions which together reveal a peculiar lack of specificity. Some of these conditions actually contradict the conceptual rigidity of the category 'infertility' itself. The 'embarrassing flexibility' of the meaning of 'infertility' is manifested particularly in relation to 'IVF' treatment in several ways: (1) the suspect etiology (origin of disease) of 'infertility'; (2) suspect indications for 'IVF'; (3) the conflation of 'infertility' and 'childlessness'; (4) the definition of 'IVF' as an 'infertility' treatment; and (5) the use of 'IVF' as a tool for the diagnosis of 'infertility'.

The Suspect Etiology of 'Infertility'

The etiologies of 'infertility', even at a strictly physiological level, are poorly understood. Hence, accounts of such 'origins' of the condition are deeply problematic. These suspect etiologies include:

1. *Idiopathic* or 'unexplained infertility' which is a common indication for a variety of 'infertility' treatments (primarily on women) despite the fact that no physiological reason for 'failure to conceive' can be found.
2. *Environmentally induced* 'infertility' which may result from exposure to pathogenic (producing illness), teratogenic (producing malformation in pregnancy), or mutagenic (producing mutations, for example cancer) substances including chemicals and radiation, either in the workplace or the general environment.

3. *Iatrogenic* (medically induced) 'infertility' which is particularly common for women. It can result from direct surgical damage; post-surgical infections as in septic (botched, usually illegal) abortions, Pelvic Inflammatory Disease (PID), the most common source of physiological infertility in women, which if not treated in time can cause irreparable damage to women's fallopian tubes; misdiagnosed or undiagnosed sexually transmitted diseases such as Chlamydia which, if untreated, can cause secondary PID; tubal sterilisation; oral and particularly injectable contraceptive drugs such as the pill or Depo Provera; and hormone (fertility) treatment which may damage women's ovaries or facilitate ectopic (tubal) pregnancy (Anderson, 1987, pp. 27–41).[14]

'Infertility' can involve either one or both partners, although both cases are commonly conflated into the category 'infertile couples' and in most cases 'infertility' investigations and treatment are carried out only on women. Significantly, 'infertility' can, particularly in the case of 'idiopathic infertility', sometimes disappear without medical intervention.

However, within the rigid, medicalised conceptual framework of 'infertility', all of these 'suspect etiologies' will constitute individualised, pathological diagnoses. As such, they will thereby rationalise equally individualistic medical intervention and treatment. This is despite the fact that environmentally induced and iatrogenic 'infertility' clearly constitute problems which do not originate in the individual casualty. 'Infertility', the medical model, eclipses or precludes social and political questions about medical (mal)practice and environmental pollution.

Suspect Indications for 'IVF'
Any and all of the etiologically 'suspect' diagnoses, plus a wide variety of other conditions called 'infertility', can be designated by practitioners as indications for 'IVF' treatment on women. 'Suspect etiologies' in particular contribute directly to the expansion of indications for 'IVF', thereby co-opting a greater number of women into the 'IVF' treatment programme. According to Françoise Laborie:

> The indications for IVF have expanded enormously . . . [to include]: *tubal damage* (61%), *male infertility* (11%), both tubal and male infertility (11%), *idiopathic* [unexplained] infertility (12%), immunological infertility [for example, women producing antibodies against their partner's sperm] (1%) and multiple causes (2%). (Laborie, 1987, p. 51, my emphasis)

With regard to the use of 'IVF' on women with tubal damage, the cause of which is not infrequently iatrogenic, Robert Edwards writes:

> The majority of patients presented with tubal disorders (81%), *Pelvic Inflammatory Disease* caused irreparable damage and blockage of the oviducts in many of them, tubal surgery having failed to restore function. (Edwards *et al.*, 1984, p. 3)

In cases of idiopathic (unexplained) 'infertility', William Walters and Peter Singer suggest that:

> Another group of *women with infertility* which may be considered suitable for IVF is that comprising women who, *although having no problems after routine infertility tests*, fail to conceive after more than one year with AID treatment. (Walters and Singer, 1984, p. 3, my emphasis)

However, Carl Wood and Ann Westmore add that:

> such couples [*sic*] may become pregnant without any treatment; 40% after two years infertility. (Wood and Westmore, 1984, p. 28)

Walters and Singer also suggest *male infertility* as a diagnostic indicator for 'IVF' on women:

> IVF and ET [embryo transfer] are being explored in the treatment of male infertility where the number, movement and structure of sperm are considered to be abnormal. (Walters and Singer, 1984, p. 3)

Thus, not only are women treated with 'IVF' on the basis of possible prior medical malpractice (as involved in many cases of damage to women's tubes from misdiagnosed or untreated PID), but, according to Laborie's statistics, at least 12 per cent undergo 'IVF' despite the lack of diagnosed pathology (their own and their partner's), and at least 11 per cent of those women in the clinics she surveyed undergo extensive medical intervention for their *male partner*'s condition.

The misleading 'gender neutrality' of the patient signifiers 'infertile couples' and 'IVF couples' (and 'pregnant couples') masks the fact that diagnosis of 'infertility' may not refer at all to women, and that 'IVF' treatment may not, in fact, be treating a *woman*'s fertility 'problem'.

The Conflation of 'Infertility' with 'Childlessness'
The terms 'infertility' and 'childlessness' are used interchangeably by

practitioners, the media and in law. Thus 'IVF' treatment has come to be known as a way of 'achieving pregnancy for childless couples' (Barker, 1981).[15] However, *'IVF couples' are not necessarily childless*. According to 'IVF' practitioners Carl Wood and Ann Westmore:

> It makes no difference to the priority given to couples if they already have children – either adopted, conceived before the infertility problem occurred, or achieved through artificial insemination or a previously successful In Vitro Fertilization attempt. (Wood and Westmore, 1984, p. 56)

William Walters and Peter Singer write, moreover, that:

> Previous childbearing suggests that factors contributing to infertility, with the exception of tubal disease, are unlikely to be present. *Women who have already had a child also have a significantly better chance of an easy ET [embryo transfer]* because the neck of the womb, having been stretched during delivery of a baby, is wider. (Walters and Singer, 1984, p. 4, my emphasis)

Thus, as these practitioners explain, 'IVF' is more likely to be successful when women have previously given birth.

The conflation of 'childlessness' with 'infertility' linguistically obscures the fact that 'IVF couples' may indeed already have children, although these may be biologically related only to one (or, in the case of adoption, neither) of their parents. It is a clear case of misrepresentation and one which fosters a categorical expansion of the use of so-called 'infertility' treatments as 'IVF' on a growing number of women (who may or may not have 'fertility' problems and who may already be parents).

The Suspect Definition of 'IVF' as an 'Infertility' Treatment
'IVF' has been represented by practitioners (by the media and in law) as an 'infertility' treatment. This representation misleadingly implies that 'IVF' treats (and attempts to cure) the *causes* or *source* of 'infertility'. This is not the case. At best, 'IVF' only *bypasses* 'infertility'. It may be a tool for medical scientists to attempt to engineer a woman's pregnancy, but it does not treat any physiological fertility 'problems' she may have, and it most certainly is not a cure. If a woman undergoes 'IVF' treatment because her tubes are damaged, her tubes will remain just as damaged during and after 'IVF' treatment. Moreover, as I have shown in my earlier discussion of 'IVF'

treatment, 'IVF' not only does not enhance women's health, but *jeopardises* it in ways that are so far barely estimated or explored. Thus, a woman undergoing 'IVF' treatment is likely to emerge in worse condition, or with more fertility 'problems' than she had before treatment (or with fertility problems she never had before).

The Suspect Use of 'IVF' as a Tool for Diagnosing Male 'Infertility'

Complicating the already suspect use of 'IVF' to treat women who are not diagnosed as 'infertile' but whose *male partners* are, 'IVF' has also been posited as a tool for diagnosing 'infertility' particularly *male* infertility. William Walters and Peter Singer suggest 'IVF' for diagnostic use particularly for women with unexplained 'infertility' (for example, women who may not have any physiological fertility 'problem', but whose male partner may or may not):

> IVF is a new technique which may be used for diagnostic as well as therapeutic purposes. In women with unexplained infertility, IVF can be used to diagnose the level of fertility defect, *that is in sperm*, eggs, fertilization or tubal transport. (Walters and Singer, 1984, p. 8, my emphasis)

Previously this type of test for sperm motility (ability to fertilise eggs) has involved the use of hamster ova, which were removed through 'IVF' procedures and then placed in a Petri dish with human sperm. The use of 'IVF' for diagnosing male 'infertility' means that women and women's eggs, in effect, replace hamsters and hamster's eggs.[16]

The Meaning of 'Infertility' and the Depersonalisation of Women through 'IVF'

The meaning of 'infertility' is clearly central to the administration of 'IVF' treatment on women. Not only is 'infertility' the categorical context of 'IVF' treatment but, as such, it is the chief means facilitating the use of 'IVF' on a growing number of women. At both conceptual and practical levels, the rigid conceptual parameters together with the specific contradictory meanings of the category 'infertility' constitute an *a priori* framework for a fragmentation, alienation and erasure of women's bodies, lives and selves. 'IVF' treatment, which shares the conceptual framework and context of 'infertility', replicates and furthers this assault on women's personhood.

'IVF': Experimentation on Women in the Medical Context

In order fully to comprehend the ontological significance of 'IVF' treatment for women, it is necessary to distinguish 'IVF' from other forms of medical treatment. 'IVF' treatment, on the one hand, shares many of the features generally characterising contemporary Western medical treatments. Because it is clinically situated in a medical context, administered by medical practitioners to medical 'patients', 'IVF' shares and is characterised by the overall conceptual framework and unequal power relations between doctor and patient implicit in general medical practice. There is a continuity between the intrinsic pathological orientation and diagnostic assumptions and imperatives of 'IVF' and those in medicine overall. There is also a continuity between the subordinated status of women in the 'IVF' context and the subordinate status of patients generally.[17]

However, 'IVF' treatment differs significantly from many other forms of medical treatment in several ways. These include: (1) the sexual specificity of 'IVF' treatment; (2) the erasure of reference to the 'IVF' patient; (3) the profound level of intervention and risk to patients in a circumstance that is not organically life threatening; (4) the characteristic vagueness and inconsistency of diagnostic indications for 'IVF' treatment; and (5) the low success rates of 'IVF' treatment.

I have already pointed out that, although 'IVF' can only be performed on women, this fact is consistently obscured both in 'IVF' nomenclature and in procedural descriptions. This erasure of the gender of the 'IVF' patient is coupled with the simultaneous fragmenting representation of women, whose body parts are identified in disembodied isolation, without reference to, or concern for, women's personhood.

'IVF' treatment also comprises an unprecedented level of intervention, manipulation and reconstitution of women's bodies. This is despite the significant absence of any organically life-threatening condition, her own or her male partner's. 'IVF' treatment on women in order to attend to their male partner's 'infertility' constitutes a most remarkable chemical and surgical alteration of one person for the treatment of another's condition. While transplant surgery (such as kidney transplants), for example, does involve the surgical recombination of one (healthy) person for treatment of another's condition, it is significantly different from 'IVF' treatment. Firstly, kidney transplant surgery is not gender specific. Moreover, it is performed in a life-threatening situation. – Additionally, the kidney donor and kidney recipient undergo comparable surgical intervention. Neither donor nor recipient is linguistically erased, to the same extent, from reference. Nor is there a conspicuous absence of concern for the health and well-being of both patients. None of the above conditions applies to the case of 'IVF' treatment of women. Regardless of the reasons used to rationalise it, 'IVF' treatment poses extraordinary and unequalled risks to women's health and personhood in the absence of any serious or comprehensive concern for women's well-being.

Despite the excessive level of intervention performed on women through 'IVF', the indications for treatment notably lack consistency. The sheer vagueness and overbreadth of the suspect category 'infertility' functions to draw an ever-increasing number of women into the treatment pool, without there being a clear, necessary and consistent relationship between the state of a woman's health and the treatment she is given.

Moreover, the low success rates of 'IVF' (the statistical rarity that women undergoing 'IVF' will actually have a live birth), compromise its status as a clinical therapy. The high failure rate of 'IVF' treatment with the concomitant extraordinary risks it poses to women's health and the fact that the course of 'IVF' treatment is not consistent, but is, in fact, always changing and incorporating greater varieties and levels of chemical and surgical intervention, together indicate that 'IVF' is, in fact, *experimental* rather than clearly therapeutic. The term 'clinical' itself connotes treatment which is not experimental, but is tried and true, accepted and safe. The administration of 'IVF' in a *clinical* (hospital or medical clinic) setting, and women's position as 'infertility patients' give clinical *credibility* to a treatment that is, in fact, a trial in progress. It is neither routine nor clinically proven and sound. While women may be labelled as 'patients' (and may, moreover, consider themselves 'patients' who are undergoing a tried, tested and proven therapy), this label obscures the fact that they are subjects of experimentation.

There is a difficulty in distinguishing 'clinical' and 'experimental' treatments that is, I would argue, characteristic of medicine in general. This is particularly true where life-threatening and poorly understood conditions are being treated (for example various cancers, or AIDS). My argument here is not that 'IVF' differs from general medical practice in treading a line between therapy and experiment. My point is, rather, that 'IVF' does *not* balance on a border-line between the two, but is clearly at the extreme – experimental – end of that divergence.[18]

Thus, 'IVF' treatment differs significantly from other medical therapies both by design and by degree. However it has not emerged in a vacuum. The well-documented history of gynaecology has comprised such wanton and over-zealous attempts to control and reconstitute women's sexuality and reproduction. This historical trend of (mal)practice toward women has been exemplified through the administration of dangerous contraceptives to women, particularly in 'third world' countries (Akhter, 1987, pp. 154–60; Kamal, 1987, pp. 146–53) and other uses of medicine for the social control of women, such as sterilisation (particularly unnecessary hysterectomies), dangerous birth control methods (for example, Intrauterine Devices (IUDs) such as the Dalckhon Shield), dangerous drugs for the management of pregnancy (such as Thalidomide and Diethylstilbestrol (DES)) among others (Corea, 1985, pp. 94–113; Direcks, 1987, pp. 161–5).

'IVF' is not characterised by an ethic of minimum intervention for maximum benefit *to the patient*, or even by the Hippocratic injunction to do no harm, or by the idea that mind and body should be regarded holistically (Rothman, 1982, p. 34). On the contrary, the ethos characterising and guiding the use of 'IVF' treatment is the maximisation of intervention and of the number of women practised upon. Moreover, the criteria for measuring success or benefits are those of practitioners' goals and expertise, and of scientific 'progress' and *not* those of how 'IVF' affects women's health, well-being and personhood.

II Defining Practice: Standards of Medical Scientific Self-regulation of 'IVF' and the Status of Women

It is a truism that there is a necessary relationship between the structure and design of any medical treatment or scientific project and those guidelines established by practitioners to administer it. Analysis of the administrative agenda of medical scientific guidelines governing practitioners' practices reveals much about the implicit objectives and priorities of the practices in question. Additionally, the congruence (and/or contradictions) between procedures and codes of practice that regulate them structure the hierarchies of medical scientific accountability that characterise relationships within the professional community and between professionals and 'patients'.

So far in this chapter, I have examined the meaning of 'IVF' for women's status by focusing my analysis on 'IVF' procedures and language. I have discussed how the depersonalisation of women is *structurally* built into 'IVF' procedures and how this structural subordination of women is linguistically reflected and (re)constructed through 'IVF' language. In this section of this chapter, I focus on a specific case-study of regulatory standards, or codes of acceptable ('IVF') practice established by the medical and scientific community in Britain. Having discussed 'IVF' *practice*, I will now discuss *practitioners' codes* of practice, their self-defined ethical standards.

The *First Report of the Voluntary Licensing Authority for Human In Vitro Fertilisation and Embryology* (1986)[19] can be seen as a case study of the necessary congruence between the implicit structure of medical scientific practice and procedures, and guidelines for their administration proposed by the medical scientific community. The code of practice regarding 'IVF' treatment articulated in the Voluntary Licensing Authority (VLA) Report establishes a regulatory framework in which women are linguistically and administratively subordinated to 'IVF' practitioners and to the procedural parameters of 'IVF' treatment. The VLA guidelines reflect and (re)construct the depersonalisation of women that is built into the design and structure of 'IVF'. Analysis of both the language and substance of the VLA code of practice further reveals the implicit objectives and priorities of medical scientists in their 'IVF' project.

The Voluntary Licensing Authority is typical of the orientation and priorities of the medical scientific community, particularly in relation to their treatment of women. It illustrates how they perceive and structure women's status within the context of projects such as 'IVF' treatment. The infrastructure of the VLA itself, both in terms of its membership and its posited system of medical scientific accountability mirrors and is mirrored by the substantive guidelines it proposes to administer 'IVF' treatment. Both this infrastructure and code of practice, moreover, are congruent with the substantive meaning of 'IVF' treatment itself. Together they constitute an assault on women's health, well-being and personhood.

The Voluntary Licensing Authority: A Model of Medical Science Self-Regulation

The VLA was established in Britain in 1985 by a joint coalition of the Medical Research Council (MRC) and the Royal College of Obstetricians and Gynaecologists (RCOG) in response to a Government committee's (the Warnock Committee's) recommendation 'that a new statutory licensing authority should be established to regulate both research and certain types of infertility services. One such service [is] IVF' (VLA, 1986, p. 6). In the absence of specificity on the part of the Warnock Committee as to *who* exactly should comprise this regulatory authority, 'the VLA was proposed by the sponsoring bodies as an interim arrangement pending the setting up of a statutory licensing authority for human IVF and research on pre-embryos' (ibid., p. 20).

The medical scientific community therefore established the VLA as a non-statutory (not legally empowered or binding) *interim medical scientific model* for the regulation of 'IVF' treatment and 'pre-embryo research' (a point to which I will return later). It not only provides a *model regulatory framework* but a potentially *incumbent* or heir-presumptive *body* for *statutory* self-regulation.[20]

Despite their claim that the VLA has been established to allay public concerns and anxieties about 'IVF', 'this new but fast growing area of medical and scientific knowledge' (ibid., p. 1), both its membership and its remit (its 'legitimate' sphere of authority) betray that the VLA is not, in fact, a consumer (-run or -oriented) protection agency. That is, it does not forward or protect the interests of women, the 'consumers' and patients of 'IVF', but, rather, reflects and seeks to protect the interests of medical scientists and their practice.

The Absence of Representation of Women's Interests in the VLA Membership

In her foreword to the VLA report, VLA 'chairman' [*sic*], Dame Mary Donaldson writes: 'Lay members now comprise half the membership of the Authority' (ibid.). This misleadingly implies that 'public' or consumer interests are equally represented (if not given priority) alongside those of medical science, simply because seven members are not doctors or research scientists. The descriptive term 'lay' person connotes a professional and ideological divorce from the interests of medical science. It suggests persons with no professional or personal ties or obligations to the medical scientific community. However the so-called 'lay' members of the VLA were nominated jointly by the MRC and the RCOG (the medical scientific community), and several have existing or prior ties with the administration of health services and research science.[21] They were clearly nominated for their professional status and experiences. Congruent with these criteria, not one of the 'lay' members of the VLA specifically represents the interests of women, the consumers and primary subjects of 'IVF' treatment.[22] The lack of representation of women's interests in the membership of the VLA betrays a lack of concern for, let alone priority, given (by the medical science community) to, the meaning of 'IVF' for women.

The VLA Infrastructural Subordination of Women

The VLA Report structures a hierarchical system of medical scientific accountability both within the medical science community and between 'IVF' practitioners and (women) patients. The VLA proposes to establish a system of internal accountability that is strictly within the confines of medical science, specifically the MRC and RCOG. To this end, 'IVF' practice, practitioners and local ethics committees are placed solely within medical scientific jurisdiction. It establishes itself as both the standard-setting body for 'IVF' practice and the central referee to whom practitioners are directly accountable through a system of licensing. The Report states that the central remit of the VLA is:

1. To approve a Code of Practice on research related to human fertilisation and embryology.
2. To invite all centres, clinicians and scientists engaged in research or in vitro fertilisation to submit their work for approval and licensing.
3. To visit each centre prior to its being granted a licence.
4. To report to the Medical Research Council and Royal College of Obstetricians and Gynaecologists.
5. To make known publicly the details of both approved and unapproved work. (Ibid., p. 3)

The VLA then delegates strictly *executive* responsibility to local ethics committees which are expected to enforce VLA standards on a day-to-day basis:

The local ethical committee is, in terms of day-to-day supervision, better placed than the VLA to ensure that only work which has been approved is being done in its centre: the VLA's role is to give more general guidance on acceptable work. (Ibid., p. 9)

Thus, the VLA establishes a restrictive system of internal, that is, medical scientific self-regulation. They *define* and *administer* 'IVF' policies and they *regulate* practitioners and their practice. Only through their primary responsibility to themselves may they be, at best, *indirectly* answerable to 'IVF patients' and to the general public. Significantly, the VLA makes no equivalent provision for practitioner's direct accountability to 'IVF patients' – women, nor, as we shall see, does it structure 'IVF' policy centrally around women's interests. Indeed, women are rarely mentioned in the VLA report.

The Substantive Erasure of Women in the VLA Standards of 'IVF' Practice

> The intention was not to draw up restrictive and rigid guidelines which might have been workable in practice, *nor to constrain further progress in areas in which research was considered essential for medical advance.* The Guidelines are intended to set the minimum acceptable standards. . . . (Ibid., p. 8, my emphasis)

The VLA intends that the 'minimum standards' for 'IVF' practice are to be dictated by the overriding concern not to constrain scientific 'progress'. Thus, *'minimum* standards' effectively mean *minimal* standards. The central index of acceptable practice is *not* the safety of 'IVF' for women, but rather facilitating and giving priority to 'medical advance' and *medical research*. This intent betrays an operating definition of 'IVF' in the VLA Report as centrally, or most importantly, a *research project*. That is, the research status, interests and potential of 'IVF' supersedes its 'clinical application' (ibid., p. 30).[23]

The specific series of thirteen policy guidelines that comprise the VLA 'minimum standards' regulating 'IVF' reflect two fundamental concerns that directly indicate the VLA's central objectives: (1) the preservation of exclusive medical scientific control over 'IVF'; and (2) the facilitation of the research potential of 'IVF'. In keeping with these priorities, the VLA standards effect a total linguistic erasure of women even as they implicitly subordinate women to practitioners and to the intrinsic objectives of 'IVF' research.

Interwoven with proposals to regulate standards of premises, that is, 'IVF' clinical and laboratory facilities and equipment, a significant portion of the VLA guidelines is concerned with the maintenance of the professionalism (and the professional exclusivity) of 'IVF' teams. Guidelines specify that 'IVF' teams must be comprised of 'appropriately experienced medical, nursing and technical staff' (ibid., p. 32). Even as the VLA Report restricts professional expertise and experience to, and defines them in terms of, themselves, it fails to make any provision in its guidelines that are specifically oriented towards 'patients'' (women's) interests. For example, in a section of the 1986 Report entitled ironically 'Involvement of non-medical staff in "IVF"' Programmes', the VLA reports that 'IVF' practitioners control nearly all aspects of treatment including the supposedly 'patient'-oriented service of counselling (ibid., p. 16).[24] The Report does not, however, point out or express ethical concern for the fact that practitioners' professional investment in the practice of 'IVF' necessarily constitutes a conflict of interest between their own and their 'patients'' (women's) interests. While the VLA applauds 'IVF' *de facto* counselling services, its guidelines do not *mandate* that counselling services be available to 'IVF' 'patients', let alone that these services, in order to serve 'patients'' (women's) best interests, must additionally be divorced from 'IVF' practitioners' interests.[25]

The two sections of the VLA guidelines proposing to monitor the professionalism of 'IVF' practitioners and premises never mention, let alone make central (the protection of) women or women's health and well-being. Likewise, the remaining eleven of the fourteen VLA guidelines betray a total erasure of women. Although classified as 'Guidelines for both Clinical and Research Applications of Human [*sic*] *In Vitro* Fertilisation' (ibid., p. 30), not one of the VLA guidelines establishes standards for the actual administration of hormones and surgeries to women which constitute the actual procedures of 'IVF'. The VLA guidelines never discuss either the so-called 'clinical administration' of 'IVF', nor by extension, any procedures women undergo, whether classified as 'clinical' or 'research'. Nor, in fact, do they ever mention the word 'woman'. Betraying the primary objective of 'IVF' practitioners and the medical science community of promoting 'medical advances', nearly all the VLA guidelines are concerned exclusively with: (1) the status of 'IVF' as a justified experiment; and (2) the status of 'the' embryo. Both concerns represent a frontal assault on the personhood and civil status of women.

Legitimacy: Defining 'IVF' as 'Ethical Research'
The central premise or objective of the VLA guidelines is stated in the first clause:

> *Scientifically sound* research involving experiments on the processes and products of *in vitro* fertilisation between gametes is ethically acceptable subject to certain provisions detailed in Sections 2–10 below. (Ibid., p. 31, my emphasis)

'IVF' is classified as an acceptable research project, which means effectively that research on women with 'IVF' procedures, or within the remit of an 'IVF' research project, is classified as acceptable.

Moreover, the ethical legitimacy of 'IVF' (research on women) is measured exclusively in terms of its 'scientific soundness', *not* in terms of its safety for the women who undergo it. This sole criterion of scientificity completely erases both that 'IVF' is performed on women and that women undergo 'IVF' nearly always as a 'clinical' 'infertility' treatment. This criterion, on its own and unmitigated by any expressed concern for the health and well-being of women, further consolidates the exclusivity of medical scientific authority in defining and regulating their own practice ('IVF').

Within the rigid framework of scientificity, the VLA defines three wider-ranging or flexible aims which it considers not only appropriate, but in fact *necessary* to justify any 'IVF' project:

> The aim of research must be clearly defined and relevant to clinical problems such as the diagnosis and treatment of infertility or of genetic disorders or for the development of safe and more effective contraceptive measures. (Ibid.)

Research on women with 'IVF' is acceptable as long as it can be defined [by practitioners] as relevant to: (1) 'infertility' diagnosis and treatment (including the use of 'IVF' on women to study *male* infertility); (2) research into and development of contraception; and (3) research into 'genetic disorders'. These aims are themselves effectively so broad as to justify study of any and all aspects of women's reproductive processes for reasons, moreover, which may have nothing at all to do with their specific health 'problems' (or with the reasons they are undergoing 'IVF' treatment). This categorical breadth of rationales for 'IVF' treatment betrays the essential falsity [bad faith] of claims that 'IVF' treatment is a sympathetic response to the distress of 'infertility'. These claims none the less constitute the central marketing strategy of both 'IVF' practitioners and the media (see Franklin, this volume).

The Treatment and Status of 'the Embryo' and the Erasure of Women

Despite the fact that 'IVF' constitutes protracted and dangerous intervention affecting women, nowhere in the VLA guidelines is there any mention of, or attention to this fact. Nor is there any attempt to establish criteria to minimise risks specifically related to 'IVF' treatment on *women*. Instead, the VLA concentrates most of its attention on setting standards for practitioners' treatment of – that is, research on – women's embryos (which the VLA calls 'pre-embryos').[26] Eight of the twelve guidelines for acceptable 'IVF' practice are concerned with the treatment of women's embryos in either a clinical or research setting (which, as I have pointed out, are not separable as both projects depend on the prior, usually labelled, 'clinical' treatment of women with 'IVF') (VLA, 1986, pp. 31–2).

The VLA's concentration on the relationship between 'IVF' and women's embryos not only excludes women by reason of the fact that women's embryos are discussed while women and the procedures women undergo are never mentioned. More fundamentally, the definition of women's embryos as entities separate from women which need separate protection has grave implications for the civil status, personhood and reproductive autonomy of women. The VLA linguistically erases women through its discussion of 'IVF' exclusively in terms of embryos. This conceptual severance of women's embryos from women erases women's original relationship with their embryos. It effectively denies that women's embryos come from their eggs which, in turn, come from their bodies. Also obscured within this framework are the ('IVF') procedures whereby women's embryos are literally severed from their bodies. Thus, as embryos are constructed and represented as *a priori* independent entities, 'IVF' appears to be a process of disembodying literally what was already disembodied conceptually.

The VLA discusses 'IVF', not only in terms of disembodied embryos, but in terms of 'embryo research'. This language misrepresents 'IVF' as a process that only treats embryos (only takes place 'in glass'). Thus, it not only erases the fact that 'IVF' constitutes recombinant and extractive treatment *of women* in order to create disembodied embryos, but that this treatment of women is *preconditional* to any *subsequent* research on women's disembodied embryos. The term 'embryo research' is a misnomer for what is, in the first order, research on women. The VLA guidelines therefore legitimate (and obscure) research on women under the rhetoric of 'embryo research'.

Moreover, intrinsic to the conceptual (and literal) severance of embryos from a woman is a consequential establishment of separate embryo 'interests'. These so-called 'embryo interests' are implicitly and necessarily in conflict with women's interests and therefore are presumptively endangered by them. This construction of embryos as having 'interests' which can be endangered sets up an imperative for the 'protection' of embryos.[27] Hence, most of the VLA guidelines not only discuss 'IVF' in terms of embryos, but do so most significantly in terms of removing them from women's control and transferring them into the presumably safer hands of 'IVF' practitioners. The VLA establishes guidelines for protecting embryos in the context of 'IVF' and appoints 'IVF' practitioners as 'embryo protectors'. This transfer of women's embryos from women to practitioners, as I will discuss later in this chapter, is effectively absolute whereas, although the VLA also establishes guidelines to protect the viability and integrity of embryos in practitioners' 'care', practitioners' research interests (their prerogative to determine how they 'dispose' of embryos) clearly supersede the 'interests' of embryos (VLA, 1986, pp. 31–2). Thus, within the VLA guidelines, embryo 'interests' effectively supersede women's interests and practitioners' interests supersede those of embryos. The VLA establishes practitioners' licence to exercise control over women by establishing practitioners' entitlement to control ('dispose' of) women's embryos (ibid., p. 31).

Finally, the VLA's exclusive (of women) concentration on setting standards for research on embryos suggests that medical scientists' fundamental goal regarding 'IVF' treatment on women is to produce embryos for research, not to relieve women's clinical 'problems'. 'Clinical IVF' is discussed only in terms of its relationship to 'embryo research':

> When human [*sic*] ova have been obtained and fertilised *in vitro* for a therapeutic purpose and are no longer required for that purpose it would be ethical to use them for soundly based research provided that the signed consent of both donors was obtained, subject to the same approval as in the preceding section. (Ibid.)

Thus, if 'IVF' treatment is the material process of manipulating and extracting parts of women's bodies for the purpose of 'creating' disembodied[28] embryos, the VLA guidelines represent an attempt to secure explicit and statutorily empowered medical scientific control over 'embryos' – which is, in effect, control over *women*. While 'IVF' may be *implicitly* a project of research on women, for the medical scientific community its *designated* significance is as embryo research. Its treatment of women is apparently incidental and not worth mentioning.[29]

Consent: The Contractual Subordination of Women

The 1986 VLA Report provides their first model of what they term a 'Specimen Agreement for *In Vitro* Fertilisation', which is in effect a model contract of prior consent (ibid., pp. 41–2). The terms of this original model contract clearly betray the primary interests of the medical scientific community to secure the material (women and women's eggs and embryos) and licence to promote the research potential of 'IVF'.

Prior consent contracts, sometimes also referred to as 'informed consent' forms may appear to be an explicit vehicle for ensuring the protection of 'patients' from medical malpractice. The VLA, however, states that the importance of prior consent is: (1) that it [the form] is a 'useful document to remind them ['patients'] of the exact terms of their consent'; and (2) that it provides 'additional security' for the doctor, giving evidence that he [*sic*] has explained 'what the treatment' involves (ibid., p. 13). Both reasons suggest that the primary function of consent forms is to *protect the practitioner* from liability, not to protect the 'patient' from injury or abuse.

The specific terms of the VLA 'Specimen Agreement for *In Vitro* Fertilisation' contractually bind 'IVF patients' both to the total discretion of practitioners and to the research objectives of 'IVF' treatment. More specifically, this form is a model for the contractual subordination of women.

Contractual Control by Practitioners over the Disposition of Women's Bodies

The contract requires that both partners of the 'IVF couple', who are referred to as 'gamete donors', agree to the procedure. The term 'gamete donors' establishes the status of the 'IVF couple' as 'voluntary', even altruistic, research participants (subjects), rather than as 'patients'. This is despite the fact that women nearly always undergo 'IVF' as a 'clinical infertility treatment'. 'Gamete donors', like 'IVF couple', conflates women with men, falsely implying that they share equally in 'IVF' treatment, thereby obscuring the fact that only women are actually treated. Moreover women are effectively subordinated to their (male) partners by the fact that the partners are required to give permission for women's medical treatment.

Practitioners' Discretion and Liability

The consent contract also establishes practitioners' absolute discretion over 'donors' (women undergoing 'IVF'). Clause 1: V, for example, establishes that the couple agrees to the 'transfer of [practitioner] selected 'pre-embryos' to the woman'. This is corroborated in Clause 5 which states:

> We accept that the decisions as to the *suitability* and number of pre-embryos for replacement at any time and whether frozen or not will be at the *absolute sole discretion* of the medical and scientific staff of the [IVF] Centre. (Ibid., p. 42, my emphasis)

Eugenic selection (quality control) is thereby defined as necessarily part of the general methodology of 'IVF' and under the discretionary authority of the practitioner.

Moreover, Clause 2 provides that 'donors' (including male partners) consent 'to the administration of such drugs and anaesthetics to the woman as may be necessary' and to 'any further operative measure which may be found to be necessary in the course of the treatment'. However, according to Clause 3, at the same time that practitioners have total discretionary control over their treatment of women, they bear no liability for a failure to 'succeed' in creating a pregnancy or a 'normal' child (ibid.).

Despite the fact that it is entitled 'Specimen Agreement for *In Vitro* Fertilisation', Clause 2 is the only section of this nine-clause contract that actually mentions the word 'women' and the procedures performed on women. Besides the establishment of the scope of practitioners' authority over the 'IVF' procedure (and over women who undergo it), by and large, the gist of this 'agreement' is concerned with the relationship of 'IVF' practitioners to embryos.

'Transferring Custody': Contractual 'Ownership' of Embryos by 'IVF' Clinics

Directly reflecting the VLA guidelines' primary objective of promoting the research potential of 'IVF', the 'IVF' consent form, with the exception of the above clauses, is almost exclusively focused on the transfer of women's embryos to medical scientific control. Clause 4:a:b:c:d:e is a detailed six-part provision for what is, effectively, a transfer of custody of embryos from 'donors' to the 'IVF' clinic. Parts (a) and (b) and (c) provide that embryos that are not 'replaced' in women should be preserved [cryogenically frozen] for 'not more than two years', within which time 'donors' may request subsequent embryo 'replacements' (only into the woman signing the contract). Ultimately, however, decisions both for the preservation of embryos and for subsequent 'replacements' remain at the prerogative and discretion of the clinic. The 'donors' may request them, but the clinic is not obliged to comply. Part (d) specifically establishes the custodial relationship of 'IVF' practitioners to embryos:

We agree that no stored pre-embryo shall be removed from the *custody* of the medical and scientific staff of the Centre without the written consent of both of us (or the survivor), such consent to be given with 28 days before such replacement or removal. (Ibid., my emphasis)[30]

Finally, clause (e) states:

We agree that after the period of two years (or such extension as may be agreed [at the discretion of the Centre]) has expired the Hospital or Centre (subject to the general terms of this agreement) may *dispose* of the stored pre-embryos at their discretion. (Ibid., my emphasis)

Effectively this means that, after two years, the 'donors'' already precarious claim on their embryos ends. Practitioners are then free, that is 'at their discretion' to 'dispose' of, that is to 'place, arrange or adapt', *to do research* on embryos without accountability to 'donors', the public, anyone but themselves and the medical science community.

As I have already discussed, 'IVF' procedures are designed to produce the maximum number of embryos (more in practice than are 'replaced' in women). This contract explicitly facilitates the stockpiling of embryos for research, a practice which is not only intrinsically predicated on prior research on women ('IVF'), but effectively supersedes and subordinates women's interests. Finally, this contract's concentration on the 'disposal' of embryos also effectively means that women who undergo 'clinical IVF' *necessarily* undergo research 'IVF'. Agreement to one is, by definition and by contract, agreement to the other.[31]

In sum, the VLA model consent form, in keeping with the VLA minimum standards of acceptable 'IVF' practice betrays three fundamental goals: the establishment of 'IVF' practitioners' discretionary authority over the practice of 'IVF' and by extension over women's bodies; the transfer of custody of embryos from women ('donors') to 'IVF' staff; and, in so doing, the establishment of a necessary link between 'clinical' and 'research' 'IVF'.[32]

Conclusion

The regulatory guidelines and specimen consent form proposed by the VLA explicitly codify the implicit values and priorities of the medical science community built into 'IVF' procedures and language. As I have discussed throughout this chapter, both the apparatus and medical scientific administrative framework of 'IVF' constitute and organise a systematic exercise of medical scientific power over women.

The apparatus of 'IVF', together with the medical scientific code of practice, articulate a double standard of accountability that constitutes an oppressive power relationship between practitioners and women. The apparatus, practice and medical scientific administration of 'IVF' at once minimise the accountability of practitioners to women (and the general public) and, at the same time, maximise the accountability of women to medical scientists and their priorities within the context of their 'IVF' project.

The structural lack of accountability of practitioners to women is constituted and protected by means of several processes and initiatives which I have described throughout this chapter. Practitioners use misleading language to name and describe 'IVF' tools and procedures such that 'IVF' appears to be a practice unrelated or, at best, inconsequentially related, to women. With 'IVF' treatment, they actively dis-integrate women's bodies and limit women's agency. Thus, women's reproduction is increasingly controlled, monitored and organised by medical scientists. Women's agency is eroded, to be replaced by the increasing power of practitioners over women's reproductive processes, bodies and lives. Moreover, the medical scientific code of ('IVF') practice explicitly structures a model of medical scientific *self*-regulation, that is, a system of *internal* professional accountability. Their model consent contract is one which, as they themselves implicitly admit, protects practitioners from accountability (and liability) to the women whom they treat with 'IVF'.

At the same time and in the same ways, 'IVF' practice and (medical scientific) regulation substantively structure the increasing accountability of women to medical scientists at physiological, ontological and regulatory levels. At a physiological level, women's bodies, body parts and bodily processes are made increasingly visible and available to practitioners for them to interpret, name, manipulate and excise. 'IVF' necessarily erodes women's physiological and social privacy, integrity and agency, an erosion which is bolstered and codified through the medical scientific (VLA) code of practice. Thus, within the context of 'IVF', there is a double standard of accountability for practitioners and women which at once empowers and structures practitioners' freedom of choice at the direct expense of women's reproductive autonomy, health and well-being.

This dual meaning of accountability is interlinked with a concomitant double standard in the meaning of choice for practitioners and women. Within the 'IVF' context, the priorities and prerogatives of scientific research and 'progress' are defined and exercised as the unrestricted practice of researchers. Hence, the simultaneous concentration of 'IVF' practitioners on the research potential of their 'IVF' project and a regulatory framework that structures minimum restrictions on the discretion and authority of practitioners.

Thus, the structural lack of direct accountability of 'IVF' practitioners to women is central to their increasing agency, an agency which is manifested as freedom of choice, expression, exercise and control. The freedom of choice, expression and exercise of 'IVF' innovators is *original* and *initiatory* at several levels. Practitioners have determined (and continue to do so) the developments, directions, methods, language and standards of their own practices. They have done so with little or no general public knowledge, let alone consent or participation. The continuing and substantively unregulated development of 'IVF' procedures and language is an example of the *de facto* freedom of choice of medical scientists *vis à vis* the persons (women) they treat and select for treatment in the course of research and development of their practices, processes and tools. Moreover, within the context of treatment, 'IVF' practitioners set the standards of eligibility for treatment. They have the freedom, final authority and discretion to choose who (which woman) will receive 'IVF' treatment. Finally, practitioners also determine the particulars of all individual treatment regimens.

By contrast, women (as women, not as professionals or practitioners) have had no directive or initiatory impact on the development and practice of 'IVF'. Choice for women in this context is, at best, a derivative, consumerist choice. Women can consent to pre-existing options which they have had no substantive role in determining. But even women's consumerist choice is limited. As I have pointed out above, women may desire to have 'IVF' treatment, but only their doctors may determine, ultimately, whether they are accepted for treatment. Moreover, women may attempt to exercise control over the course of their 'IVF' treatment, but again, treatment regimens are ultimately not up to women. Indeed, if women attempt to intervene too strenuously, they may be judged by practitioners as unco-operative and jeopardise their access to treatment (be dropped from the programme, or not be permitted to try again in the (likely) event that treatment does not result in (their) pregnancy).

At present women have the choice not to be treated with 'IVF'.

For many women, however, this may mean that they are 'choosing', in effect, to remain biologically childless (or live with husbands who are) in a social context which stigmatises 'infertility'. The choice between 'IVF' and social stigmatisation is not one which empowers women. Moreover, we live in a (Western) culture which is increasingly promoting (and legally mandating) medical intervention into (women's) reproduction, in large part on the basis of 'protecting' the so-called interests of ('unborn children') embryos (Corea, 1979; Rothman, 1982). As I discussed earlier in this chapter, under the rubric of 'infertility', 'IVF' treatment is administered to an ever-increasing pool of women who have no fertility problems themselves, and/or who are not childless. It is, therefore, not unreasonable to foresee that these trends are likely to continue and that, as a consequence, the opportunity to refuse this sort of intervention may become eradicated. Forms of 'IVF' treatment may become, for the 'protection' of their offspring, a mandatory part of reproduction for all women.

This chapter has mainly concentrated on the structural nature and meaning of 'IVF' for women. My focus has not been on women's experiences or resistance *per se*. However, in decoding the implicit (medical scientific) values and power structure of 'IVF' language, procedures and administration, this chapter outlines the conditions with which women must come to grips in order to resist the increasing medical scientific definition of, and control over, women's reproductive processes and agency. Clarifying and understanding the projects and processes of medical science which depersonalise and disempower women is also preconditional to challenging and changing the values that made and make these processes thinkable.

Notes

For their invaluable support and assistance while I wrote this chapter I would like to thank: Annette Burfoot, Joyce Canaan, Christine Crowe, Maureen McNeil, Ian Varcoe and Steven Yearley, (who have given me feedback on countless drafts of this chapter, and particularly Sarah Franklin who assisted in the difficult project of structuring the ideas in the first part of the chapter and gave me feedback and support throughout.

1. By 'ontology' I refer to *processes of being* in the sense of *living experience*. The processes of erasure and recombination of women in the

context of 'IVF' treatment, I will argue in this chapter, impose conditions which, to a great extent, structure particular sorts of living experience for women, a living experience which works to the detriment of women's personhood. I will argue that 'IVF' treatment constitutes a structural series of *parameters* which constrict women's reproductive agency and which abridge what Mary Daly calls women's 'Be-ing', that is, women's (potential) living experience *free* from patriarchal possession. 'Be-ing' in Daly's sense of the word is compromised, eroded, if not totally pre-cluded, by the ontological constraints placed on women within the design, structure and function of 'IVF' treatment (Daly, 1979, pp. 2–7).

2. Human chorionic gonadotrophin (HCG) is a hormone produced by pregnant women and can be extracted from their urine. Human meno-pausal gonadotrophin (HMG) (Pergonal) is a term used to describe a form of follicle stimulating hormone extracted from the urine of post-menopausal women (Barker, 1981, p. 172).

3. Moreover, Mary Anderson reports that women may additionally be administered 'Gonadotrophin Releasing Hormone (GnRH)': 'Pulsed doses are given at 90-minute intervals and the equipment for injecting subcutaneously can be worn by the patient in the form of a small box not much bigger than a cigarette packet.' She adds that a Prolactin sup-pressant drug called 'Bromocriptine' may also be administered to women who 'fail' to ovulate owing to 'high levels of the hormone prolactin.' Bromocriptine causes 'side-effects' such as dizziness and nausea (Ander-son, 1987, p. 68).

4. In fact, the word 'women' itself is rarely used at all, despite the fact that the procedures discussed at the 1986 ESHRE Conference are nearly all performed on women.

5. 'Hydatidiform mole' or 'molar pregnancy' is the term used to describe a cystic mole which 'looks like a bunch of grapes' that grows in a woman's uterus and gives the appearance of a normal pregnancy (Crook, 1986, p. 5).

6. According to Mary Anderson, as regards fertility treatments that are limited to hormone therapy, 'With the use of Clomid, multiple preg-nancy, especially twins is a possibility (15–25 per cent); with gonadotro-phin therapy it is a real risk (over 50 per cent . . .)'. Thus, women who conceive before completing the rest of the 'IVF' procedure which follows 'superovulation' can run the risk of a multiple pregnancy, particularly in the case of women diagnosed (as part of a couple) as having idiopathic or unexplained infertility and treated with 'IVF'. As Wood and Westmore report, 'such couples [sic] may become pregnant without treatment . . .'. Moreover, as discussed later in this chapter, many or all of women's superovulated eggs can be reimplanted (Anderson, 1987, p. 68). How-ever, evidence that hormone treatment is not safe for women does not preclude its use by medical practitioners. (See also Klein and Rowland, 1988, for a detailed documentation of the adverse affects of Clomid and other hormones on women and their offspring.)

7. The fact that certain parts of one's body are expelled as part of body functioning (for example blood, tears, eggs, endometrial tissue, etc.) does not mean that they are any less a part of one's body than stationary organs such as kidneys.

8. 'Transducer' is the term for the hand-held instrument practitioners use to aspirate women's eggs. Bruel amd Kjaer, describing the 'oocyte collection' technique using a vaginal transducer add: 'The patient is premedicated approximately 45 minutes prior to the aspiration with 10mg dixyrazin (Esucos, UBC, Brussels, Belgium) and 100mg pthidine hydrochloride (Pethedin, ACO Solna, Sweden) given i.m. [intra muscular]. The patient is placed in the lithotomy position [on her back with her legs in stirrups] and *the* vagina is carefully cleaned with saline and culture medium. For apprehensive patients a local anaesthesia can be injected paracervically' (Bruel and Kjaer, pp. 4–5, my emphasis).

9. Similar footage of this procedure appears in the television film 'Soft Cell' which was screened on 11 January 1988 on Channel 4, Great Britain and produced by The Steel Bank Film Co-operative.

10. It might be argued that expressions such as 'the uterus' *imply* women, as only a woman has a uterus. I would argue, however, that, while this language denotes a female organ, it neither defines that organ as necessarily *part* of a woman's *whole body*, nor places that part as necessarily within a female *person*. As only women undergo 'IVF' treatment, such disembodied language as 'the uterus' contributes significantly to the erasure and consequent subordination of women in the 'IVF' context. Moreover, the use of disembodied terminology to discuss organs and tissues of the human body is a central characteristic of medical scientific language. I would argue, as others have before, that this language contributes to the general objectification and subordination of patients (male and female) within medicine (see Illich, 1985).

11. The term 'suspect classification' refers in USA constitutional law to those categories (such as race, age and so on) which are associated with discrimination and civil or personal injury. The United States courts 'developed the term "suspect classification" to denote occasions where a law or act adversely discriminates against a particular group (classification) of people and where, that law is therefore 'suspect' – that is suspected of being arbitrarily discriminatory and therefore in violation of equal protection and due process. In the case of "suspect classification", the Court strictly scrutinises the law to determine that it does not arbitrarily infringe on "fundamental" (constitutional) rights' (Steinberg, 1986, pp. 24–25). In this chapter, I use both the terms 'suspect classification' and 'suspect' to indicate categories (such as 'infertility') or practices which, I argue, require strict scrutiny as to their potential discriminatory and injurious effects on women.

12. 'Vagueness and Overbreadth' refers (in US law) to a law or standard (for example) which is unconstitutionally unclear and/or over-inclusive (too sweeping), such that a person's (or class of persons') civil rights (of equal protection and due process under the law) are violated. In this instance, I use the concept of 'vagueness and overbreadth' to describe the sweeping inconsistency of the system of classification 'infertility'. I argue that the 'vagueness and overbreadth' of the category 'infertility' contributes directly to the increasing treatment of women with dangerous and experimental techniques such as 'IVF' and the consequent erosion of women's reproductive autonomy, integrity and privacy.

13. By extension, this model also constructs men's feelings and experiences of 'childlessness' in terms of their pathological and diagnostic significance. This is not to suggest, however, that men's feelings and experiences of 'childlessness', nor their experiences of 'infertility' investigations and treatments (most of which are performed on women) are in any way equivalent or comparable to women's, particularly in the context of 'IVF' treatment.

14. Mary Anderson explains two causes of iatrogenic infertility:

Infection [PID] can distort the tube, pin it down to surrounding structures, damage its fimbria, block its canal and destroy the specialised lining cells and their hair-like projections. Such infection is, unfortunately, not infrequently seen nowadays. Bacterial infection associated with abortion, the use of the coil or from surrounding structures such as appendicitis may result in damaged tubes. Gonococcal infection [gonorrhoea] may be the cause and there are several other implicated organisms. (Anderson, 1987, p. 36)

Anderson also points out that hormone therapy in the treatment of 'infertility' can also *cause* 'infertility' in women:

Another risk of Gonadotrophin therapy is excessive stimulation of the ovaries with cyst formation and in the worst cases 'blowing up' of the ovaries, producing acute abdominal pain. (Ibid., p. 68)

15. The title of Dr Graham Barker's book is characteristic of this conflation of 'infertility' and 'childlessness'. It is: *Your Search for Fertility: A Sympathetic Guide to Achieving Pregnancy for Childless Couples* (my emphasis).

16. Walters and Singer go on to write:

Because normal IVF and embryo growth rates are less than 50 per cent, a control system is needed when testing the sperm–egg interaction in unexplained infertility. This control is applied by placing one egg with fertile matched donor sperm cell as well as another similar egg with the husband's sperm. (Walters and Singer, 1984, p. 8)

Thus women (for whom, along with their partners, practitioners have been unable to diagnose a physiological cause of their biological childlessness) undergo 'IVF' in order that practitioner's can test 'sperm–egg interaction'. Practitioners place one woman's egg in a Petri dish with donor sperm and one in a dish with her husband's sperm. Obviously this test requires that practitioners extract at least two eggs from women; if not, the cycle of hormone stimulation and extraction procedures on women must be repeated.

Walters and Singer posit several extremely dubious interpretations of the results of this diagnostic test:

Successful fertilisation with the husband's sperm followed by pregnancy after ET [embryo transfer] would indicate that some immunological, chemical or physical barrier is preventing pregnancy. Failure to initiate pregnancy following ET may indicate abnormal uterine function which prevents implantation. (Ibid.)

A far less risky, though hardly unproblematic, test for this 'immunological, chemical or physical barrier', also called 'cervical mucus hostility' already exists; the 'post-coital test', where a couple is required to have sexual intercourse, after which the mixture of sperm and the woman's cervical mucus is removed and examined. Walters and Singer do not explain why 'IVF', a risky and highly unreliable series of procedures should be considered a suitable replacement for the old test. (That is, why should a problematic test be replaced by a much more problematic one?) The suggestion that 'failure to initiate pregnancy' (whose initiative is being referred to here?) may indicate 'abnormal uterine function' is not a particularly warranted or meaningful conclusion. 'Embryo transfer' is the least 'successful' of all 'IVF' procedures, particularly when only one embryo is transferred into a woman. The 'failure' here says much more about 'IVF' and ET than it does about women's uteri. However this conclusion can, of course, be used by practitioners as an indication for 'IVF' treatment.

The only definitive interpretation diagnostic 'IVF' on women offers is regarding the quality of men's sperm:

Fertilisation with donor sperm but not with husband's sperm indicates sperm abnormalities in the latter. (Ibid.)

Walters and Singer conclude:

Finally, in cases where eggs cannot be fertilised by either the husband's or donor's sperm, abnormalities of the egg may be responsible. (Ibid.)

By this logic, it could equally indicate 'abnormalities' in both men's sperm. And much more likely (an interpretation Walters and Singer never consider, but which could explain all 'failures' they describe) it could indicate problems with 'IVF' (both as test and treatment).

17. See Illich, 1976, for a discussion of doctor/patient power relations and how Western medicine constitutes one of the greatest contemporary threats to health.

18. See Christine Crowe's chapter in this volume for her discussion of the history of women as test-sites in the course of research and development of 'IVF'. See also Klein and Rowland, 1988.

19. This report has since been updated in the *Second Report of the Voluntary Licensing Authority* (1987) which is substantively similar to the first report and again in the *Third Report of the Voluntary Licensing Authority* (1988) in which certain minor changes have been made.

20. I suggest that the aim of the medical scientific community to establish an incumbent and *model* body for self-regulation regarding 'IVF' and related research projects has since been realised as reflected in the Government White Paper issued by the Department of Health and Social Security (DHSS, 1987). In this proposed framework for legislation, which, as of 1989, is still pending for discussion in Parliament, the government has outlined provisions for establishing a statutory licensing authority which are substantively similar to the current VLA code of practice.

21. Of a total of fifteen nominated members, four were nominated by the Medical Research Council (MRC). They include a professor of medicine (a doctor), a director of medical research, a director of veterinary research and a hospice medical director. The four members nominated by the Royal College of Obstetricians and Gynaecologists (RCOG) are doctors, all of whom specialise in obstetrics and gynaecology. The remaining seven, who were nominated jointly by the MRC and RCOG, comprise the so-called 'lay' membership. These include the former Health Service Commissioner for England, Scotland and Wales, a magistrate, a theologian, an actress who is also on the Executive Committee of Population Concern, an editorial director of IPC magazines and on the General Advisory Council to the Institute of British Advertising and a research psychologist and research consultant for the International Centre for Child Studies.

22. While there were, in fact, several women, including the 'chairman' (*sic*) who were/are members of the VLA, they were not chosen to represent women's interests in particular. For example, none of the women chosen are described as having experience working in women's reproductive rights organisations or advice centres on women's health matters, or counselling women and so on. While I would accept that it is not an obvious or simple task to articulate what women's interests are and to represent them, I nevertheless, would argue that the exclusion of feminist and other groups of women who have explicitly worked to secure women's reproductive autonomy reflects a definite lack of concern for women's reproductive rights.

23. The *Third Report* of the VLA (1988) attempts to make a distinction between experimental and clinical 'IVF' as if they are separate projects. However, as I have pointed out, the VLA minimum standards of 'IVF' clearly give priority to and implicitly define 'IVF' as an embryo research project. Moreover, as discussed in this chapter, an average of five women's eggs are extracted from women with hormone treatment and egg recovery techniques and only three or four of their fertilised eggs are replaced in women. Moreover, as set out in the specimen consent contract, once extracted, women's eggs (and embryos) become the *de facto* (and soon to be *de jure*) property of practitioners, who may 'dispose' of women's embryos at their discretion (see my discussion of the VLA contract above). Thus, 'clinical IVF' produces research embryos.

24. The VLA wrote up this finding under the misleading heading, 'Involvement of Non-medical Staff in "IVF" Programmes' (VLA, 1986, p. 16). The VLA goes on to report that some 'IVF' clinics employ 'specially trained' counsellors so that 'patients who fail to achieve a pregnancy have the opportunity to discuss their problems and decide on future treatment with either the medical or nursing staff'. The VLA does not however, say whether this special training should be medical or of some other kind.

25. The subsequent *Third Report of the Voluntary Licensing Authority* (1988) does recognise the conflict of interest inherent in 'IVF' practitioners' control over counselling, but only when the counsellor is the *prescribing* doctor:

Proper counselling is possible only if space and time are available to the *couple* in a neutral atmosphere with a fully-trained counsellor, possibly a member of the team, who is not the prescribing doctor. (VLA, 1988, p. 15, my emphasis)

They do not consider that a 'neutral atmosphere' is, by definition, compromised if counsellors are members of the 'IVF' team and, thus, are effectively allied with and co-opted into the professional community, even if they themselves are not 'IVF' practitioners *per se*. Moreover the (1988) *Report* continues:

Pre-treatment counselling may have the effect of *screening out* some couples who, when they fully consider the low success rate and invasiveness of treatment, may decide not to continue with treatment. (Ibid., my emphasis)

In one sense, this passage does reflect an explicit recognition of the fact that 'IVF' is invasive (albeit they only refer here to 'couples') and that success rates are low and that it is, therefore, important to inform 'patients' of these facts before they embark on treatment. However, this 'screening out' procedure does suggest that, effectively, practitioners can use this process to *select* more co-operative 'patients'. While I believe that 'pre-treatment' counselling is a necessary factor that makes in-formed consent possible, I would argue that this process alone does not ensure that 'patients' are fully aware of the ramifications of treatment. In order to have informed consent, there must be information available. While the VLA does, here, acknowledge that 'IVF' is invasive, there is, as I have pointed out in this chapter, very little investigation of, or concern about, the full (potential and likely adverse) effects of 'IVF' treatment on women. Moreover, the question of informed consent should not beg the more fundamental question of whether 'IVF', given the way women are necessarily treated (and subordinated) by these procedures, quite apart from, or in spite of their knowledge of or consent to these conditions, is in itself desirable, or acceptable or beneficial for women.

Finally, as in the original (1986) Report, the 1988 Report, despite acknowledging the importance of counselling to *'patients'* does not *mandate* the provision of counselling services in their guidelines (ibid., pp. 29–32).

26. In response to public criticism and (so far) unsuccessful legislative attempts – The Unborn Children (Protection) Bill: proposed by Enoch Powell in October 1984 and reintroduced in November 1985 by Kenneth Hargreaves with minor amendments (both Bills failed, through lack of time, to pass in Parliament) – to forbid embryo research on the basis of the assertion that an embryo, from the moment of conception, has full human and civil status (civil personhood), the VLA coined the term 'pre-embryo' in order to protect the freedom of 'IVF' practitioners and embryologists to continue doing embryo research. The term 'pre-embryo', which refers to the first fourteen days of 'embryo development' establishes the embryo as a *separate entity* from the woman, but one without civil status or 'rights', thus allowing medical scientists to con-tinue their research without criminal liability (for the treatment of embryos) and, they hoped, with allayed public concern and objections.

Thus, while the term 'pre-embryo' side-steps the pressures of the 'embryo rights' lobby, it does not, in effect, challenge their fundamental pre-supposition that embryos do have inherent rights of personhood. It simply posits *when* (at which time or stage of development) embryos can potentially be considered 'persons'. After fourteen days, when the 'pre-embryo' becomes the embryo, presumably it can then be regarded as having 'rights'.

Assigning 'rights' or civil personhood to embryos, before or after fourteen days, constitutes an implicit attack on women's civil rights and status. Because it explicitly subordinates her interests to those 'interests and rights' of her embryo, it can make her (legally) accountable for her conduct during pregnancy and provides the basis for the criminalisation of abortion. The establishment of civil status to an embryo, moreover, effectively subordinates women to those persons and professionals (such as doctors or the state) who claim to represent the 'best interests of the embryo/foetus/child'. For further discussion of the construction and significance of the term 'pre-embryo', see Crowe in this volume.

27. This ethic of presumptive endangerment also is clear, for example, in the related context of political opposition to abortion on the basis of a perceived embryonic personhood. In this context, a woman's pregnancy is constructed *not* as her whole body, but as a vessel carrying an independent being. Hence, her desire to terminate her pregnancy is construed as an imposition of her self-interests on those conflicting (right to life) 'interests' of her foetus. When a woman is denied abortion on this basis, her reproductive rights and autonomy are subordinated to the presumed 'rights' of her embryo. In this case, both the state (by criminalising abortion) and medical scientists exercise control over women's reproduction and abrogate her bodily and civil autonomy under the rubric (and rhetoric) of 'protecting embryos' (from women).

28. *The Oxford English Dictionary* defines disembody as 'separate from body or concrete form'. My specific usage of disembodied emphasizes removal from a body, referring to an action rather than a state of being.

29. The only concern about women's health and well-being expressed in the VLA Report as a whole is regarding the number of 'pre-embryos' transferred and the risks to women of multiple pregnancy (VLA, 1986, p. 16). While the VLA *Report* (1986) *recommends* that no more than three, or occasionally four 'pre-embryos' be transferred, it does not establish this as a prescribed *standard* for 'IVF' treatment, and this concern is not mentioned in the guidelines. This provision has since been incorporated into the 1988 guidelines – particularly in relation to the derivative 'IVF' procedure: 'GIFT' (gamete intra-fallopian transfer), where the risks to women of ectopic and/or multiple pregnancy are higher than in the original 'IVF' procedure since women's eggs and (partner's) sperm are injected by practitioners directly into women's fallopian tubes (where practitioners hope they will fertilise – but not implant).

30. While the clause may be interpreted as offering protection to 'donors'' claim on their embryos, suggesting perhaps that the Centre may not have them destroyed or given to someone else, the prior establishment of practitioners' absolute discretionary authority over *and sole access to*

embryos does not guarantee that 'donors' can reclaim their embryos for reimplantation into the woman who signs the contract. Nor does it provide specific safeguards against the clandestine 'replacement' of a woman's embryo into another woman. Additionally, this clause does not necessarily preclude practitioners' destruction or other use of 'unsuitable' embryos.

31. The original 1986 version of the VLA specimen consent form provided a deletable clause (6) which states:

> We understand that pre-embryos not used for replacement or storage and any pre-embryos remaining after the agreed period of storage *may be used for the advancement of medical and scientific knowledge* and *we welcome such use*. We realise that the development of such pre-embryos cannot proceed for long outside the [*sic*] body and the period of survival will be brief. (VLA, 1986, p. 42, my emphasis)

This clause not only establishes the intrinsic relationship between so-called clinical 'IVF' treatment and embryo research – that agreeing to one is agreeing to the other – but represents this relationship as the intent of patients (women and their male partners) rather than as the prerogative and intent of practitioners. Significantly, while this clause may be deleted by patients, its provisions (the transfer of custody of women's eggs to practitioners to be 'disposed' of (researched at their discretion) has already been firmly established in the rest of the contract. Thus deletion of this clause in no way affects or severs the substance of the contract. This clause, while appearing to offer choice to patients *not* to participate in embryo research, does no such thing. Interestingly, and perhaps as a result of external (public) or internal (medical scientific) criticism, this unnecessary clause was dropped from subsequent versions of the contract (VLA, 1987; VLA, 1988).

32. The 1988 version of this specimen contract was reworked. In this version, information about 'IVF' procedures performed on women is explicitly acknowledged. However, no information regarding possible adverse effects is included. Thus, while this version of the contract appears to be more sensitive to the issue of *informed* consent, the information provided is so limited that it could hardly be said that signing this contract is a substantive exercise of choice. While I agree that informed consent is a necessary factor protecting the autonomy and agency (health and well-being) of patients, it is not, in and of itself, tantamount to free choice and does not, by itself, preclude the subordination or endangerment of patients. The question of consent is a secondary concern to the overriding question of whether a treatment is acceptable under any circumstances regardless of patient's consent. That a patient may truly consent to any treatment does not render that treatment *ipso facto* appropriate, harmless or justified, nor should patients' consent be the first (or only) measure of the legitimacy of any treatment.

While the letter of this version of the contract is somewhat different, its spirit remains consistent with the original. The 1988 contract, like the original, provides for the transfer of custody of women's eggs and embryos to practitioners' control and thus intrinsically interlinks 'IVF' treatment with embryo research as an overall project.

5 The Management of Uncertainty in Obstetric Practice: Ultrasonography, *In Vitro* Fertilisation and Embryo Transfer

Frances V. Price

Introduction

The extent and significance of the paradox in the rapid proliferation of technologies in obstetric practice is only now apparent. By increasing the options available such technologies address 'needs' which, although disputed, are familiar both to those who are fertile and those who are not. Typically, women who want a child seek, in the first instance, to become pregnant. Those who are pregnant appreciate reassurance about foetal well-being. Techniques for manipulating fertilisation and monitoring the foetus have advanced apace. These technologies facilitate not only the diagnosis of certain reproductive risks but, in some cases, also the action necessary to minimise them. Nevertheless the emergence of new kinds of risk and uncertainty has been a corollary, which has been masked by features of the institution of medicine which promote confidence and by increasing medicalisation of all aspects of reproduction.

One graphic dimension of the enlargement of the range of technologies in reproductive medicine is the fact that conception can be accomplished, and the unborn foetus visualised, outside the female body. The 'intrauterine inmate' (Saling and Arabin, 1988, p. 5), whose 'formidable inaccessibility' was bemoaned by clinicians in earlier years (Dobbs and Gairdner, 1966, p. 453), is conveniently 'released' from the pregnant woman as an image: a visible second patient for monitoring and, perhaps, therapy. This facility to use technology to externalise conception and embryonic and foetal development, has extended scientific knowledge, and thereby enhanced the role and power of associated bodies of medical and scientific expertise.

But it has also sharpened the problems and criticism surrounding expert practices in this ethically sensitive area. That the limits and contradictions of expertise in this field are not always acknowledged is a source of feminist and more general political concern (Department of Health and Social Security, 1987; Stacey, 1988). Medicine occupies a privileged position in relation to decisions about the risks and benefits of therapeutic and diagnostic procedures. But, on various fronts, confidence in expertise, including medical expertise, has been shaken.

Expertise embodies social relationships premised on trust, with its legitimacy presumed to rest on a body of established knowledge. However, in recent years, the pronouncements of scientific and professional experts have become the subject of increased public scrutiny. For instance, the role of the expert in decision making was central to the analysis of what had gone wrong in the mismanagement of technology in three recent momentous disasters: the chemical plant at Bhopal, the space shuttle Challenger and the nuclear reactor at Chernobyl. Conflicting expert assessments concerning these disasters received worldwide publicity and caused genuine upset and bewilderment: clearly what was presented as established fact was rife with unstated qualifications, assumptions, limiting conditions and other uncertainties.

For more than ten years, Dorothy Nelkin and others have documented the declining trust in science and in the regulation of scientists, and also the demands for greater scientific accountability and for public participation in technical policy decisions (Nelkin and Swazey, 1979; Nelkin, 1979; Nelkin, 1984). The great optimism of the 1950s and 1960s about the future benefits obtainable from technology has been qualified. Both the monitoring and the control of technologies in everyday use are seen to be problematic. There is an awareness of the risk of unanticipated adverse outcomes, and concern that the scientifically recommended conditions for a technology in use may not be enforced.

In the early 1980s the complexity of risk assessment was the subject of a study group report from the Royal Society (Royal Society, 1983b). This report drew attention to the many aspects of risk, its assessment, perception and management. The extensive literature in the technical field of risk analysis indicates that such analysis is presumed to take place as a scientific process of quantification, and to be free of institutional interests and constraints (Wynne, 1987). Risks as probabilistic adverse outcomes, for which there is some measure of outcome magnitude, are distinguished from uncertainty. Quantified risk assessment in relation to bounded engineering systems such as chemical plants is markedly different from consideration of risk in relation to technologies in clinical practice, where it is unlikely that probabilities can be attached to future 'states of the world' because there is insufficient information. Here it is more appropriate to refer to uncertainty than to risk (O'Brien, 1986, p. 6). In medicine, typically, risk problems are not well structured. There is not a high degree of consensus on the definition, measurement and comprehension of the probabilities to be attached to outcomes. In this area there is a paucity of research, especially in the United Kingdom (O'Brien, 1986, p. 41).

Two apparently dissimilar reproductive technologies – diagnostic obstetric ultrasonography, and *in vitro* fertilisation and embryo transfer (IVF and ET) – are considered in this chapter to explore issues surrounding the management of uncertainty in obstetric practice. These two technologies are outlined and then situated in the context of medical authority relations and the discourse about risk in which they feature. At the heart of the matter is a model of the doctor–patient relationship. Supported by claims to expertise, medical practitioners are accustomed both to being authoritative in decision making and to having autonomous control of their activities. The limits of their expertise in relation to these technologies is suggested by an examination of the prevailing knowledge about issues of safety, efficacy and conditions of practice. However, the focus of the chapter is not only the extent of expert knowledge and the medical management of uncertainty, but also the changing locus of social and political control. There are public and professional constituencies concerned to monitor such knowledge and conditions of practice; and there are also efforts to shift the locus of control.

The Two Technologies: Diagnostic Obstetric Ultrasonography, and *In Vitro* Fertilisation and Embryo Transfer

Using diagnostic ultrasonography, implanted embryos and developing foetuses can be visualised externally on a screen, as if separate from the pregnant woman (Petchesky, 1987). A beam of very brief pulses of high-frequency sound, generated by a transducer placed in contact with her skin, is directed through her body and partly

reflected by soft tissues and follicular, embryonic and foetal structures. The echoes from the reflections are visualised as an image on a
screen for the operator to interpret. The developing foetus thus
becomes observable and measurable and, thereby, manipulable. In
some sense the foetus becomes 'knowable' and foetal images, and
information disclosed about them, may be of profound significance in
the lived experience of the pregnancy (Stewart, 1986). With image as
outcome, captured perhaps on photograph or video, diagnostic ultrasonography since the late 1970s has become the most routinised of
the reproductive technologies in the United Kingdom. North American references to the sonogram as 'a new pregnancy ritual' have some
resonance on the eastern side of the Atlantic. No written consent is
required. Typically, without counselling, women are 'sent for a scan'.

Prior to X-radiology, the information about a foetus required for
obstetric decision-making could only come from clinical observations
and from the pregnant woman's report of her condition. With
developments in radiology, imaging the foetus as a diagnostic procedure became feasible. The possibility of harm to the foetus from
exposure to ionizing radiation was recognised over sixty years ago
(Dorland and Hubeny, 1926). Restrictions on foetal irradiation in
antenatal care followed much later, accelerated by the findings of the
Oxford Survey of Childhood Cancer which linked antenatal radiography with childhood cancer deaths (Stewart *et al.*, 1958). An alternative means of viewing the foetus using diagnostic ultrasound
techniques was introduced into obstetrics following Donald's pioneering work with tumours in the mid-1950s (Oakley, 1984, pp.
156–61). Such techniques are not associated with ionizing radiation
and are used as a non-invasive professional resource for monitoring
both pregnancy and the foetus(es). This is mainly to ascertain due
date, to detect anomalies and to anticipate complications in delivery.

By contrast, many years of intermittently controversial research
with animals on both sides of the Atlantic preceded work on human
in vitro fertilisation (IVF) by a handful of pioneers (Rock and
Menkin, 1944; Edwards, 1965). From 1968 onwards, with the help of
scores of women who came to his Oldham Clinic, Patrick Steptoe, an
obstetrician and gynaecologist, co-operated with Robert Edwards, a
physiologist, and with Jean Purdy, their scientific assistant, to develop the reproductive technology of IVF and ET. Their work with
human embryos met with intense ethical criticism (Edwards and
Steptoe, 1980). They did not receive either the funds or the ethical
guidance that they requested from the United Kingdom's Medical

Research Council (MRC). In the early years in Oldham no woman became pregnant after embryo transfer. Later, just a few experienced early pregnancies which aborted, or ectopic pregnancies which had to be terminated. Not until 1978 did their efforts culminate in the pregnancy of Leslie Brown and the safe delivery of her daughter, Louise Brown, hailed as the world's first 'test-tube' baby. Since then, the procedure of IVF and ET, and its analogues such as gamete intrafallopian transfer (GIFT), have been rapidly developed and implemented throughout the world. Thousands of babies have been born following such 'assisted conception'. Written consent is required for each stage of the procedure and most centres offer some form of counselling, which, however, may not be independent of the medical team involved (Pfeffer and Quick, 1988).

Over ten years after the birth of Louise Brown, the success rate of the technique is still low. Live births resulted from only 8.6 per cent of treatment cycles in Britain in 1985 and 1986 (Voluntary Licensing Authority, 1988, p. 19). However, together with the psychosocial objective of alleviating childlessness, there is also the avowed intention of both scientists and clinicians to continue to improve the technique; to explore both early embryo development and the causes of human infertility; and to develop techniques for the diagnosis of genetic disorders in the early embryo prior to transfer.

The first technology, diagnostic obstetric ultrasonography, developed to facilitate diagnosis by imaging the foetus, is surgically non-invasive, of clinical utility, in widespread use and presumed to be benign. The second, IVF and ET, developed to bypass infertility and alleviate childlessness, is surgically invasive, of low efficacy, associated with high-risk outcomes and controversial. Both technologies were developed to provide a service in reproductive medicine and neither has been rigorously evaluated. The extent of scientific indeterminacy about the risks and benefits of each has become visible, to a greater or lesser extent, in the course of public controversies, in which the context of medical authority has loomed large.

The Context: Medical Authority and the Discourse about Risk and Uncertainty in Obstetric Practice

Historically and institutionally, medicine is a system of authority. Self-regulating procedures concerning responsibilities to patients, to the profession and to other registered practitioners are integral to the organisation of the profession. Strong institutional pressures protect the privileged status of clinical judgment, which is used to control the discourse about risk in treatment.

Medicine is one area of risk management in which the politics of public participation has had a low profile. Even the idea of partici-pation, as purposive action taken to influence plans and programmes, seldom features except in relation to debates about the doctrine of informed consent. Doctors are responsible, not only for clinical judgment about whether to proceed with a treatment, or diagnostic examination, but also for how much information to convey about risk. The idea of consent to treatment is harnessed to evaluations of risk by the clinician involved: ' . . . treatment risks are voluntary only to the extent that the individual doctor sees fit to disclose risk information to the patient' (O'Brien, 1986, p. 37).

The expectation is that practitioners will maintain standards 'rightly' set by experienced and skilled medical opinion (*Bolam* v. *Friern Hospital Management Committee*, 1951). In law, the standard of practice required is determined by 'the broad limits of acceptable medical practice', in line with judgements about medical competence and negligence. In English law, patients must be told of the substan-tial risks involved in medical treatment (*Sidaway* v. *Gov. of Bethlem Royal Hospital*, 1984). How much a doctor should disclose, however, remains a matter of clinical judgement. Doctors are assumed to employ their medical expertise as the agents of their patients in the attempt to maximise the benefits of treatment. They are presumed to be aware of the range of patients' preferences – one such preference being that regarding risk. This presumption may take on a height-ened significance in relation to infertile women who, as Naomi Pfeffer and others have emphasised, are commonly represented as 'desperate' and willing to go to any lengths to have a baby (Pfeffer, 1987; Pfeffer and Quick, 1988).

Beyond this, the double standard in medical innovation in the United Kingdom contributes to the broad context of uncertainty in relation to the two technologies of interest here. New pharmaceuti-cals have to undergo an extensive programme of stringent tests concerning their safety before they can be approved for release by the Committee on Safety of Medicines. Comparable restrictions on the introduction of new techniques and technologies into clinical practice do not exist in the United Kingdom. Nor is the clinical utility or safety of such procedures routinely monitored, as is the case with drugs. In a short space of time an innovatory technology may be incorporated into widespread practice without definite evidence of benefit. Quite apart from any individual medical outcome or adverse bio-effect, unintended outcomes may occur repeatedly and there may be highly significant social consequences.

For a disconcertingly large number of clinical procedures, trial and error play a significant part, and there is uncertainty about their efficacy and safety. In the quest to minimise risk a randomised controlled trial (RCT) may be set up, in a way that is recognised as scientifically valid, to try to resolve the uncertainty as to whether a technology is likely to be of greater benefit than harm (Chalmers, 1986). In a movement away from a style of clinical investigation which relies on crude and uncontrolled comparisons between different medical practices, RCTs have identified unnecessary surgical procedures – in relation to breast tumours, for example (Fisher *et al.*, 1985). However, in order to obtain the necessary sample sizes, such trials depend on the co-operation of large numbers of people, and there is an apparent lack of public and professional support. In particular, concern that the randomisation procedure compromises the doctor–patient relationship continues to prove an obstacle to participation. Despite controversies surrounding what is to be regarded as evidence of the benefits of innovative procedures, confidence in the clinical activities of medical practitioners persists. The image encouraged is of control, confident practice and adequate regulation by the profession. This is a source of deep confusion, which shows up in malpractice suits.

However, the construction of what is taken to be 'adequate knowledge', on which the claim to expertise and authority legitimately rests, differs amongst specialities in medicine. So does the nature of the work being done, the social relations involved and the extent of disclosure of uncertainty to those seeking medical assistance and intervention. Controversies surround technologies in use in obstetrics, a medical speciality to which, some ten years ago, the late Archie Cochrane, a prominent medical epidemiologist, awarded the wooden spoon (Cochrane, 1979). In terms of evaluating practice, either by utilising the methodology of the RCT or by heeding the results of those that had been conducted, obstetrics was, for him, the least rigorously grounded speciality in medicine. In 1984, in a paper entitled 'Confronting Cochrane's Challenge to Obstetrics', Iain Chalmers wrote: 'There is a dearth of scientific evidence with which to assess either the efficacy or safety of most of the various things that obstetricians do' (Chalmers, 1984, p. 722).

Decisions about obstetric procedures and practices are further complicated by the legal position of obstetric attendants and by the presence of a foetus without the capacity to consent. Legislative developments in the early years of this century granted a monopoly over obstetric practice, to be shared by obstetricians and midwives, as a 'licence to represent the state as the ultimate guardian of the nation's children' (Eekelaar and Dingwall, 1984, p. 259). State resources come into play here but parents have to face the consequences of what happens to their child(ren) during pregnancy, labour and childbirth, and to live with these consequences for many years. Moreover, it is the mother who takes responsibility in most instances. Caroline Glendinning has drawn attention to the extent of 'unshared care', even 'within the family', where the child is handicapped (Glendinning, 1983). With gamete and embryo donation and surrogacy, forms of motherhood and fatherhood have become differentiated and these questions of responsibility more complex (Stanworth, 1987b; Stacey, 1988).

There is now greater public and professional recognition of the lack of research evidence to justify not only recent obstetric innovations, but also many routine procedures. Obstetric expertise was publicly paraded in 1986 at a lengthy enquiry about the case of the consultant obstetrician Wendy Savage who was suspended from clinical practice in East London after allegations of malpractice made by her colleagues (Savage, 1986). Subsequently she was reinstated. The decision that the enquiry should take place in public was most unusual and her case received extensive publicity. The disputed evaluation by her peers of her competence and expertise raised fundamental issues. Detailed discussions about the management of childbirth and about professional reluctance to acknowledge the uncertain efficacy of specific obstetric practices underlined the extent to which conditions of appropriate care in the field are contested.

In the highly-charged medico-legal climate surrounding the enquiry, the contradictions in obstetric expertise were all too visible. The appropriateness of exclusive medical decisional authority was also challenged. Pregnancy and delivery are not intrinsically medical events – although complications requiring medical treatment may arise. Nor are they just physiological processes. Both are also social and psychological events in which there are various options available. In the past, the essential skill of the midwife lay in knowing how to judge the boundary between what promised to be a normal, and what a complicated, pregnancy and delivery, and deciding when to summon the further medical aid of a doctor (Donnison, 1977). In the distinctive vocabulary of risk prominent in the obstetric literature, normal pregnancies are now designated 'low-risk'. For some obstetricians, however, even the concept of 'the low-risk obstetric patient' is regarded as risk-laden and therefore untenable, given the range of perceived hazards for childbearing women (Wilson and Schifrin, 1980).

A particular perception of biomedical risk is encoded in contemporary obstetric practice. Pregnant women are encouraged to comply with the prevailing antenatal care practices, which may include monitoring by ultrasound. The focus of directives about such practices is the safety and health of the foetus(es), thereby transferring clinical attention from the pregnant woman. When 'sent for a scan', women can dissent, but, in fact, the rates of non-compliance are very low. The expectation of risk-free clinical practice is tacitly encouraged.

By contrast, IVF has been the subject of much media attention, primarily as the procedure of last resort for the involuntarily childless. There is evidence that the procedure is very stressful and that it has become invested with unrealistic expectations by those who hope to achieve a pregnancy. Women may acquiesce in the face of what are acknowledged to be high-risk strategies to achieve this goal (Leiblum, Kemmann and Taska, 1989; Williams, 1988) and clinicians claim the freedom of clinical judgement to aid them (Craft, Brinsden and Simons, 1987b). From a consideration of the uncertainties about the use of diagnostic obstetric ultrasound this chapter moves to a consideration of the uncertainties about IVF and ET.

Uncertainty Surrounding the Use of Diagnostic Obstetric Ultrasound: Safety and Efficacy

Half-way through Beverley Hyde's 1984 interview study of pregnant women's attitudes to antenatal scanning, a television news item reported the possibility of harm from a scan (Hyde, 1986). Following the broadcast, some women who had already been scanned expressed to Hyde their anxiety about safety, whereas none had done so before. No unscanned women appeared to have been upset by the news item. For all of these women, Hyde reports, 'this was the first time that the question of risk had been suggested by any doctor or scientist' (Hyde, 1986, p. 591). She reflects on their confidence in medical judgement: '. . . . women who had never been scanned probably assumed that future scans would take place only after the posited danger had been discounted, whereas some of the previously scanned women were anxious about the ultrasound they had been exposed to before (as they thought) any potential for harm had been considered' (Hyde, 1986, p. 591). The power of the institution of medicine is seen here as both minimising the fears of risk and also cultivating confidence in its control. The aura of medical authority is bolstered by an ideology of professionalism and a widespread trust in the effectiveness of institutional control.

That ultrasound can have biological effects is not in doubt. In the main, these effects have been described with reference to mechanical (cavitation) or thermal (heating) mechanisms, although other indirect mechanisms are also believed to operate (Wells, 1986; Wells, 1987). There have been experiments on insects, plants, cell suspensions and intact small mammals (National Council on Radiation Protection and Measurements, 1983). Evidence that foetal abnormalities and growth retardation are more common in mice after experimental exposure to ultrasound has provided grounds for caution (O'Brien, 1983; Takabayashi *et al.*, 1981).

The debate within the medical profession about risk associated with diagnostic ultrasound has centred on evaluations of data relating to the issue of safety in the use of equipment: scientific data on biological effects following certain exposure conditions and technical data relating to the definition and measurement of exposure conditions. Periods of great concern and controversy about bio-effects have coloured the history of the technology. As it turns out, early fears have not been substantiated by the available evidence (Macintosh and Davey, 1970; Liebeskind *et al.*, 1979). On the other hand, two studies, frequently cited as providing evidence for the safety of ultrasound, are both based on clinical series without a comparison group and are therefore difficult to interpret (Bernstine, 1969; Hellman *et al.*, 1970).

In the early 1970s, at a time when antenatal ultrasound imaging was not yet in widespread use, questions about hazards to the mother or foetus were raised within the MRC, following the receipt by the MRC Cell Biology and Disorders Board (which includes among its responsibilities advice to the MRC on biophysics and cell and molecular biology) of a number of proposals for RCTs. A pilot study was completed and a prospective RCT with MRC funding anticipated (Mole, 1986; Oakley, 1984, pp. 169–70). Subsequent deliberations by the Cell Board led to the conclusion that possible bio-effects would be too subtle and difficult to distinguish from other effects of the post-natal environment. The decision in 1973 not to proceed with the RCT was justified on grounds of cost and also because the Board had doubts as to whether the trial could yield valid scientific conclusions (Mole, 1986; Oakley, 1984, pp. 170–1). Thus, an early opportunity to conduct a prospective RCT was forgone.

The section of the population which has been exposed to ultrasonography in pregnancy is now very large indeed. Figures available in 1985 indicate that 85 per cent of pregnant women in England, more than 85 per cent of women in Scotland and 95 per cent in Northern Ireland were scanned at some time during their pregnancy (Whitfield, 1986). These figures are certainly higher now as the use of diagnostic obstetric ultrasound for routine screening in antenatal care is widespread in health authorities in the United Kingdom, although not accepted clinical practice elsewhere. In the United States, for instance, the National Institutes of Health (NIH) Consensus Development Conference decided in 1984 that the available data on clinical efficiency and safety did not allow a recommendation for routine screening (NIH, 1984).

The Royal College of Obstetricians and Gynaecologists (RCOG) Working Party was set up to review the available experimental and epidemiological data and to deliberate on a policy of routine ultrasound scanning of pregnant women. Whilst acknowledging the need for more research, they issued the reassuring statement that there are cogent reasons to expect benefit to all mothers and babies from 'a well performed scan between 16–18 weeks of pregnancy' (RCOG, 1984, p. 21). The criteria for 'a well performed scan' are not specified. Doubts about the scientific credibility of the report were publicly voiced. Reviewers drew attention to confusing errors and commented on the reliance placed by the Working Party on the work of one team of clinical researchers: '. . . it relies heavily on the results of studies conducted at King's College Hospital, while ignoring much of the less flattering literature' (Roberts *et al.*, 1983; Hibbard *et al.*, 1985; Lilford and Chard, 1985, p. 435).

In March 1985, prompted by a request for an assessment of obstetric ultrasound from the Department of Health and Social Security, the MRC saw it as timely to reconsider a range of issues concerning this imaging technology. They convened an *ad hoc* meeting and invited experts in epidemiology, genetics, medical physics, physics, obstetrics and developmental biology, together with representatives of the RCOG, the Royal College of General Practitioners and the Royal College of Radiology (MRC, 1986). It is of interest that at least one invited speaker commented on the lack of any clear hypotheses about the harmful effects of *in utero* exposure to ultrasound (Beral, 1986). Val Beral identified four areas of concern in the literature: first, *in utero* ultrasound exposure might 'affect the special senses, causing hearing or visual defects'; second, it might 'disturb neurological function, leading to disorders of learning, perception or behaviour'; third, it might 'induce structural changes, (if exposure occurs early), causing malformations or a reduction in birthweight'; and fourth, it might 'cause mutations, predisposing to cancer or genetic defects in the next generation' (Beral, 1986). The basis for concern, she observed, was not always obvious.

Other speakers made specific reference to the potential risks associated with developments in techniques and equipment. The linear array scanner dominated discussion, although it was acknowledged that the use of Doppler scanning and sector scanning techniques involve higher output levels. Studies in developmental biology indicate a greater potential risk to the foetus up to about eight weeks after fertilisation, and the practice of scanning early in pregnancy, characteristic of pre-natal diagnosis by chorionic villus sampling (CVS) and of IVF and GIFT programmes, for instance, was also of concern.

The report of the summing-up of this MRC meeting suggests that those present regarded the practice of scanning at about sixteen weeks of pregnancy as likely to be advantageous. However, the lack of definitive data to support this view was also acknowledged. The effectiveness and possible hazards of diagnostic ultrasound used in a routine way in obstetrics have never been fully evaluated by RCTs (Thacker, 1985). It would be difficult now to mount a prospective trial. In the first place, this is because very large numbers of women would have to be recruited; secondly, because women in the control group would be denied a scan, recruitment would be limited by ethical difficulties; and thirdly, because of the great cost of any such trial. In addition, it appears that the professional mood has changed. The concern and confusion surrounding the scientific evidence about the biological effects of ultrasonic devices, evident in earlier years, has subsided among clinicians, at least in the United Kingdom. There is a widespread belief that, at a scientific and technical level, the contentious issues have been resolved, and that there is consensus within the medical profession that the scientific evidence is good enough to close the debate about risk of harm from exposure to ultrasound. No review body or other mechanism exists to ensure that guidelines and safety standards are met.

In the late 1980s, few would dispute the view that 'no independently confirmed study has demonstrated any deleterious effect following *in vivo* diagnostic examinations' (Kossoff, 1986, p. 4). However, the scientific debate about safety is not dormant. Any bio-effects are likely to be subtle in expression. Delayed or infrequent events cannot be ruled out. In such circumstances, complacency is clearly not justified. To minimise the risk of harm there are limiting conditions for the exposure to ultrasound and strictures about prudent use are in order (Andrews *et al.*, 1987). A disconcerting problem is the limited state of knowledge about the risks and standardisation of ultrasound in obstetrics (Kossoff and Barnett, 1986). A picture of confusion is presented by a recent review of contemporary reports on diagnostic ultrasound (Wells, 1987). Researchers evidently do not have the necessary knowledge of physics and biology and may fail to understand key aspects of prior work in the field. Wells criticises published research, not only for being disparate in objective, but also for being based on poorly designed and controlled experiments which are then inadequately reported (Wells, 1987).

Human epidemiological data to date do not suggest that exposure to ultrasound, in itself, is detectably detrimental. However, this cannot be taken to mean that current diagnostic practices using ultrasound are 'safe'. To assess the risk of harm, information is required about exposure conditions. However, there is no consensus about what aspects of exposure to ultrasound might be of significance, and both the definition of exposure conditions and the establishment of quantitative exposure recommendations for obstetric ultrasound pose problems. The standards, recommendations and guidelines published in the form of national or international documents which address the safety of ultrasound do not deal with methods of measurement or the labelling of parameters. Only since 1986 has the National Physical Laboratory (NPL) produced an instrument, the NPL ultrasound beam calibrator, routinely able to measure all aspects of acoustic output to enable checks of safety standards. At the moment, there is no source for pressure to have equipment which is in use in hospitals accurately calibrated. In a diagnostic procedure, it is not usual for either the output powers of the equipment in use or the exposure times to be recorded (Frizzell, 1986; Preston, 1986;

Andrews *et al.*, 1987). Exposure to obstetric ultrasound is not deter-mined by 'scientifically-established levels related to risk, but by the amount of energy convenient for equipment design for good diagnos-tic performance' (Wells, 1986). The information available on the output powers and other physical parameters of a growing range of ultrasonic equipment is sparse. Large variations are evident between different types of equipment (Wells, 1987).

High-resolution obstetric ultrasonography features in almost every aspect of obstetric practice. Obstetricians regard the ultrasound scan not only as an integral part of antenatal care for visualising the foetus and placenta, but as a professional resource in IVF and its analogues, and, in the management of infertility, for monitoring ovarian func-tion and follicular development. IVF and CVS and other pro-grammes which incorporate early scanning of the foetus have been greatly expanded. Ultrasonic methods for making dynamic measure-ments of foetal condition and of blood flow in the foetus and uterus, using higher output Doppler ultrasound, are assuming a rapidly increasing importance in the work of certain clinicians at the fore-front of the field (Campbell *et al.*, 1983). Clinicians consider such examinations of value in antenatal care and they are likely to become more widespread.

Many questions about the safety and risk of ultrasound are clearly not settled. A mismatch is evident between the state of the scientific and technical knowledge in the field and authoritative medical asser-tions. Prominent obstetricians, experienced practitioners in the field, offer unqualified assurance to mothers. For instance, Stuart Camp-bell, Professor of Obstetrics and Gynaecology at King's College Hospital and special adviser to *Mother and Baby*, was quoted in that magazine: 'We are sure the process is absolutely safe and carries no risk at all to either the mother or her baby. All our knowledge of ultrasound and the ways it affects tissues indicates it is totally safe' (Steven, 1987b). Two sorts of function may be ascribed to such confident pronouncements. On the one hand, they serve an external function in helping to persuade and to reassure women in order to maintain professional authority in the use of routine ultrasound scanning in pregnancy. The second and internal function is to under-line cognitive orthodoxy about diagnostic ultrasound in the pro-fession. Limiting conditions do not feature. Nor are diagnostic uncertainties which may arise in everyday clinical practice using ultrasonography accommodated in such pronouncements.

**Uncertainties Surrounding the Scanning Procedure: Interpretation
and Communication**

The production of visual displays is such a characteristic feature of
scientific activity today that the task of interpreting the display, which
is the intended outcome of the activity, is often relegated to the
background. A combination of a particular social organisation of
technical skills enables instruments to produce images – Lynch's
'docile object' or 'material template' – which can be worked on, and
with, by experts (Lynch, 1985, p. 38). In diagnostic ultrasonography
there is typically a significant division of labour between the operator, who is presumed to possess the crucial skills to produce numerical and interpretational data, and the medical consultant. In the
United Kingdom, radiographers are central to the procedure (Witcombe and Radford, 1986). Skills derived from training and practice
are required to perform a scan and to interpret the results. The
arrangements for training and certification of operators, of concern in
the RCOG Report in 1984, are still not satisfactorily resolved (Meire,
1987).

For the radiologist Margaret Furness 'the sonologist walks blind-
fold in tiger country' (Furness, 1987, p. 675). Rapid developments in
ultrasound equipment yield not only more and more data but also
uncertainties about interpretations. Newly identified features extend
both the range of normality at each stage of gestation and the stock of
knowledge about the natural history of developmental conditions.
Margaret Furness remarks: 'Some conditions now being demonstrated have not previously been recognized at a stage when management decisions were required' (Furness, 1987, p. 675).

New observations, she cautions, contribute to an already sizeable
list of 'artifacts and red herrings'. A misdiagnosis or an intervention
following diagnosis may lead to the termination of a wanted and
normal pregnancy. Overdiagnosis of foetal abnormality is but one
example of the cascade effect in clinical care where one medical
intervention leads to another with an unwanted outcome for the
woman (Mold and Stein, 1986).

The widespread introduction of ultrasound scanning to obstetrics
has been accompanied by changes in the social relations of expertise between pregnant women and obstetricians. The technology is
usually operated by paramedical staff (radiographers, medical physics technicians or midwives) who are required to interpret the results

of the technical procedure, generally without disclosure to the woman being scanned. In fact, most obstetric ultrasound scanning is carried out by radiographers who report both numerical and interpretational data to referring clinicians (Witcombe and Radford, 1986). It is they who have to deal with the pregnant women in interaction with the machine. If radiographers choose to communicate their findings, to explain and to reassure, they are contravening the guidance given by the Disciplinary Committee of the Radiographers' Board in consultation with the Council for the Professions Supplementary to Medicine: 'No registered radiographer should knowingly disclose to any patient or to any unauthorised person the result of any investigation . . .' (quoted in Witcombe and Radford, 1986, p. 113).

The social organisation of the technology and the uncertainties surrounding diagnosis by ultrasound complicate decisions about what the pregnant woman should be told about observations, about the 'meaning' of measurements and about what interventions are to be recommended. The attempt to minimise patient anxiety, Furness suggests, has become a major concern to radiologists. She provides an example of such anxiety after a scan:

> A general practitioner rings to ask what he should tell Mrs Smith: she has just seen a report saying her fetus has a 32-week-size head and a 34-week femur, and she is convinced she has a long-legged mentally retarded child.
> An anxious nurse is told she needs a repeat scan at 16 weeks, because her 12½ week fetus may have exomphalos; and she cannot be dissuaded from immediate termination. (Furness, 1987, p. 675)

There is much to suggest that most women regard a scan as more than a medical procedure. Hyde's study illustrates the significance of the social and psychological implications for the woman concerned. Those women who expressed a wish to be scanned, but for whom there had been no clinical indication to scan, told her it would be interesting, reassuring or 'good to see the baby'. The contemporary practice is to allow women to participate to the extent of viewing the image of their foetus. This was not always the case. Stuart Campbell's work is often cited as a turning-point (Campbell *et al.*, 1982). In the early 1980s his research team at King's College Hospital demonstrated pregnant women's preference for seeing, rather than not seeing, their foetus on the screen and receiving, rather than not receiving, information from the scan operator as to foetal age, shape and movements. Those women who both saw the scan and received descriptive information from the operator were afterwards found to be more positive about the scan procedure and about themselves.

The same research team used the findings of a subsequent study to promote the idea that the pregnant woman's positive attitudes to scanning may be used to benefit her foetus by encouraging compliance with health care recommendations, and particularly directives to stop smoking and to limit alcohol consumption (Reading *et al.*, 1982).

Where the scan is a routine antenatal procedure women are encouraged to regard it as a positive process and they expect to receive reassurance. However, a prominent theme in letters about the experience of scanning solicited in 1984 by the National Childbirth Trust (NCT) was of disquiet at the operator's lack of communicativeness or at their distant attitude: 'She ran the scanner over my stomach while discussing last Saturday's party with someone else' (Smith, 1985, p. 6).

In more than a third of the cases reported to the NCT, the result of the scan was discussed either later by another person or not at all. A few women could not see the screen. Following their survey, the NCT wrote to the Royal College of Radiographers to suggest that guidance be given to radiologists as to how to react towards the pregnant woman should their interpretation of the scan indicate that there was a problem with the pregnancy (Smith, 1985).

The division of labour and of diagnostic responsibility between operator and consultant may cause extraordinary stress when an anomaly is found but not directly communicated. In this situation, several strategies to obtain information have been reported which highlight the incongruous ways in which such a state of uncertainty may be created for the woman being scanned that she may resist the professional conventions regarding diagnostic disclosure:

> Four other scan operators came in and had a look. The radiographer at first told me a letter would be sent to my GP and for me to make an appointment to see the GP in ten to fourteen days' time. This I could not accept and made a fuss until I was told there and then. I knew something was going on as a total of five people had been in to see the screen, but not me. It was only when I became rather upset by the lack of information given to me that they decided to tell the truth. A cup of sweet tea followed. A horrendous experience!
>
> I was scanned by a radiologist at the first scan – told to come back the next day by a nursing officer. On asking why, was told couldn't tell me – come back tomorrow to be scanned by a doctor. I refused to move and was then told.[1]

The pregnant woman may also be distressed that her medical attendants may respond entirely to the image on the screen and completely

The Management of Uncertainty

ignore her presence: 'the fact that I was even involved and upset seemed irrelevant'.

It is not the medical profession which has brought to the fore issues about current knowledge and different forms of practice, and kept open the debate about the balance of possible benefits and hazards of routine ultrasound screening in obstetrics. Nor was Margaret Furness by any means the first to highlight these issues. In the United Kingdom it is the paramedicals, in the main radiologists, midwives and consumer groups such as the Association for Improvements in Maternity Services (AIMS) and the NCT who have taken the lead. For instance, in 1982, the consumer group AIMS made enquiries at the Department of Health and Social Services about the need for a randomised controlled trial to establish the benefits and hazards of routine ultrasound scanning. They were informed that the MRC considered it unnecessary. AIMS subsequently published a critique of the 1984 RCOG Working Party report on routine ultrasound examination in pregnancy (Squire, 1984).

These concerns go beyond the debates about risk of harm from exposure to ultrasound, on which the RCOG Working Party and the MRC Ad Hoc Meeting found a limited consensus. They address the uncertainties of everyday practice: the risk of heightened anxieties and stress from the conduct and interpretation of routine scans, and the effects of diagnostic disclosure. The radiologists Margaret Furness and Hylton Meire are forceful about such concerns (Furness, 1987; Meire, 1987). It is clear that there are clashes of values, interests and perceptions involved, between scan operators and consultants, and between operators and pregnant women.

Uncertainty and *In Vitro* Fertilisation: Safety and Efficacy

To those seeking medical assistance to become pregnant, IVF has featured as a costly clinical service of last resort. There is a lack of Health Service funding. In addition, the investigation and management of infertility has been accorded a low status in medicine for a very long time and the provision of services has been given low priority. Few of the estimated 5 to 10 per cent of couples in the United Kingdom who cannot conceive spontaneously have access to the full range of infertility services available in the National Health Service (NHS) (Mathieson, 1986; Pfeffer, 1987; Pfeffer and Quick, 1988).

Even if access to these conventional services is secured, their effectiveness is in doubt. A review article in the *British Medical Journal* estimated that, despite the many advances in the management of infertility, 'less than eighteen per cent of the infertile population may conceive as a result of medical intervention' (Lilford and Dalton, 1987, p. 155). If IVF were widely available, the article suggests, controversially, that around 23 per cent of the same population might conceive. The authors urge, therefore, that more emphasis should be placed on IVF and ET, and also on GIFT, when treating infertility. This suggestion has been strongly contested by other clinicians for whom IVF 'remains (and will remain for some time) the most disappointing and expensive of all treatments' (Winston and Margara, 1987). Moreover, few can afford to attempt to circumvent the inadequate conventional NHS services by recourse to the latest techniques available, in the main, only in the private sector. In addition, these techniques are only appropriate for a comparatively small number of women.

For the majority, IVF is unlikely to provide the desired solution. The vigour of research and the considerable publicity surrounding births following IVF and ET and GIFT belies the low success rate in establishing clinical pregnancies (VLA, 1988, p. 19). The high rates of oocyte recovery and of fertilisation are not paralleled by the rates of implantation. Pregnancy is what is wanted by the woman contemplating IVF. Private IVF clinics are in business to achieve as high an incidence of pregnancy as possible and there is competitiveness about claimed pregnancy rates which may confuse and mislead patients (Fishel and Webster, 1987; Blackwell *et al.*, 1987).

In 1981 it was predicted that the pregnancy rate in IVF would increase with the number of embryos replaced in each intervention (Biggers, 1981). Early reports from IVF centres worldwide supported this prediction (Muasher *et al.*, 1984; Webster, 1986; Seppala *et al.*, 1985). Such data encouraged the transfer of three, four, five or six embryos in clinical practice. The register of all notified IVF and ET pregnancies in Australia and New Zealand indicates between 1979 and 1985 a gradual increase in the proportion of pregnancies in which at least three embryos were transferred. However, the issue of multiple embryo transfer received considerable attention as it became known that IVF centres worldwide were reporting an enhanced multiple pregnancy rate where large numbers of embryos are transferred (Lancaster, 1987a; Muasher and Garcia, 1986).

In the various hearings and deliberations of advisory bodies on IVF, questions of safety and efficacy have been central. Possible harmful effects on the resultant child(ren) are the primary concern. For the women involved there is consensus that the major clinical risks of IVF and ET, and the more recent GIFT procedure, are ectopic and multiple pregnancies: late miscarriage, pre-term delivery and neonatal mortality and morbidity may be some of the consequences of the latter. Several factors in combination may put at risk such pregnancies as do result: maternal age, nulliparity, the context of infertility and factors associated with the IVF and ET or GIFT technique (Cohen, 1986). Such discussions of risk relate to an acknowledged pregnancy.

Assessments are complicated by the lack of standardisation in the way centres report data and their very different clinical practices:

> Different methods of follicular stimulation, oocyte collection, patient monitoring, and embryology are used; some clinics replace only a few embryos while others replace six or more; some offer freezing to reduce wastage of gametes and cleaving embryos, but many still do not have this facility. (Fishel *et al.*, 1986)

Trounson has called attention to 'the strong tendency to report observations usually by retrospective analyses of data generated through clinical services'. These observations then form 'the basis for comparison and then definitive conclusion as to the methods used or outcome achieved' (Trounson, 1986). RCTs to evaluate the effectiveness of IVF and GIFT procedures are few, as are the reports describing the outcomes of the resulting pregnancies. No RCT has yet used childbirth as the end point and there is little data on patients who defer treatment or who choose alternative treatment.

The current state of the art only permits embryos to be assessed for transfer on the basis of their morphology and development in culture. Both are imprecise methods (Leese, 1987). Early review papers listed possible factors which might lead to an increase in the risk of congenital abnormalities among children born following IVF (Biggers, 1981; Angell *et al.*, 1983; Edwards, 1983). Too few have been born as yet to calculate any increased risk from the procedure. A greater than expected prevalence of spina bifida and transposition of the great vessels was evident in the analysis of data from the register of IVF and GIFT pregnancies in Australia and New Zealand (Lancaster, 1987a). Although the interpretation of this finding is controversial and based on insufficient data, the probability that it occurred by chance is low. In the United Kingdom information is awaited from the In-Vitro Fertilisation Register, a centrally maintained register of

IVF births, set up by the MRC. The original protocol specified that every child born as a result of IVF and resident in this country should be followed up for one year. Funding restrictions have required a reappraisal of the programme: only one thousand children born as the result of IVF have been followed up. More data are awaited on children born following IVF and ET (Mushin *et al.*, 1986; Wirth *et al.*, 1987).

'Judgements under Uncertainty' and the Limits of Expertise

All stages of the IVF procedure may cause distress. Marie Johnston and her co-workers have investigated the stress and 'judgements under uncertainty' experienced by couples on an IVF programme (Johnston, Shaw and Bird, 1987). Their findings substantiate the hypothesis that both women and their partners in such programmes overestimate the likelihood of becoming pregnant and having a baby. They emphasise the impact of media reports of successful outcomes. Discussions of failed attempts seldom feature in popular accounts. Patients face uncertainty at each stage of the procedure: at assessment interviews for selection onto the programme, at laparoscopic oocyte recovery, at fertilisation, at embryo transfer to the uterus and after return home if the embryo(s) fail to implant. The financial and time costs of undergoing further treatment cycles may have to be faced. All the consequent absences from home and work and disruption of social obligations may be difficult to explain both to friends and to relatives: 'Each stage carried low predictability and low control in achieving a highly valued objective, factors that contribute to stress in other situations' (Johnston, Shaw and Bird, 1987, p. 26). The evidence of high anxiety levels at all stages of the procedure was likely to be, quite literally, counter-productive. As many as 55 out of 91 couples who left an IVF programme after one attempt said that anxiety was their reason for not attempting another IVF cycle (Mao and Wood, 1984, p. 532).

The extent to which a woman can know what it means to consent to an IVF treatment is difficult to assess. Her 'need' or desire for a child may overwhelm her experience of the realities of the treatment. Beth Alder has reported that twelve out of twenty women who had completed at least one treatment cycle in a research-based IVF programme without becoming pregnant, were not fully satisfied with the opportunities for asking questions and for discussion during the treatment (Alder and Templeton, 1985). In a more recent study,

Paula Shaw and Marie Johnston refer to the desire for 'more information throughout the waiting and treatment programme from medical staff, in written form and in greater access to a nurse counsellor who would respond to telephone calls, questions and requests for meetings' (Shaw and Johnston, 1987).

Because it is perceived as having profound societal implications, the extent of medical control of human reproduction permitted by procedures such as IVF raises ethical questions. Proposals for action to monitor and regulate all scientific and clinical procedures involving embryos have been on international agendas for some time. In the United Kingdom, the Warnock Committee recommended opening up non-medical participation in such matters and the eventual establishment of a statutory review body, complete with an inspectorate supported by the full might of the criminal law. Subsequently, as an interim measure, the Voluntary Licensing Authority (VLA) was set up jointly by the RCOG and MRC in 1985, to license and monitor centres undertaking either IVF and ET, or research involving human embryos. All such work has to have prior vetting by a local Ethics Committee. The VLA's negotiated guidelines are intended to 'set the minimum acceptable standards required' and 'to offer a basis on which local ethical committees can agree their own house rules' (VLA, 1986, p. 8). Membership of the VLA is by invitation and is intended to be equally balanced between professional and lay members. In 1987, therefore, when it was considered appropriate to include another scientist (a reproductive endocrinologist) and a paediatrician, two new lay members were also included – Rabbi Julia Neuberger and Sir John Osborn.

The original VLA guidelines were based on those already in use amongst the pioneering teams, but also incorporated recommendations from the Warnock Committee, the MRC and the RCOG. The VLA has no power to enforce them, beyond withdrawal of licenses. Nevertheless, aberrant teams may continue to practise, unlicensed. Peer group pressure was expected to be as effective a check on clinicians as it is presumed to be on the scientific research community. It was not envisaged that clinicians would flout the guidelines nor that they would challenge the legitimacy of the VLA. However, this was to be the case.

In 1987, to meet and attempt to control rapid developments in the field, the VLA revised and expanded its guidelines (VLA, 1987; Price, 1988). Certain practices were censured as a matter of public policy. A few clinicians vociferously contested these revisions, protesting that they infringed their freedom of clinical judgement (Craft *et al.*, 1987b). The dispute, amplified by the media, centred on three issues: how many embryos or eggs to transfer, selective foeticide on grounds of number, and gamete donation by known donors (Kanhai *et al.*, 1986; Gillie, 1987; Ferriman, 1987; Veitch, 1987; Fraser, 1987).

The IVF team at Humana Hospital, Wellington, one of the VLA's licensed centres, refused to provide a written undertaking that they would adhere to the new guideline restricting the number of embryos that were to be transferred in any one procedure. They argued for the flexibility to continue their clinical practice of transferring up to twelve embryos. Ian Craft, the director of the Humana's infertility unit kept a high profile throughout this much publicised dispute, asserting publicly that the VLA had 'moved the goal posts' (Craft *et al.*, 1987b), that clinical freedom was at stake and that the VLA guidelines must permit a flexible approach to treatment (Craft *et al*, 1988). In September 1987, the VLA withdrew their licence of approval from the Humana Clinic (Laurance, 1987). This centre subsequently agreed to abide by the guidelines and again obtained the VLA's licence. Nevertheless Craft and his team of clinicians continue to urge the safeguarding of clinical freedom – particularly with reference to replacing more than four eggs in the GIFT procedure (Craft *et al.*, 1988).

Controversies involving certain IVF clinicians on the one hand, and members of the VLA and other interested parties on the other, turn first on what is to count as evidence and, second, on who can directly or indirectly obtain a 'hearing' for their views and/or exert countervailing power. There is reluctance by IVF clinicians and scientists to acknowledge the authority of, and by some influential members of the VLA to receive expert advice from, those who are neither scientists nor clinicians. This, in fact, is a major issue in a fast-developing field which is said to be 'consumer-led'.

The appreciable risk of multiple births, and the ensuing consequences for neonatal care, following multiple egg or embryo transfer after IVF or in the GIFT procedure, received the attention of neonatal paediatricians in 1986 and 1987 at national and international conferences. Paediatricians chided their obstetric colleagues, expressing their concern that, while the initiation of pregnancy through IVF and GIFT was to be financed largely in the private sector, no provision at all had been made for the additional costs of neonatal care in the public sector. It appears that in the early IVF programmes no allowance was made for the consequences for the NHS of these privately-funded programmes. It is likely that it was believed that, since the number of babies anticipated was small, the extra costs could be ignored. However, at least one regional centre reported in 1986 that there had been a disproportionate number of multiple pregnancies, premature deliveries and very low birthweight infants associated with IVF programmes.[2] Letters in professional journals and in newspapers in the United Kingdom called attention to the incidence, risks, and consequences for care of multiple births (Anderson, 1987; Richards and Price, 1987). The neonatal care issue was dramatically highlighted in the summer of 1987 by the publicity surrounding the premature delivery and early deaths of all the septuplets born to Susan Halton in Liverpool.

By 1987, IVF centres world-wide were successfully initiating pregnancies with the transfer of no more than three embryos. Provided with this clinical data, the VLA reacted to the concern about multiple births by issuing a guideline to restrict the number of eggs and embryos transferred in clinical practice in GIFT and IVF: 'Consideration must be given to ensuring that whilst a woman has the best chance of achieving a pregnancy the risks of large multiple pregnancy are minimised' (VLA, 1987, p. 35). On this contested issue, neonatalogists and paediatricians were able to mobilise through their professional organisations. The President of the British Association of Perinatal Medicine received widespread publicity for his letter to the Minister of Health and to the Secretary of State for Social Services about the serious shortage of neonatal nurses, which drew attention to the impact of such births on the workload of neonatal units.[3] Questions to the Secretary of State for Social Services in the House of Commons drew attention to the incidence of multiple births and to the extent to which infertility treatments and IVF may have contributed to the rise in the rates of multiple births.[4] Moreover the VLA could use data from leading research teams to support their guidelines restricting large multiple transfers of eggs and embryos (Testart *et al.*, 1987).

By comparison, there is no equivalent constituency regarding the other two contested issues, selective foeticide and gamete donation by known donors. However, clinicians have been provided with a legal reason for hesitancy about the procedure in the aftermath of the debate among lawyers as to whether or not selective foeticide is permitted by the 1967 Abortion Act (Keown, 1987; Brahams, 1987; VLA, 1988). Even with the knowledge that the clinical prognosis for a higher order multiple birth is unfavourable, selective foeticide in such cases is a difficult option for the women involved and poses a complicated challenge to the accepted notions of motherhood (Rothman, 1985). The long-term social and psychological consequences for the mother and her resultant child(ren) are unknown. There are no published follow-up studies.

Oocyte donation involves the donor in the discomfort and risks of a surgical procedure. Moreover, in the absence of a freezing programme, the organisation of an anonymous oocyte donation programme is problematic, especially if donor and recipient cycles are to be synchronised, for it is then difficult to maintain confidentiality. In the GIFT procedure, both the donor and the recipient are likely to have their operation on the same day and, in the absence of any informed debate about the wisdom of the practice, clinicians have used relatives and friends for both sperm and egg donation in IVF and GIFT procedures (Veitch, 1987; Fraser, 1987; Steven, 1987). Media interviews with these clinicians suggest that their perception, narrowly defined and without any supporting evidence, is that these are situations involving minimal risk:

> They're all situations where sisters would wish to help sisters. You can understand that you might wish to have the same genetic background to an egg donated to you as you had of your parents. Why not? It doesn't necessarily mean to say it is going to be bad. Some of the adversaries have suggested that children will have some conflict of identity later or emotional crises when they are seventeen or eighteen going through their difficult years. They can equally have them with anonymous parents. It would be no different, I think.[5]

As yet there has only been speculation about the wider implications of such facilitation, for the individuals concerned and others (Price, 1988). Clinicians admit that they are 'testing the water'. When the donation is not anonymous, it is likely to be imbued with ideas about the continuity of the relationship which led to the donation in the first place. In this sense, it is not an outright gift like that of a body part such as a cornea or kidney. Depending on the stage in the life course and degree of dependency, this may put pressure on relatives to donate.

At the time of publication of the White Paper on Human Fertilisation and Embryology in November 1987 there was unease about the fact that forthcoming legislation might endorse donations by known donors by default, in the absence of 'scientific' evidence of harm. Those who disputed that the contested issues are solely matters of clinical judgement, covered by the ethics of the doctor–patient relationship, could not cite contrary evidence. The VLA has received criticism from, and been put under pressure by, clinicians at several of its licensed centres about its discouragement of the use of close relatives for gamete donation, particularly in the face of the difficulties of obtaining anonymously donated oocytes. The social, legal and broad political consequences of the development and outcome of such donations for parents and children are novel and not yet subject to systematic appraisal. The VLA has neither the remit nor the funds to initiate follow-up studies. Nevertheless, in September 1988, it convened a conference jointly with the King's Fund Centre to promote discussion on egg donation, after the Authority had been approached 'by a number of experts in the fields of anthropology and child development asking that it should take a wider view' (VLA, 1988, p. 10).

In 1978, the year of Louise Brown's birth, an advisory group set by the MRC, and concerned with the ethics, rather than the science, of IVF research, concluded: 'in the context of female infertility due to tubal occlusion, in vitro fertilisation with subsequent embryo transfer should be regarded as a therapeutic procedure covered by the normal ethics of the doctor–patient relationship' (MRC, 1985). The MRC endorsed this view. The phrase 'covered by the normal ethics of the doctor–patient relationship' was apparently unproblematic. This presupposes that there are no unresolved issues of ethics in the doctor–patient relationship, and that this constitutes a sufficient guarantee against the risk of an adverse outcome in a field where there is not only dissent about 'good practice', but also enormous pressure to establish as many pregnancies as possible.

Conclusion

Medical practice directives traditionally centre on the doctor–patient dyad, to the relative exclusion of other relationships and wider social issues, and with the terms of this relationship and its boundaries ill-defined (Kennedy, 1986). Until relatively recently, professional self-regulation was unchallenged. The idea that law had a place in regulating any field in medicine was not even canvassed. Except in relation to malpractice, medical law is in its infancy and there are few statutes in Britain which relate to obstetric practice.

One consequence of the emphasis on the doctor–patient dyad is the focus on clinical judgement in relation to the individual clinical

case. The process of individualising what might otherwise be regarded as institutional issues encourages the neglect of the social and
political dimensions in risk perception. This is illustrated in this
chapter by the controversy surrounding the VLA's stipulation about
the maximum number of eggs or embryos to be transferred in the
IVF procedure, because of the concern about the risk of a multiple
pregnancy. The IVF team at the Humana Hospital, Wellington,
argued that this restriction would affect many women's chances of
achieving a pregnancy.

Particular problems of risk management in medicine are mediated
by the doctor–patient relationship. Although the professional directives 'to do no harm' and beyond that to promote 'the best interests'
of the patient are seldom unproblematic, clinical judgement is privileged in law and used to control the discourse about risk. The
hermetic nature of, and presumptions about, this dyadic relationship
serve to foster rather than minimise uncertainties in contemporary
practice. The case that doctors be accountable for their clinical
activities to a far wider audience than their peers is a recent and, it
seems for some clinicians, still a novel theme. Nevertheless the
development of the discipline of medical ethics has opened up a
debate about medical authority, and clinical practice has come under
increasing scrutiny.

The limits of expertise and of the management and control of
disturbing uncertainties may only become obvious when practices
and procedures spark controversy, and when management disputes
between clinicians are conducted in public. So it has been with IVF.
Vociferous dissent about what constitutes 'good practice' in the field
turns, in part, on different evaluations of acknowledged clinical risks
and on the professional priority to be given in each clinical case to
establishing and maintaining a pregnancy. There is an additional
concern: as it stands, because the GIFT procedure involves clinical
work with gametes, not embryos, monitoring the use of this procedure is not covered by the remit of the VLA. Clinicians do not
require to be licensed by the VLA to offer GIFT as a service in
district hospitals.

The focus on the authority of 'the doctor' in the dyadic model is
also misleading. The social relations of modern medicine seldom
involve one-to-one doctor–patient care, except perhaps in primary
care. Technological advance has eroded the uncontested authority of
the consultant (Cockburn, 1985). When complex medical technology
is involved, the labour process may include many 'third party' health

professionals with appropriate skills, and sometimes multidisciplinary teams. (There are, as yet, only anecdotal accounts of how, and from where, teams are recruited in rapidly developing complex innovatory services in medicine such as IVF.) A differential distribution of skill and knowledge in the allocation of work responsibilities is characteristic. The scientific and technical knowledge of, for instance, medical physicists, radiologists, endocrinologists and embryologists enters into the decision making surrounding one or other of the two technologies considered here and, in important respects, the consultant does not control the labour process in relation to either. Drawing on expertise from various disciplines, research is efficiently coupled to innovatory clinical services using these technologies, encouraging a multidisciplinary approach to both research and clinical practice. Inevitably, the growth of multidisciplinary practices has led to the need for greater intra-profession accountability, and the acknowledgement of uncertainty.

The double standard which operates in medical innovation in the United Kingdom is bound to generate unease. Until the efficacy and safety of new drugs have been assessed during formal procedures set up in the public interest, and fortified by the introduction of a restricted drugs list, doctors, in effect, do not have the clinical freedom to prescribe them. This is not the case for non-drug interventions such as surgical and diagnostic procedures. Typically, members of the profession who have pioneered an innovative technology are centrally involved in deciding what constitutes 'adequate knowledge' about the benefits of such an innovation: on what issues consensus can be negotiated; what are the risks associated with it; and what procedures are appropriate to minimise them. Emerging practices thus come to define early guidelines in the use of a new technology which are subsequently developed on an *ad hoc* basis as problems are identified. Given the power and social significance of medical authority, it then becomes a political issue as to which aspects of expertise are challenged.

From improvised early applications in the 1950s the low-cost technology of obstetric diagnostic ultrasound has now been highly developed and brought into widespread use in the public sector. It provides a useful illustration of the way scientific and technical uncertainties are identified and managed in this medical speciality. The technology is capable, not only of enabling the detection of many foetal structural and functional abnormalities, but also of guiding clinicians as an adjunct to techniques of prenatal diagnosis (such as amniocentesis), IVF and GIFT, and as they attempt to treat the foetus-as-patient *in utero*. It does not appear to be perceived as remote from public understanding.

The 'safety' of a scan is a sensitive and much discussed issue, particularly in relation to early pregnancy. The absence of any unambiguous demonstration of adverse effects in humans has led to the assumption that ultrasound is benign. The dearth of authoritative guidelines stems from the lack of a scientifically adequate data-base for developing reasonable estimates of possible bio-effects and of risk. Several hypothetical mechanisms by which ultrasound can affect biological material are acknowledged but readily discounted as unlikely 'under the intensity levels of current diagnostic conditions'. However, no consensus exists on what aspects of exposure might be important. Typically, output intensities are neither standardised nor recorded and, as midwife Margaret Andrews and her colleagues emphasised in the *British Journal of Obstetrics and Gynaecology*, there are few exposure time measurements in clinical conditions. Their intention was to stimulate discussion on the minimisation of exposure during ultrasound procedures (Andrews *et al.*, 1987). International guidelines for the use of ultrasound exist, but no special regulations have been laid down in the United Kingdom.

This is all the more surprising because the advocacy of the procedure for all pregnancies and the adoption of the technique into routine use have taken place without firm evidence of clear beneficial effects on perinatal outcome. There is still no firm scientific basis for believing that routine ultrasound scanning and obstetric practice is more effective in decreasing morbidity and mortality than is the selective scanning of women whose pregnancies are regarded as high-risk.

However, unheeded concerns about ultrasound go beyond the fears about risk from exposure. Since the mid 1980s, consumer groups and paramedicals (radiologists in particular) have published articles voicing concern about conditions of practice, about adverse psychological effects and patient anxiety and deficiencies in ultrasound services. In December 1987 Hylton Mcire, a consultant radiologist, urged that there was a need for firm guidance from a national body to ensure a co-ordinated and planned approach to obstetric ultrasound (Meire, 1987, p. 1122). As yet no political constituency has taken up these issues.

Obstetric ultrasonography enables the diagnostic interpretation of the image of an embryo or foetus which remains physically within the pregnant woman. With few exceptions her agency in reproduction must be acknowledged in decisions about any action subsequent to the diagnosis. By comparison, the embryo, after conception *in vitro* and prior to transfer in the IVF procedure, is available to be examined as a physically separate entity and may be frozen for later use. The woman whose egg has been fertilised is not generally involved in the decision-making about the quality of the consequent embryo. Decisions about which embryos to transfer and, up to a point, how many, have been regarded as matters of clinical judgement. This contrast is highly significant in the debate about the regulation and control of these two technologies and the uncertainty associated with them.

Public and published disputes in relation to IVF are not, in essence, about technical risks or about safety or efficacy. They are about perceived and potential social risks and 'slippery-slope' arguments. Existing guidelines have been flouted and the experience of the VLA illustrates the fact that voluntary self-regulation by the profession is inadequate. The IVF procedure raises fundamental ethical questions about the control of human reproduction and the grounds for limiting clinical freedom. IVF clinicians and their scientific colleagues cannot legitimately claim any special skills to make ethical and social decisions, and there are demands, not only for accountability to a statutory body, but also for public participation in the form of representative lay membership of such a body.

The malaise surrounding contemporary reproductive technologies has a political, rather than a technical, focus. It must be located in the wider context of public concern, not only about risk and uncertainty, but also about social relationships. In particular, there are clear and worrying gender dimensions to these scientific innovations which have yet to be properly addressed. Attempts to bring pressure to bear have challenged traditional bases of medical authority and the power of clinicians to take decisions of social import in relation to 'the individual clinical case'. The limits of expertise and the desirability of unrestricted freedom of clinical judgement in reproductive medicine are now under review.

Notes

1. This and the preceding quotations are from written descriptions provided by mothers of triplets in the course of early preparatory work which I undertook for a national study involving the parents of triplets, quadruplets, quintuplets and sextuplets in the United Kingdom. This study, funded by the DHSS Small Grant Scheme and the Doris Bott Fund as one of a series of integrated studies, is still going on.
2. Communication from P. M. Dunn, Professor of Perinatal Medicine and Child Health, University of Bristol.
3. Letter from C. Robertson, President of the British Association of Perinatal Medicine, dated 11 February 1987.
4. See *Hansard*, 27 January 1986, Col. 389; 19 December 1986, Cols 792–3.
5. Ian Craft, 'Antenna' Programme, BBC2, 30 September 1987.

6 Recreating the Family? Policy Considerations Relating to the 'New' Reproductive Technologies

Erica Haimes

Introduction

The new reproductive technologies have raised the issue of how much a child should be told about the circumstances of her/his conception and birth. This has led to widespread discussion, much of which has focused on what to tell a child who was conceived with the aid of gamete donation (that is, through donated sperm using artificial insemination and/or a donated egg, using *in vitro* fertilisation). This child is not wholly the genetic child of the adults who (s)he might regard as her/his parents. The question is whether the child should be told this and, if so, whether further information about the donor should also be made available to the child. Arguments both for and against this have been made, based on the common grounds of the importance attached to the relationship between parents and child and how this can be protected when that relationship involves a third and even a fourth party, the donor(s). The individual's sense of personal identity is thought to be at risk when issues about her/his parentage are not clear. Contributions to the discussion have come from various quarters: from those who draw parallels with adoption (Brandon and Warner, 1977; Haimes and Timms, 1985); from clinicians and medical scientists who have practised in and researched the technical aspects of these issues (for example, the Royal College of Obstetricians and Gynaecologists) and from those involved in policy discussions, who have had to review the range of technologies and the consequences of their application. The last group includes the Committee of Inquiry into Human Fertilisation and Embryology, chaired by Mary Warnock.

My own interest in these issues stems from my earlier research on adoption and from explorations of the similarities and/or differences between this and artificial insemination by donor (Haimes, 1988). In this chapter I review discussions which emanate from the fields of medical science and policy. My review covers both accounts of current practice and contributions to the continuing debate on what to tell the child, as contained in a series of prominent reports. These include the aforementioned *Warnock Report* (1984; 1985), the Royal College of Obstetricians and Gynaecologists' *Report on In Vitro Fertilisation and Embryo Replacement or Transfer* (RCOG, 1983), the Council for Science and Society Report on *Human Procreation* (CSS, 1984)[1] and the Board for Social Responsibility Report, *Personal Origins* (BSR, 1985).[2] These represent (along with other contributions mentioned in the text and the bibliography) the voices of expertise on medical, scientific and related ethical issues.[3] I shall argue that current practice is directed at discouraging any contact between the donor on the one hand and the receiving couple and resultant child on the other. The reports reviewed here either seek to continue such practices or to modify them only slightly. In examining why this position is consistently advocated and why such separation is thought to be beneficial to all parties, I argue that an explanation might be derived from the accounts themselves. That is, the way in which such accounts divide the debate into straightforward and difficult issues is significant here. Such distinctions act also to categorise these actual families constructed by the application of the new reproductive technologies into difficult and straightforward types. I suggest that the distinctions convey a set of assumptions about 'normal families' against which those produced through the use of reproductive technologies are compared. The analysis indicates that, although critical concern is expressed with reference to issues of identity in children conceived through sperm or egg donation, the discussion is conducted with reference to the full range of technologies available. The use of artificial insemination by husband (AIH) and *in vitro* fertilisation (IVF) using the couple's own gametes, as well as the non-technical (or, not necessarily technical) procedure of surrogacy are drawn into the debate. By analysing the grounds for these comparisons I hope to contribute to an understanding of the way reproductive technologies, though 'new' in their technical aspects, are assessed with reference to established notions about the norms of family life.

Mechanisms of Separation in the Practice of Gamete Donation

First, what evidence is there that the social separation of donor and resultant family is either likely or intended? It could be argued that there are three possible modes of interaction. These can be referred to as: complete separation; mediated links; direct contact. The current practice of gamete donation, guided by standards of professional practice rather than legal regulation, follows a line of complete separation. Donors are anonymous. There is little shared knowledge about donor recruitment between practitioners and none between practitioners and lay persons. The registering of the husband (and male partners if a settled relationship is apparent) as the father is not discouraged (although illegal). The mixing of the husband's sperm with donor sperm is not unheard of, leaving some ambiguity about who might be the genetic father. It is also significant that egg *donation* occurs, thus permitting the receiving woman to become pregnant and to give birth, thereby minimising the role of the donor by disguising her existence through the mimicking of an 'ordinary' birth. The alternatives of adoption or surrogacy would have no such effect (Wood and Westmore, 1984 p. 122). Finally, the most obvious element of separation and one which therefore is the least visible, is that the whole procedure occurs by means of artificial insemination and/or *in vitro* fertilisation rather than sexual intercourse.This is not to suggest that intercourse is necessarily more or less desirable than artificial means of impregnation, merely that such artificial means inevitably result in a further distancing of the donor. That, of course, is their attraction to many of the parties involved.

These are the practices which, it should be noted, are recommended by medical scientists and practitioners, such as Carl Wood, an established and much published IVF researcher, and the British Agencies for Adoption and Fostering (BAAF) Medical Group, as well as policy makers. They involve a distancing, almost a denial of the donor's role, which is likely to continue if the recommendations of various investigative committees are accepted. Of these the two likely to be the most influential, on policy makers and clinicians respectively, are the report of the Warnock Committee (1984) and the report of the Royal College of Obstetricians and Gynaecologists (1983). The RCOG advise their members regarding artificial insemination by donor (AID) that:

(i) neither donor nor couple should know the other's identity; and that

(ii) donors should have the same physical characteristics as the husband (1983, p. 6).

The latter recommendation is presumably, 'to make the sort of rough match which is generally thought desirable' (British Agencies for Adoption and Fostering, 1984, p. 13).

Similar recommendations can be found in the *Warnock Report:*

(i)   the law should be changed to permit the husband to be registered as the father legally (Warnock, 1985, p. 85);
(ii) the woman giving birth should be regarded as the mother of the child (ibid., p. 85);
(iii) neither sperm nor egg donors should have any rights or responsibilities towards the child (ibid., p. 85);
(iv) anyone donating gametes should be unknown to the couple before, during and after the treatment (ibid., p. 82);
(v)   similar provisions should apply to embryo donation (ibid., p. 86);
(vi) the AID child should be treated in law as the legitimate child of its mother and her husband, where both have consented to treatment (ibid., p. 85).

These recommendations do not have the status of law, but they are the only systematic appraisal so far of policy needs arising from the application of the whole range of reproductive technologies. Although the subject of much debate and criticism since publication, these recommendations have been formally reviewed and were subject to further comment in a consultation paper on infertility services (Department of Health and Social Security, 1986). In this more recent document it is argued that there is likely to be a broad measure of agreement (ibid., p. 4) on most of the above recommendations. This has since been confirmed by the inclusion of these recommendations in the DHSS White Paper, *Human Fertilisation and Embryology: A Framework for Legislation* (1987, pp. 13–16).

The only recommendations which appear to be against current practice and advice are those from the Warnock Committee suggesting that the child should be informed of her/his method of conception and that, at the age of eighteen, she/he should be able to obtain further 'basic information' (non-identifying) on the ethnic origins and genetic health of the donor (Warnock, 1985, p. 82). Also, the Committee suggested, presumably as a prerequisite for the previous recommendation, that a centrally-maintained register of these births should be considered (ibid., p. 81). I shall be considering these additional recommendations in more detail later, but it should be noted that these are the only suggestions advocating anything other than complete separation, in this case *mediated* links. In this instance, the donor's existence is acknowledged, but the only link advocated is still very much at a distance, mediated by officials operating the register and passing on only the basic information specified. No *direct* contact between child and donor is envisaged.

These distancing mechanisms are thought to be necessary because they are said to be in the best interests of, variously, the donor, the child and, finally, the receiving couple. I shall review the reasons given in each case, to see how they are presented and defended. For the moment I shall not attempt a critique of these views, except to point out where they appear to contradict themselves on their own terms. However, it may become apparent to the reader that this deliberately naive approach leads inevitably to a series of questions about what is behind these arguments. Those are questions to which I turn in the final section of this chapter.

The Donor

Anonymity of the donor is assumed to be in her/his best interests. According to one report, such a policy 'favours the donor' (Council for Science and Society, 1984, p. 8). However, the reasoning behind this often remains unexplicated (see, for example, Brandon and Warner, 1977). When explanations are provided they usually revolve around the concern that donors do not wish to incur any parental responsibility. This coincides with recommendations to remove any legal obligation regarding parental resonsibility (see above), yet the recommendation for anonymity remains (Warnock, 1985, pp. 82, 85; Council for Science and Society 1984, pp. 38–9).

A second reason for retaining anonymity, it is argued, is that, even without risk of incurring parental responsibility, donors will not want to be identified and therefore will not come forward. In the DHSS Consultation Paper, evidence from Sweden is cited to support this claim (1986, p. 7). (Since 1983 Swedish sperm donors' names have been registered; the right of an AID conceived person on reaching the age of eighteen to seek access to that identifying information has been established.) It was claimed, however, by the Swedish Insemination Committee (1983, pp. 14–15) that, although doctors feared the decline of donations, this would only be a temporary setback, since a number of donors interviewed had said they did not object to their names being registered. Singer and Wells (1984, p. 74) register a similar finding. Nevertheless, there is not sufficient evidence in favour of either argument since there have been few studies of donors and they have surveyed only small numbers. The fears of practitioners may, in fact, be justified. However, assertions like Reilly's that the number of donors would 'diminish drastically' (1977, p. 202), when set against the Swedish confidence, do not really go far enough. This begs the question of why it is such an issue for donors to 'admit to' being donors. Both sets of arguments assume the problem without explicating its nature. The Swedish Committee begins to suggest the nature of the problem in its reference to 'public attitudes' towards AID, which see it as a 'questionable method' of correcting childlessness (1983, p. 14). Until further studies of donors have been conducted we can only surmise attitudes to being named. However, our conjectures come from the same pool of knowledge as the assumptions mentioned above, that is, the suggestion that donors would be embarrassed if their status were generally known. It is assumed that embarrassment would arise from the method of donation (masturbation in the case of sperm donations) plus uncertainty about the attitude of others to the practice of gamete donation. Clearly the practice of distancing cannot be linked to the legal obligations arising from being a donor, since, as Reilly points out, 'it would be relatively easy to resolve most of them by formulating specific rules to define the legal relations among the child, the parents, and the donor' (1977, p. 4). This is exactly what the *Warnock Report* tries to do.

The Child
Whilst much of the professional literature (that is, from doctors or medical practitioners, scientists, social workers and policy makers) acknowledges, in keeping with the Warnock Committee, the need for the child to know her/his method of conception, it also argues that information about the donor should only provide a 'pen-picture'. This might cover ethnic grouping and genetic health, but nothing to identify the donor by name. Sometimes the appropriateness of this is assumed (for example, in the British Agencies for Adoption and Fostering's recommendations to the Warnock Committee, 1984). At other times, it is seen as the only possible outcome of trying to balance the donor's interests with those of the child (Council for Science and Society, 1984, pp. 8–9). Once again, the Swedish legislation provides a contrast, based on the notion that it is in the child's best interests, in the case of AID at least, to know all that is available about her/his biological origins. Why might possessing this

information be seen as going against the child's interests? The above literature cites several reasons, amongst them the stigma of illegitimacy, under current law (see, for example, Council for Science and Society, 1984, p. 45). However, this neglects two factors: the proposed changes in the law mean that an AID child would not be illegitimate (Warnock, 1985, p. 85) and second, stigma is more likely to arise from the knowledge of gamete donation than from the knowledge of the donor's name. Similarly, the stigma experienced simply by being different is said to be an important consideration (for example, Royal College of Obstetricians and Gynaecologists, 1983, pp. 9–10). However, once again, this comes from being a child of gamete donation, not from knowing the donor's name. Finally, it is argued that the child might simply be confused about her/his parentage (Board for Social Responsibility, 1985, p. 45), but this too would arise from knowing about her/his conception. In fact, knowledge of the identity of her/his genetic parents may, as the Swedes argue, help to resolve this confusion. These arguments about the child's best interests centre upon the general issue of secrecy about the whole process of conception rather than about the identity of the donor. Once it is accepted (as it has been by the *Warnock Report*) that the child's conception should not remain a secret and once the legal issue of the child's legitimacy has been resolved, the basis for preserving the donor's anonymity, from the child's point of view, on the face of it seems weak. In the specific case of egg donation, the risk of illegitimacy does not even occur, so there are even fewer arguments in this instance for maintaining such distance.

Therefore, it could be argued that, rather than all parties being protected by the anonymity of the donor, it is, in fact, the donor who is protected, at the child's expense. Whilst this is one possible interpretation, the limited evidence which exists, and which was cited earlier, appears to indicate that donors themselves do not see such a conflict, since they may be willing to be identified. Clearly further empirical studies are needed to clarify this point. The lack of such research is itself part of the problem, since access is usually through medical practitioners who tend to support the need for anonymity.

From a systematic review of the arguments cited in the literature it becomes clear that, as with the preceding section on the donor, such arguments are derived from a different set of concerns to those stated. The inconsistencies and contradictions which have been identified are not a failure of logic on behalf of those advocating them but are, rather, an indication of more fundamental issues which tend to remain unstated precisely because of their foundational qualities. This will become more apparent as we turn now to consider the third party said to be of concern, the receiving couple.

The Receiving Couple
One recurring feature of these discussions is the relative 'invisibility' of the couple receiving treatment. This is akin to the situation which arose in adoption. When the adopted person's right of access to her/his original birth records was discussed at committee and parliamentary level, concern was expressed primarily for the child's interests and the natural mother's interests. The adoptive parents who clearly had a stake, having raised the child, were not given a central place in the discussion, either because their interests might be deemed selfish if openly expressed or because the legislation was simply not perceived as affecting them (Haimes and Timms, 1985). Similarly, the receiving couple tend to be forgotten during discussions on the anonymity of the donor. Once the husband's position as the legal father has been established and once it has been acknowledged that his infertility (and the woman's infertility in the case of egg donation) cannot be hidden at the price of keeping the child in the dark about her/his conception, there remains no legal reason for the anonymity of the donor. However, it has been argued by Robert Snowden and his colleagues, that 'conflicting emotional ties between the family of the recipient and the family of the donor would also be likely to arise' if the identity of the donor were to be known (Snowden *et al.*, 1983, p. 103). Certainly this was the feeling of the *Warnock Report*: 'our general view is that anonymity protects all parties not only from legal complications but also from emotional difficulties' (Warnock, 1985, p. 15). Once again, those difficulties are not fully explained.

These are the arguments for retaining the anonymity of all parties: donors from families and vice versa. However, they contain inconsistencies which suggest that we need to look further to understand why anonymity is considered appropriate. Prior to this, I shall recapitulate those inconsistencies. First, legal difficulties have been cited as one reason for anonymity but these are resolvable through the implementation of suggestions which establish the legal rights of the receiving couple as parents, and also legitimate the child. Moreover, those difficulties arise from the initial acknowledgement of gamete donation, rather than from the subsequent divulging of the donor's name. Yet, anonymity is still advocated. Secondly, emotional difficulties have been cited but not explored. There is no clear evidence on this issue. Donors might well feel embarrassment, but we do not know this to be the case. The child might be considered better off in not knowing the donor's name, but the Swedes think otherwise. Again the evidence is limited and the possible lessons to be learnt from elsewhere, including adoption, remain controversial (Haimes, 1988). The most consistent indication of potential emotional difficulties comes from the receiving couple, if their apparent insistence on secrecy about the whole process can be read in this way. Successive studies have found this reaction (Owens, 1982/3; 1984; Humphrey, 1984; Alder, 1984) but again there has been little exploration of *why* couples feel this way.

So can anonymity be said to be in the interests of all the parties concerned? Despite the poor quality of the evidence in support of this view, the main contributors to the debate feel that it is appropriate. A further examination of the material is necessary, therefore, to understand why that view is so firmly established. One possibility is to investigate the wider context of the debate. From this we find that issues about anonymity in gamete donation are, in fact, embedded in a broader discussion about the application of the complete range of new reproductive technologies. This broader discussion provides further data on the way gamete donation is perceived in relation to these other techniques, especially in their family-building capabilities. Within that discussion we can begin to understand more clearly the issues surrounding donor anonymity.

Reproductive Technologies and the Family

We need to begin by surveying the complete range of technologies available, rather than just those considered so far. The technologies are artificial insemination by husband (AIH), artificial insemination by donor (AID), *in vitro* fertilisation (IVF) using (a) wife's egg and husband's sperm (embryo replacement), (b) wife's egg and donor sperm, (c) donor egg and husband's sperm, (d) donor egg and donor sperm (that is, embryo transfer or donation), and embryo lavage. Additionally, surrogacy can occur through the use of AID and IVF (Warnock, 1985). A review of the literature indicates that, as far as the scientists, clinicians and policy makers are concerned, the technologies *qua* technologies, present little or no problem. The Royal College of Obstetricians and Gynaecologists for example, concludes: 'so far there is no evidence that children born following in vitro fertilisation and embryo replacement have a higher risk of physical abnormality than children conceived naturally' (RCOG, 1983, p. 2).

One exception is the Warnock Committee's uncertainty about the reliability of embryo lavage (Warnock, 1985, p. 40). However, in the same literature there is also a tendency to classify the *application* of the technology into three forms. The first form covers those described as the 'simple cases' (Singer and Wells, 1984), the ones where there is 'no moral objection to its practice' (Warnock, 1985, p. 18), that is, AIH and IVF without donation. Such practices, it is argued, are simply overcoming 'nature's defects . . . nature's errors' (Wood and Westmore, 1984, p. 97). The technology is considered to be effective and the social and moral standing of the couple is established, so the application is acceptable and unproblematic. The second form covers those applications of the techniques involving donors: distinguished in the literature from the 'simple cases' because of the issues already discussed. Ultimately the form is acceptable, it is argued, because it represents the opportunity for couples to have a family, at least partly genetically related (ibid, p. 30; Warnock, 1985, p. 23). It allows them to fulfil the 'natural desire' for parenthood (Council for Science and Society, 1984, p. 45). The final form covers those cases which are technically possible but considered socially undesirable: in particular, cases involving surrogacy and single parenthood. In such cases, the scientific and medical experts tend to seek recourse to ethical committees for guidance (Wood and Westmore, 1984, p. 114). Those contributing to policy decisions are clearer about their views: 'we are all agreed that surrogacy for convenience alone . . . is totally, ethically unacceptable' (Warnock, 1985, p. 46); 'it violates the dignity of motherhood that a woman should be paid for bearing a child by proxy' (Board for Social Responsibility, 1984, p. 15); ' . . . we believe that as a general rule it is better for children to be born into a two-parent family, with both father and mother' (Warnock, 1985, p. 11). It might be argued that this final form could be sub-divided, a point which will be discussed later.

From the sketch above, two further threads of analysis emerge. The first is that it is evident that there are different elements which make up the notion of 'the family' as it is being used here. These apparently have different degrees of importance in relation to each other. The second thread is that 'families-by-donation' are in an anomalous position as an intermediate category of 'problematic but allowable'.

To take up the first thread: if the three forms and the family configurations within each are examined more closely it is apparent that there are at least three important constituent elements to the family, as it is featured in this context. First there is the ideological component. To what extent are the different family types produced by use of the new reproductive technologies supportive of a particular (that is, the dominant) ideology of family life? That is, to what extent do they reflect assumptions about the inherent worth of such families and the values they display? Second, there is the structural dimension. To what extent do such families reproduce the grouping assumed in the ideal family type, that is, two parents, plus children? Finally, we must consider genetic composition. To what extent do these families reproduce the biological relationships assumed in the 'normal family'? Whilst the distinctions between these three elements are perhaps not absolute, they none the less provide a useful heuristic device to gain a purchase on the presuppositions embodied in the perceptions of clinicians and policy makers. What is important for this discussion is the relative value placed on each of the three elements identified above.

The relationship between each of the family forms and these three elements needs to be considered in turn. First, there are the configurations created through the 'simple cases' of AIH and IVF between husband and wife. All three elements of the 'normal family' are satisfied: the ideology of the family is not only demonstrated, but also enhanced by the efforts these couples are prepared to expend to become parents. The structure of the conventional form of two-parents-plus-children is satisfied and the genetic composition begs no questions since the social, nurturing parents are also the genetic parents, so the resultant child is indubitably linked to her/his parents. However, when we consider the configurations which emerge from the range of families-by-donation, it is clear that only two out of three key elements are satisfied. In AID, IVF with donated gametes and embryo lavage this is consistently the case. Once again, the value of family life is demonstrated and each family has the appearance of an ordinary structure, of two parents and child(ren). However, in three of the cases, AID, IVF with donor sperm and IVF with donor egg, the child is not genetically linked to both parents. In the other two cases, embryo donation and embryo lavage, neither nurturing parent is a genetic parent. Opinions vary as to whether, in families-by-donation, it is preferable for at least one parent to be genetically linked to the child, thus, nearly resembling an ordinary family, or whether, because of the unevenness this is said to create between the two parents, it is preferable for neither parent to be a genetic parent. However, for our concerns, it is more relevant to ask why this emerges as a question in the first place and what stress is laid on this element in comparison with the other two being discussed. Part of the answer can be found by completing the survey of family configurations, by examining the third group of families: that is, those families thought to be undesirable by the policy makers. These require a slightly more detailed consideration and possibly a further sub-division.

First there is the use of AID by a single woman and also the use of artificial insemination and a form of surrogacy by a single man wanting to become a parent. Neither of these possibilities is condoned under the Warnock Committee's recommendations (Warnock, 1985, p. 11). In fact, the case of the single man was only superficially considered, but it is covered by the general embargo on creating single-parent families set out by the report. Then there are the possible variations associated with surrogacy: using artificial insemination of the husband's sperm; using artificial insemination of donor sperm, so neither nurturing parent is a genetic parent, and finally surrogacy using IVF. In terms of the three elements, this last set of surrogacy configurations can be divided off from the single parent families, thus splitting this third group into two sub-groups.

First, I shall consider single-parent families. It could be argued that the ideology espoused by single people wishing to use the new reproductive technologies relates more to one of 'rights' than of 'familyness'. In this instance, the right to be a parent is essentially individualistic and is contrasted with the shared group characteristics of the wish to 'have a family'. The failure to satisfy the appropriate ideological characteristics of the family is further reflected in the structure (and, of course, the label) of this configuration: one-parent families. In discussions about the use of the new technologies by single people (see the earlier quotations) the issue of whether or not the parent is a genetic parent to the child is not raised, since that is apparently irrelevant, given the other 'failings' of such families.[4] Neither is there objection to the 'intrusion' of a donor, since these instances are not seen as having anything upon which a donor could intrude, that is, a marital relationship. In this case, it is the ideology of individualism, seen as undermining the ideology of the family, which raises most objections.

There is then a distinction to be drawn between these and the other group of technically possible but socially undesirable families: those involving surrogacy. Other than the case of the single man, which belongs to the previous sub-set, cases of surrogacy can be seen as placing the highest possible value on the desire to have a family. This also involves a family which satisfies the requirement of the two-parent structure as well. However, the practice of surrogacy can amount to a questioning of the role of motherhood, depending ultimately on the surrendering of a child by a woman who has given birth to it. Not only does this bring into question views which place a high regard on the value of pre-natal bonding between a woman and the child she is carrying, it also places obstacles in the path of attempts, such as those made by the Warnock Committee, to define who constitutes the real mother in other uses of the new reproductive technologies. For example, in the case of egg and embryo donation, the woman giving birth is to be regarded in law as the mother of the child (Warnock, 1985, p. 85). If the birth experience is given primacy in defining motherhood, then surrogacy undermines motherhood. Since motherhood is at the centre of 'familyness', to subvert mother-hood is to subvert the family. Once again the question of the genetic composition of the resultant family receives little attention, although the 'role' of the surrogate is obviously similar to that of the sperm or egg donor (though this, of course, is not to equate their levels of involvement). The genetic composition of families created by the different types of surrogacy is similar to that found in the families-by-donation, but the process by which this is arrived at is, neverthe-less, less acceptable than for families-by-donation. This is demon-strated in the case of surrogacy-for-convenience in which the genetic and social parents would be the same, but it is this form of surrogacy which is most clearly rejected. The surrogate's role is too immediate, too long in terms of time and too threatening to the concept of motherhood. Yet it should be noted that the case against surrogacy is not fully established in professional and policy-making circles (see, for example, the note of dissent in the *Warnock Report* and Blyth, 1987). This suggests the tension between the apparently legitimate desire for a family and the risk this entails to established conceptions of motherhood.

Emerging from the analysis above is a conceptual framework with which to compare the range of possible outcomes of applying repro-ductive technologies, without losing sight of the normative assump-tions contained within the literature. Those assumptions carry within them a form of ranking whereby the ideological orientation of the family/individual initiating the application appears to be the most important feature. The ideological and structural features are closely related, though not, as the case of surrogacy shows, entirely overlapping, since appropriate structural features are apparently not sufficient to justify challenging ideological appropriateness. The issue of genetic composition seems to be the least important of the three, although not unimportant. It would appear that most accounts attend to genetic links only when the ideological and structural features are uncontentious. When those features are contentious the issue of genetic links gains little attention.

This conclusion leads us to examine the second thread to emerge from the debate: the anomalous position of the family-by-donation, in being both acceptable to these discussants, but also perceived by them as problematic.

To recapitulate, it is clear that families which are 'simple cases' are so because they conform to some notion of the normal family in which marriage, sex and reproduction are grouped together (Mac-Intyre, 1977). On the other hand, families which subvert these conventions are seen as at the opposite extreme and are, as a consequence, unacceptable (Leathard, 1986). However, the ambiguous position of families-by-donation lies in the fact that the use of donors can be both threatening to, and supportive of, the ideal of the family: 'The initial motivation toward IVF is pro-family – to produce a child for an otherwise incomplete family. But is IVF anti-family in the broader view because it, *and its possible variants*, will decrease or blur traditional bondings among mother, father and off-spring?' (Grobstein and Flower, 1985 p. 880, my emphasis). By what criteria therefore are these families acceptable and by what criteria are they problematic? As the above quotation indicates, families-by-donation are considered acceptable because they conform to the ideological and structural requirements of normal families: that is, they represent both the wish to have a family and the assumption that an ordinary family includes children. An even greater advantage is the opportunity they provide for social eugenics: " . . . the AID child should be born into a stable marriage or heterosexual relationship in which there is an expectation that both parties will be able to provide for the emotional, social, familial, educational and economic needs of the child until he or she reaches maturity' (BAAF, 1984, p. 14). Although such families lack the full biological linkage of ordinary families, this is the least visible and thus, to an extent, the least important of the criteria involved. As Carol Smart argues, the biological link between donor and child is overriden, in the case of AID, in favour of attaching the child to a social father in a two-parent family (Smart, 1987, p. 114). Consequently, the family resulting from gamete donation can 'pass' as a normal family.

On the other hand, there are several problematic features in such families indicating that genetic composition, though perhaps less important is not unimportant. These families are seen as having, for instance, the constant potential of being exposed as something other than an ordinary family, in everyday interaction. They can give themselves away or others can make connections which suggest there is something not quite right because of a particular mix of eye colour, for example, or perhaps blood groups. They are, in Goffman's terms, seen as discreditable (Goffman, 1968, p. 14). Members of families that do not conform are seen to run the risk of being stigmatised in several ways: the infertile parent runs the risk of individual exposure; the child risks stigmatisation through not being 'placeable' socially by reference to biological ties (Harris, 1983; Blank, 1984); and the whole family could be seen therefore as an 'artificial family' (Snowden and Mitchell, 1981), with reference to their particular grouping as much as to the technical procedures involved in its construction. There are other problems too: should exposure occur, the structural elements of the family would also be exposed. That is to say, the role of the donor(s) as a third (and possibly fourth) party in the marital relationship would become apparent.[5] These then are perhaps the 'emotional difficulties' through which members try to conform to 'normal' families. If such problems are not to be perceived as outweighing the advantages of such families solutions need to be found.

What are the possible solutions to the above problems? The family's discreditable status could be dealt with by advocating absolute and complete secrecy. But this is inadequate on two counts: first, too many people (at *least* the couple, the medical team and the donor(s)) know already, so the risk of exposure cannot be entirely eradicated; secondly, the idea of secrets within the family as a recommendation for the family's social survival undermines the pro-family ideology that gamete donation can be said to represent. Part of the rhetoric of 'a proper family life' is openness and trust (Board for Social Responsibility, 1985, p. 53). The solution arrived at by the *Warnock Report*, therefore, was that parents should tell the child about the gamete donation, thus preventing damage being caused accidentally and, at the same time, celebrating the honesty and intimacy of a family that can cope with such issues. However, this leaves the problem of how the child's genetic identity is to be resolved. Harris argues that: 'Recognition of parentage . . . has the consequence of enabling the child to be attributed not merely to the society, but to a *position within* the society. Both of these attributions are quite properly called placement' (1983, p. 26). So this is perceived by discussants as being far from a trivial problem. Again, the *Warnock Report* offers a solution to this by recommending that information about the child's genetic origins should be given to her/him, either by the parents or from official records, from age 18.

However, once it has been established (a) that secrecy is not possible, nor desirable and (b) that the child should have a right to genetic information, the structural non-conformity of the family is fully apparent. None the less the consequences of this can be contained by glossing the details of that non-conformity. Therefore, if the donor is not named the non-conformity cannot be manifested in the form of a real, living person. The donor is simply that: her/his role as a third/fourth party in the marital relationship remains limited, vague and shadowy. A named donor implies the continued presence of an actual individual in those family relationships.

Anonymity can therefore be regarded, perhaps, as an exercise in damage limitation, by those who wish both to accept gamete donation and to resolve some of the problems it represents to notions of the 'ordinary family'. It helps to preserve as many as possible of the conventional features of the family by setting a barrier around the unit. No routes exist to provide a way through that barrier: the donor has no way back into the family, post-donation, and no member of the family has a route back out, to reach the donor. Each remains anonymous to the other. Explicable *perhaps* in terms of donors' wishes not to assume any sort of parental role, anonymity is also explicable by the desire to prevent donors *claiming* any such role and thus risking a distortion of the family structure and ideology.

Conclusion

I have considered a range of reports contributing to the debate on the possible applications of the new reproductive technologies. I have argued that those reports draw upon normative assumptions about the family, which then inform their discussion about particular issues: in this case, the issue of how much information to pass on to the family and child about the gamete donors. I have shown that the recommendation to retain the anonymity between donor and family can only be understood by reference to the desire, imputed by the reports to the parties involved, to conform to the 'ordinary' family as far as possible – ideologically and structurally, if not genetically. This analysis should not be read as an attempt to give a functionalist account of the role of the family. Rather, it is an attempt to uncover the presuppositions which exist in the debates reviewed here. Likewise, I am not assuming that policy makers and clinicians contributing to this literature actually experience reality and live their lives only within such apparently narrow possibilities. Rather, this analysis illustrates David H. Morgan's point that: 'Persons involved in the framing and enacting of legislation both draw upon conventionally held notions of familial relationships (or more complicatedly, upon notions of what these conventional notions are . . .) and, in so doing reinforce these notions through their public pronouncements or through their deployment in law and judgement' (D. H. Morgan, 1985, p. 72).

In fact, there is further evidence of this in the latest policy-making stage, the DHSS White Paper on *Human Fertilisation and Embryology* (1987). This has been published since the period during which discussion of the consultative document took place came to an end and it is therefore an indication of the speed with which views on these subjects emerge. As mentioned earlier, the bulk of the recommendations of the *Warnock Report* have been adopted in the White Paper, including the view that only non-identifying information on donors should be made available. However, an important note has been added:

> Attitudes to the anonymity of donors, however, may well change over time as happened with adoption. The Government therefore proposes to keep the position under review. The Bill will include powers to amend the categories of information to be made available to children born following donation, so that the possibility of granting access to identifying information in future remains open. (Department of Health and Social Security, 1987, p. 14)

What would be the effect of removing anonymity of donors? As this chapter has shown, anonymity serves as a device to protect the anomalous family and to promote the ideology of 'family life'. For the latter purpose it is only one device amongst many (Smart, 1987, cites others) and, thus, the impact of its removal would perhaps be minimal. However, its other purpose, to protect the anomalous family from potential damage, is, as I have suggested, perhaps more important. The form and extent of that impact is not obvious though, since the evidence from adoption (Haimes, 1988) suggests a range of possible outcomes:

(i)   Access to donors' names will not necessarily mean direct contact with donors, since requests for information are likely to be highly mediated through professional structures such as counselling. Thus the anomaly is in less danger of being exposed than might first be thought.

(ii) Requests for donors' names might be framed as representing a pathological need, such that the individual making the request is deemed marginal and in need of other kinds of help. The problem of the anomalous family thus becomes transformed into the problem of the particular damaged individual.

(iii) Requests for donors' names might cause damage to families-by-donation or donors' families, perhaps simply through the exposure of being such. This could lead to a re-categorisation of families-by-donation as being undesirable. That is, the anomaly is removed by a curtailment of the practice.

(iv) Adults conceived through gamete donation may recognise the threat to their own and their parents' social identity from the exposure mentioned above, and so contain their interest to minimise the threat of exposure.

(v)   Donors could recognise the threat to their social identity and discontinue donations. This would be the equivalent of (iii) above, in re-designating donation as undesirable.

(vi) Adverse outcomes may not arise from the loss of anonymity and the links formed between donors, couples and adults conceived through donation may instead help to break down the assumptions surrounding 'ordinary' and 'extraordinary' families. That is, the removal of anonymity could lead to changes in the notion of the normal family and of its presumed desirability.

These outcomes are highly speculative and they are not mutually exclusive or exhaustive. However, they suggest that, whatever happens regarding anonymity, it is difficult to understand any particular outcome without reference to assumptions about the 'ordinary' family. Decisions on how to apply or regulate the new reproductive technologies are only intelligible in terms of 'the family'. What is significant about the debate is not so much the positions taken regarding the release of donors' names, but how these reinforce established ideological notions about 'the family'.

Notes

I should like to thank the editors of this volume for their encouragement and comments. Maureen McNeil, in particular, has given much valuable advice. I should also like to thank Frances Price, Christine Crowe and Robin Williams for their support and advice. Finally, I should like to thank Rachel Haigh for her tolerance and skill.

1. The Council for Science and Society describes itself as 'composed . . . of experts in the respective fields together with lawyers, philosophers and others who can bring a wide range of skills and experience to bear on the subject' (Council for Science and Society, 1984, p. v).
2. The Board for Social Responsibility is a Church of England organisation which describes itself as being 'fortunate in being able to find from within its own membership the knowledge and expertise required to enable it to submit evidence' to the Warnock Committee. The Working Party comprised a professor and a reader in genetics and two professors of moral theology (Board for Social Responsibility, 1985, p. iii).
3. This group of medical and social work practitioners, medical scientists and contributors to policy-making have, in many ways, come to be the 'owners' of this issue (Gusfield, 1975, cited in Parton, 1985); that is, they have had the greatest impact on defining the problem and proffering solutions. Others, feminists in particular (Finnret, 1984), have contributed to the discussion, but have been accorded only limited legitimacy by these groups.
4. It is technically possible, for instance, for a single woman to receive a donated embryo, in which case she would not be the child's genetic mother.
5. The families of donors could also be threatened by the extension to their membership. Hence, the recommendation from some quarters that the donor's spouse should be required to give consent to donations.

7 Conflicting Concerns: The Political Context of Recent Embryo Research Policy in Britain
Edward Yoxen

Introduction

On the night of the 1987 British General Election, the BBC sent its interviewers onto the streets to ask electors what they expected from the next government. In Trafalgar Square this important task fell to Esther Rantzen. One of her interviewees was an earnest young man, who was given a few moments to utter the passionate plea that the next government ban experiments on human embryos. For him, at least, this was the most important issue on the legislative agenda. Six months later, in debate in the House of Lords on a government White Paper, published in the autumn of 1987, which promises the statutory regulation, but not the banning of such experiments, the Earl of Lauderdale, a Scottish peer and a devout Catholic, compared such investigations with those conducted at Auschwitz: 'Like it or not, pleasing or offensive to the progressive children of the Enlightenment as it may be, I say that this is darkness all day: it is not light. This is a licence to kill without even trial for a crime. We must not allow it' (*Hansard*, 1988, p. 1487). His sentiments, if not his wild and imprecise language, were echoed by several other peers, Lord Longford amongst them.

Real antipathy to the continuing practice of research on human embryos is unmistakable at present in certain quarters, as is the corresponding desire for legislation to bring it to a halt. It might seem obvious that this should be so, given that, for example, some people are firmly committed to the doctrine that the life of individual human beings begins and becomes morally significant at conception. But the mere fact that such views exist in British society, as they have for many years, tells us very little about their political significance and impact at present. It might be, for example, that people holding such views can only influence legislation in very specific political circumstances. Nor does the enduring presence of such beliefs explain the pervasive concern about human embryo research, which will be considered in more detail below. In particular, it leaves unexplained that concern felt by people who explicitly do not share such doctrinal views about the embryo. Most importantly, it does not account for the remarkable way in which the issue of research using human embryos has gained prominence in a great deal of public discussion, as the most problematic question posed by recent innovations in reproductive technology.

One of the more striking instances of the construction of the agenda for political debate over this question occurs in the commentary on the *Warnock Report* by the Oxford-trained moral philosopher and educational theoretician, Mary Warnock, who between 1982 and 1984 chaired the committee which produced it: 'All other issues we had to consider seemed relatively trivial compared with this one, concerned as it is with a matter which nobody could deny is of central moral significance, the value of human life' (Warnock, 1985, p. xvi). This comment highlights one of the more interesting undiscussed aspects of this Report, and Warnock's role in its production, which is the recurrent references to teaching people how to think about moral questions. In a sense the Report is advice to government and instruction to us all. That the moral status of human embryos can be related to such a fundamental issue is indeed undeniable. But what is it about the cultural context of the early 1980s that has allowed this issue to be given such salience, and to be used to structure the agenda for debate?

The anxieties referred to above all relate to a variety of procedures, based on the fertilisation of human eggs outside the body. The product of the complex and extended process of fertilisation in which two germ cells unite and two sets of genes are brought together is an embryo, that organises itself into increasingly complex structures and systems, as each of its constituent cells divides in two. With *in vitro* fertilisation (IVF), this process occurs in a culture medium, where the embryo can be inspected as it grows. If the embryo is to be transferred to a woman's uterus the interaction with it will be minimal. An increasing number of human embryos are being used instead for a variety of research procedures, which involve their immediate or eventual destruction. The term 'research' is used to cover many different activities here.

These include investigations that may throw some light on the genetic and medical circumstances of a particular couple attempting to begin a pregnancy through *in vitro* fertilisation, by examining embryos created with their gametes; studies of the media in which human embryos grow, of general relevance to *in vitro* fertilisation as a procedure; and studies of human development at the earliest stages, held to be of general relevance to embryology and medical science. The ends, then, differ considerably. So do the means. Some embryos may become available when a woman seeks assistance from an *in vitro* fertilisation centre. For example, they may come to be 'spare' embryos, that will not be returned to her uterus or donated to another woman. There is already anecdotal evidence that permission to use any such embryos for research is not always sought by those running IVF programmes. Research here, then, is intended but undeclared. Alternatively, embryos may be obtained via surgery specifically arranged to remove eggs from a woman being sterilised. There are indications here too that permission to remove ova for research purposes is sometimes used to bargain for an earlier operation.

It should be obvious, then, that human embryo research is not just a lab-bench procedure, involving a cluster of human cells, the moral status of which is in dispute. It has significant medical, psychological and moral implications for the woman, without whom it could not take place. Yet the conventional focus on the embryo on its own obscures and marginalises this question.

I believe that much recent debate has been based on what I call an 'over-individualised notion of the embryo'.[1] Commentators have concentrated on those genetic and developmental properties that confer individuality, to the virtual exclusion of those that concern the necessary continuing relatedness to another being, the mother. Thus human embryos, even when they are fertilised *in vitro*, derive from ova which are formed within a woman's body and must be replaced within a woman's body to develop beyond a certain point. Her feelings, or their feelings, if one woman donates the embryo to another, are, I believe, much more important than the moral status of the embryo cell-system itself. That is not to say that the human embryo has no moral status; I am not suggesting that any act with a human embryo would be acceptable. Nor am I suggesting that we simply ignore the moral sentiments of those who believe in the sanctity of human life from the earliest phase of fertilisation. My statement is about priorities.

It follows that human embryo research may be opposed or criticised by people who are not particularly worried about the status or fate of human embryos *per se*, but who are actively concerned about various possible risks to women posed by *in vitro* fertilisation and by the acquisition of research material from them. One might, for example, be in favour of abortion on demand but against human embryo research, in the belief that such stands will increase women's freedom. If one focused simply on the embryo, then this combination of views is rather paradoxical.

This then forces us to consider why, in the recent debates in Britain, and elsewhere, the questions have often been posed in terms of this 'over-individualised conception of the embryo'. What was it about the context that required or enabled this to happen? Whose interests did it serve? What political tensions led to issues being framed and ranked in this way?

This chapter is an attempt to explore the sociology of 'concern', about an area of the life sciences. By 'concern' I mean critical comment appearing in the mass media, made in terms which imply that popular sentiment exists on this issue.[2] It also endeavours to relate the administration of research to conflicts of political ideology at the national level. It draws on a growing literature on the 'new Right' in British politics, by arguing that, in this area at least, the influence exerted by this political formation has been more to change the terms of debate than to bring about new legislation. This in itself is, of course, significant. As I shall argue, in such a climate it has been difficult, though not impossible, to ask questions about the power relations implicit in new reproductive technologies.

The Emergence of Concern with Human Embryo Research in the 1980s

There is evidence that the use of human embryos for research purposes has become a preoccupation in general moral debate. For example, there was the symposium on human embryo research run by the Ciba Foundation in London in November 1985, the proceedings of which appeared in 1986 (Bock and O'Connor, 1986). The following year saw the organisation of four lectures on this topic to inaugurate a new Centre for Social Ethics and Policy in the University of Manchester. In addition, it is significant that the first issue of a new journal, *Bioethics*, carried two articles on this topic, one of them by Mary Warnock (Fleming, 1988; Warnock, 1987). These examples, of course, relate to academic discussion. Instances of press comment are mentioned below. These developments indicate particular pre-occupations in certain circles, but they only really show what few would deny, that this question has been under debate recently.

I want to claim more, that this issue has had increased visibility and perceived significance over the last few years. This can be illustrated with fairly crude data from the index to *The Times*, which classifies all news reports, features and correspondence in *The Times* and its three supplements. It appears monthly and is cumulated annually. In 1985, there were no entries at all under 'Embryos', 'Infertility', 'Fertilis-ation' or 'Ethics'. Nor did any of the hundreds of items under 'Science and technology' refer to embryo research or *in vitro* fertilis-ation. Instead, the heading which designates the relevant material is 'Birth and pregnancy'. In 1985, the entries under this heading took up a whole two-column page. Those under the sub-heading 'Re-search' virtually all related to human embryo research and to Enoch Powell's Private Member's Bill, to be considered below, which would have proscribed it. These entries alone occupied approximately ten column inches. By contrast, in 1984, whilst the total space devoted to 'Birth and pregnancy' was the same, the section on 'Research', again almost exclusively concerned with human embryo research, occupied four column inches. In 1983, it was two column inches, and in 1978, the year in which the first person conceived by *in vitro* fertilisation was born in Britain, there were no items indexed under this sub-heading, although yet again a page of entries related to 'Birth and pregnancy'.

The *British Humanities Index* lists articles appearing in a wide range of general periodicals, in some theology, philosophy and non-specialist law journals, and in the political weeklies. The listing gives complementary results. In 1985, there were sixteen items under 'Embryology', all of which related to human embryo research. These included two articles in *The Times*, one by the polemical journalist, Paul Johnson, and the other by Cardinal Basil Hume. In 1984, there was one such item, an article by James Le Fanu, 'Experiments that we do not need' in the *Daily Telegraph*, the gist of which later appeared in the *Lancet*. In 1983, there was no entry under 'Embry-ology'.

Now there are obvious problems with data generated like this. The column inch is a very imprecise unit and it would be foolish to use it as much more than a device for cross-checking impressions. How-ever, I would claim that in 1984 and 1985 the issue of human embryo research achieved a prominence in the press it had not had before, and that such attention resulted from a belief shared by journalists, editors and contributors that this was a new issue requiring serious comment.

More interesting is the finding that the topic of human embryo research dominated reports on *research* relating to birth and pregnancy in *The Times* and its supplements. This may be partly a distortion created by the indexing process, which can cause the clustering of some items under one convenient heading, to the exclusion of others, which have no obvious theme. But if this is so, it only supports my contention that human embryo research has been perceived as an important issue in its own right since 1984.

It is quite easy to construct a plausible account of how this issue came to receive such extensive attention. An invention (human *in vitro* fertilisation) was taken up initially in 1978 by a very few doctors, then, by the early 1980s, by rather more. This led, first, to debate within the institutions of the medical profession. As the questions became more complex and the technical achievements more intensively publicised, the British government established a committee of inquiry chaired by Mary Warnock in 1982. The appearance of its report in 1984 inevitably excited public interest, and criticism of its methods, assumptions and conclusions. This created an opportunity for an astute populist politician – Enoch Powell – with particular constituency and ideological interests, to seize the political initiative. His action in itself broadened the scope for public comment, both for and against *in vitro* fertilisation and its related research procedures. On this view there is nothing particularly remarkable, or indeed interesting, about an increase in reporting and analysis in 1984 and 1985. It reflects the media response to political conflict.

But, whilst this account outlines the temporal succession of activities, such a mechanistic version of events, as stimuli that lead to the next response, is a misleading and simplistic representation of the way political agendas develop and particular issues are brought within the scope of the institutions of parliamentary and party politics. For example it is not obvious from the above account why there should have been conflict or, indeed, commitment to particular positions. Why should what is ostensibly a rather esoteric technical consequence of a medical procedure have produced such sharp and varied disagreements?

My belief is that we cannot give a full account of this phenomenon without considering the new, more explicit reliance on morality within political rhetoric and the use of it in political mobilisation, primarily by groups and individuals on the Right in British politics, evident in the 1980s. This has emerged in attacks on liberal social legislation passed in the 1960s, such as that relating to abortion and sexuality, and in the re-emphasis on the importance of the nuclear family in welfare, legal and economic policy. What is interesting about the debates on all these issues is that they have exposed differences of approach, priority and ability to respond *within* organisations across the political spectrum. These differences have also been obvious around the issue of human embryo research.

My approach in trying to provide an account of events that 'failed to happen' will be through a series of negative questions. The first is to ask why concern about the use of human embryos as research material did not surface earlier. It leads one to ask why there was no government action on the moral questions raised by 'artificial reproduction' for so long. It might seem an odd question, depending on one's time-frame, but there is evidence that several governments were reluctant to act in this general area. This raises, in turn, the more specific questions as to why the Conservative government of 1983–7 did not act on more of the Warnock Committee recommendations after 1984; why several Private Members' Bills, including that from Enoch Powell in the 1984/5 session, have failed to reach the statute book; and why the present government is still moving slowly towards legislation.

Why did Concern not appear Earlier?

The question of why concern about research did not surface earlier can be addressed in four overlapping ways. These are the different foci of earlier critical comment, the rapid expansion of *in vitro* fertilisation from 1983, the general increase in attention given to involuntary infertility in the 1980s and the greater political and cultural influence of groups campaigning on particular moral issues in the 1980s.

Firstly, there was, in fact, some critical discussion of IVF as a research-based procedure before the 1980s. The achievement of human *in vitro* fertilisation was first claimed in 1944 by John Rock and Miriam Menkin in the United States, using ova obtained in a hysterectomy, which were not transferred back to the uterus (Rock and Menkin, 1944). Their published results were criticised in Boston, Massachusetts, where they were produced, and John Rock, himself a

Catholic, moved on to other projects, including his more controversial work on the oral contraceptive pill (McLouglin, 1982). No
claims to have repeated this now discredited achievement were
made, in Britain at least, until 1969. Then, Robert Edwards, a
physiologist at Cambridge University, Patrick Steptoe, a gynaecologist working in Oldham, and their colleague, Donald Bavister, announced the results of their work with ova removed from some of
Steptoe's patients in 1969 (Edwards *et al.*, 1969). They claimed that
some of the ova could be shown under the microscope to have passed
through the earliest phases of fertilisation, although some experts
disputed this interpretation.

This work was widely reported, as was the more striking claim, the
following year, to have facilitated the development of human embryos *in vitro* through several cell divisions, such that, within a
woman's body, they could have begun the process of implantation in
the lining of the uterus (Edwards *et al.*, 1970). This was harder to
dispute technically. The results provoked rather more moral criticism. However, Jon Turney's detailed analysis of the press coverage
of the research indicates that the main objections were that it made
possible embryo transfer and, thus, novel forms of surrogate motherhood, and that the handling of embryos *in vitro* might lead to serious
developmental abnormalities (Turney, 1978). The latter view was
taken by the Medical Research Council, which refused to fund the
research planned by Edwards and Steptoe (Edwards and Steptoe,
1980). But the separate, more metaphysical objection to using human
embryos as research material, because of their status as entities
within the human species, did not attract much attention in Britain at
this time.

Secondly, until the early 1980s, few people seem to have expected
that IVF would become widespread, or that, were this to happen, it
would do so very quickly. Until then, there was no public sign that
ancillary or unrelated research with human embryos would expand.
The success rates of the few groups working on IVF were extremely
low and the risks to the developing foetus unknown. Many doctors
took the view that it had no immediate future as a medical procedure.

By the 1980s, much has changed. The diffusion of the technique
has been very rapid, as physicians concerned with infertility have
overcome their earlier scepticism. For example, in 1983, Clifford
Grobstein, reviewing the results of attempts at *in vitro* fertilisation,
could only consider data from twelve different teams in seven countries
(Grobstein *et al.*, 1983). In Britain only one group had reported any

results at this time. In Australia there were published data from four hospitals. But, by 1985, a survey for the international congress on IVF in Helsinki revealed that 200 teams were offering IVF in twenty-five countries (Seppala *et al.*, 1985). Since the latter was not a count of published results, this may exaggerate the contrast, but the general pattern is still clear. Similarly, in 1986, Simon Fishel, a physiologist and sometime colleague of Robert Edwards, published data showing an enormous increase in the number of publications on IVF from around thirty in 1978 to over 300 in 1985 (Fishel, 1986). The source of these figures is not given. His figure for the number of clinics offering IVF in Britain alone is twenty-eight, whereas in 1978 it had been one. Edwards's own account of this change, made in a lecture in the series in Manchester mentioned above, is that there was 'an explosion of energy around the world'.

But even such an increase in scientific and medical activity is not in itself sufficient to explain the appearance of moral concern in the public media. The question of *research* with human embryos could have remained a relatively minor and esoteric one, as is research with foetal or placental tissue today. That it has not done so must depend on other contributory factors.

This brings me to the greater public attention given to infertility in the 1980s. It is not easy to document this from sources such as the *British Humanities Index* or the *Social Sciences Index*, because 'infertility' is used very sporadically as an indexing term and covers so many different kinds of report that it is far from obvious which subset of entries to use for comparison over time. But there are other indications. The number of people who are diagnosed as involuntarily infertile has been increasing since the 1960s, for reasons that are being debated by demographers. Moreover, the numbers seeking help have been increasing, at least in the USA (Aral and Cates, 1983). Recently attempts have been made to gather statistics on these trends, which at least suggests a greater professional interest (Mosher and Pratt, 1985; Hull *et al.*, 1985; Johnson *et al.*, 1987). Only one doctor specialising in this field has gone on record on several occasions criticising the kind of care and medical assistance that is generally available in Britain. It is also striking that the most systematic published attempt to survey the provision of infertility services has come from the Labour MP, Frank Dobson. This suggests a certain official lethargy and an active non-professional concern with what is considered to be a new medical problem (Mathieson, 1986).

Furthermore, voluntary and involuntary infertility has captured the attention of feminist writers. Naomi Pfeffer's and Anne Woolett's book *The Experience of Infertility*, was an early feminist exploration of the issue (1983). More recently, Lesley Doyal has written of a feminist strategy to allow the more open discussion of the needs of infertile women and of the development of campaigns by the women's movement touching these issues (Doyal, 1987; see also Berer, 1985). More articles and programmes of all kinds have been appearing in the mass media on the general topic of infertility in the last five years than was previously the case. Thus, people are now more likely to have a view about the relevance of new technologies to the allevi- ation of such problems, even if this has no connection with their personal experiences.

Given the sensational publicity that innovations in technique and the resulting births continue to receive, one could reasonably assume that many people believe that techniques like *in vitro* fertilisation will soon, appropriately or inappropriately, be in relatively common use. One might then expect that research with human embryos would also come to be seen as a likely consequence, but one which people view less favourably. This would be consistent with the findings of opinion surveys that have frequently shown that, whilst people tend to be very much in favour of medical innovations, they are much more likely to be opposed to the related medical or biological research (MORI, 1985). An assumption here is that IVF and embryo research are, in fact, linked in the popular imagination.

In reality, the evidence from opinion surveys suggests that the picture is more complicated. Even though interest in IVF as a procedure grew throughout the 1980s, the particular concern with human embryo research, indicated at the beginning of this chapter, seems to be a preoccupation of certain communities. Surveys of attitudes to human embryo research and other issues raised by innovations in reproductive technology suggest that a relatively small proportion of people are particularly concerned about this question. Elizabeth Alder and her colleagues found in March and April 1985 that, in three groups of women in Edinburgh, seeking medical or contraceptive assistance, and representative of the general popu- lation, 67 per cent approved of research on human embryos up to fourteen days after fertilisation in order to improve IVF treatment (Alder *et al.*, 1986). In a series of more detailed questions, the percentages of women strongly opposed to embryo research in differ- ent forms was generally around 5–8 per cent. Their reasons for holding these views were not explored in any detail.

One interpretation of this study is that, whilst it is a majority view that human embryo research is acceptable, if subject to some kind of regulation (which is what Alder and her colleagues seek to demonstrate), there are people none the less, who strongly dissent from this view and who are prepared to act on these views if given the opportunity. Thus, in 1985, the supporters of Enoch Powell's Unborn Children (Protection) Bill, which sought to ban human embryo research as part of a general mobilisation of sentiment against abortion and antenatal procedures which destroy the embryo or foetus, were able to gather two million signatures on a petition to Parliament. Lobbying on this scale requires considerable local and national organisation, which suggests that the activists involved believed that such sentiments could be mobilised and that it would be worthwhile to expend the effort in doing so. This raises the question of the political context within which people are motivated to act on particular questions.

This leads me to the fourth factor in accounting for the current preoccupation with embryo research – that is, the ideological cross-currents in British politics in the 1980s. One important development is indicated by the recurrent attempts by groups opposed to abortion to exploit new issues in reproductive medicine and to renew their campaign in a less liberal and pluralist political climate. Various commentators have written of a 'new' debate on abortion evident in recent years (Callahan, 1986; Paige and Karnofsky, 1986; Lovenduski and Outshoorn, 1986). More generally, one of the striking features of much neo-conservative moral rhetoric is its absolutism and unwillingness to compromise on questions of conscience (Zaner, 1984; Rayner, 1986). One would certainly expect such organisations to take up issues like human embryo research and that they would go beyond disapproval to active lobbying for its prohibition.

In fact, as will be shown below, not only those groups very specifically concerned with stopping legal abortion, but also other organisations and individuals within what has been called the 'moral Right' have taken up the issue. That is not to say that criticism has only come from conservatives or anti-progressives, since there has also been significant feminist criticism of human embryo research.

Which brings me to the principal question of this chapter: whether the particular salience of human embryo research as an issue has also arisen because of the influence of the loose coalition of traditionalist and neo-conservative groups on the Right in British politics. Is there evidence that such organisations have espoused this question and pressed for action on it? In so doing, have they provoked others to express views that otherwise would have remained unstated? Can one also argue that the terms of the debate have largely been set by sections of the so-called 'new Right'?

The New Role of Morality in British Politics

Miriam David has argued that one of the things that makes the New Right *new* is its reassociation of morality and politics: '. . . [T]he moral issues . . . are not new except insofar as they are what makes the political parties of the right the new, rather than the old right. They are new to the extent that they are explicitly on the agenda for some kind of policy resolution' (David, 1983, p. 31).

This is a characterisation of political parties, such as the Conservative Party in Britain under the influence of peripheral pressure groups and loosely associated centres of opinion within the party. Despite their organisational diffuseness, an important result has been a change in political and economic discourse, with a new stress on values, ideals and questions of morality. This is epitomised by the phrase 'a return to Victorian values', with its conscious allusion to different modes of self-reliance, respect for traditional authority, patriotism and sexual inequalities.

Linked with this important shift of rhetoric, but still a separate phenomenon, is the growing political influence accredited to organisations concerned with specific moral issues, such as the sale of pornography, the depiction of sex and violence in the mass media, the provision of contraception to girls under the age of sixteen, the role of the nuclear family and the legality of abortion. On these issues the links with the established political parties in Britain tend to be much looser: 'Although the moral right's adherents are likely to be Conservative supporters, this cannot be assumed. This British moral lobby is politically non-aligned and thus cannot unproblematically be defined as part of the new right, let alone of Thatcherism' (Bland, 1985, p. 21). Here the label the 'moral Right' is more appropriate, to denote separate non-party organisations, whose members wish fervently for a change in social standards and mores.

Tessa ten Tusscher has also argued that it is important to understand the changing position of women in the last twenty years, with more women drawn into the paid workforce, more women in trade unions, more women entering higher education and a greater degree of personal and sexual autonomy being possible for women. She indicates the threat that such changes represented to patriarchal social relations, as a crucial element in explaining the growth of the New Right:

It was this crisis of patriarchy which promoted the birth of the moral right. Both inside and outside the Conservative Party, lobbies, organizations and groups of 'concerned adults' were reacting against the tide of feminism. Mary Whitehouse and her National Viewers and Listeners Association . . ., the Festival of Light, elements within the National Association of Freedom and other middle-class associations and the organized church were recoiling with horror against the growth of the so-called permissive society and the sexual revolution. Working women were blamed for juvenile delinquency and the rising crime rate. The media capitalized on the theme of 'latch-key' children, social scientists bemoaned the breakdown of the family and predicted the concomitant breakdown of order and morality. The anti-abortion lobby started its campaign against 'a woman's right to choose' and launched a virulent defence of the 'Right to Life'.
(ten Tusscher, 1986, p. 75)

The particular conditions of economic crisis in the late 1970s provided an environment within which groups promoting such ideas enjoyed new political opportunities and renewed influence. None the less, in Britain, there is no coalition with the political profile of 'the Moral Majority' in the USA, where the concerted action of hitherto disparate single-issue and fundamentalist religious groups was a crucial factor in the election of a Republican president and in the removal of important liberal politicians from the US Congress (Wolfe 1981; Durham, 1985; Shapiro, 1985). Moreover, commentators like Rosalind Pollack Petchesky have argued that, in the USA, action against abortion was central to the general political programme of neo-conservative strategists, both in mobilising electoral support from a wider base and in breaking up the structure of welfare provisions created in the 1960s and 1970s. In the process, gains made by feminists in the United States over this period were deliberately and consciously eroded (Petchesky, 1986).

By contrast, analogous moral right organisations in Britain seem significantly weaker, their funding markedly less and their impact on the party in government less certain. But this is not to say that they have not been important in creating and influencing public debate, particularly on issues relating to the family, reproduction and sexuality. At the same time, their success in bringing about changes in legislation has been mixed.

Organisations of this general anti-liberal character have been very active in lobbying Parliament on the issues raised by the *Warnock Report* (South, 1985). The Welsh Labour MP, Leo Abse, has identified the Society for the Protection of the Unborn Child (SPUC), LIFE (also an organisation opposed to legal abortion), CARE (formerly known as the Festival of Light) and the Order of Christian Unity (OCU) as important in this respect (Abse, 1986). The OCU, for example, has produced two editions of its publication, *Test Tube Babies: A Christian View*, from a conference organised at the Royal Society of Medicine in May 1983. Amongst other contributions this features an article from the Catholic philosopher, Teresa Iglesias, which is an absolutist attack on human embryo research as a violation of a fundamental right to life that such entities are said to possess (Iglesias, 1985).

Other organisations, usually identified as part of the 'moral Right', such as the Responsible Society, presented documents to the Warnock Committee, although whether specific reference to embryo research was made in them is unclear. Similarly, a whole range of groups opposed to abortion are also listed in the *Warnock Report* as having offered their views. Whilst it is a reasonable supposition that these were hostile to embryo research, the political orientation of these organisations is not a foregone conclusion. Abse has indicated that SPUC was already critical of the Warnock exercise before its conclusions appeared, and was organising its supporters and sympathisers inside and outside Parliament during this period. He also states that the controversial nature of the Warnock Committee recommendations and the forthright way in which they were presented was a valuable opportunity for an organisation, 'that was in danger of becoming a lobby without a cause', from which otherwise sympathetic MPs had been distancing themselves (Abse, 1986, p. 211).

The 'moral Right' has been active in criticising the use of human embryos as research material. Arguably this has had the effect of focusing more attention on this issue than it would otherwise have had. Their concern with human embryo research as an issue, made public by the *Warnock Report* itself, provided a context within which new initiatives to question the legality of abortion could be conceived.

Perhaps the clearest illustration of this is the Private Members' Bill introduced to Parliament by Enoch Powell in December 1984. This proposed a complete ban on the use of human embryos for any research purposes and a registration system intended to ensure that all viable human embryos were re-implanted. It recognised that IVF should be used as a medical procedure to alleviate infertility, although the Bill was attacked as likely to create very severe constraints on the practice of IVF. Leo Abse has argued that the parliamentary debates on the *Warnock Report* in the autumn of 1984, first in the House of Lords, and then in the House of Commons, revealed the weakness of the forces broadly supporting its recommendations. What Abse calls 'the fundamentalist lobby' was then keen to act and awaited the results of the ballot for Private Members' Bills with interest, in the hope that one of the MPs gaining access to Parliamentary time could be persuaded to take up this issue:

> Enoch Powell . . . proved to their surprise to be the answer to their prayers: his considerable reputation as a Parliamentarian did not rest upon his contributions to past debates which had heralded in what is now pejoratively referred to as permissive legislation: nor had he hitherto publicly concerned himself with the rights of children, born or unborn. And indeed he had no history or formal association with the fundamentalist lobby: his religious views and political philosophy have a different flavour, permeated as they are by the Manichean fallacy, seeing the universe divided into good and evil. Warnock was seen by him as satanic, the dark side of the universal dualism. When announcing or defending his intention to stop effective embryo research he insisted that it was a 'gut reaction': he did not rest his statements on religious conviction or, as indeed he could not have, on rationality. Unashamedly he asserted his instincts demanded his action: . . . [At the same time]. . . To champion the anti-Warnock movement afforded him a singular opportunity to gain support both of his Catholic electorate and those stricken with Ulster's primitive brand of Presbyterianism. (Abse, 1986, p. 211)

Whilst Powell is not of the 'moral Right' in the sense of being close to evangelical or highly traditionalist single-issue organisations, his unusual political idiom is certainly moralising. His extreme nationalism is offered as grounded in a set of obscure but powerful intuitions. The stern warnings to the British nation and his increasingly barbed attacks on Tory policy have the quality of academic sermons from a populist preaching in the increasingly archaic language of an older cultural elite. However, the particular local advantages aside, one could hardly imagine he would be hostile to, or even wary of, the dogmatic crusading of the 'moral Right' groups. Their stance resembles precisely that kind of repudiation of liberality that he exploited and led so effectively earlier in his political career.

However, the opportunities that his calculated generosity opened up for the anti-abortion lobby produced, in turn, an opposing reaction from well-organised liberal pressure groups. This eventually stopped his Bill, in the Parliamentary maze through which Private Members' Bills must pass. This is Leo Abse's analysis of the relevant events in Parliament through 1985, which is described in more detail below. It is also consistent with other analyses of Private Members' legislation. Before discussing these developments, it is necessary to consider the attitudes of ministers and leading Conservative politicians on these questions from the early 1980s, since the lobbying just described was a response to what was seen as a lack of action on the part of the government. Moreover one factor in the demise of Powell's bill, as also in that of its successors, was the lack of government support. This leads to my second question: Why did the government not establish an inquiry, like that eventually chaired by Mary Warnock, sooner?

Why did the Government only establish a Committee of Inquiry in 1982?

The question used in the above heading is awkward in several respects. There is the question of time-frame. One could argue that four years, from the first birth after *in vitro* fertilisation in 1978 to the establishment of an official governmental inquiry in Britain, is not a long time. But one can also view the achievement of IVF in a longer perspective. In the USA, where *in vitro* fertilisation in general and human embryo research in particular were under an effective moratorium throughout the 1970s, official hearings were arranged in 1978 to generate a policy for the Department of Health, Education and Welfare (which would have been the major public sponsor of research in this field). The explanation for the disparity between the USA and Great Britain may lie in the 1973 decision by the American Supreme Court to change the law on abortion, which made the question of any research with foetal material extremely sensitive (Fletcher, 1985). This extended to any work with human embryos. Thus, in the aftermath of a very controversial legal decision, government departments had to anticipate possible criticisms from anti-abortion groups. In Britain, the corresponding change in abortion law occurred in 1967. Although the use of foetuses obtained from abortions soon became a controversial issue that was reviewed by a committee chaired by Sir John Peel in 1972, by the late 1970s no one felt it appropriate to link the new procedure of IVF with foetal research (Peel, 1972).

However, if one does take the longer view, then the inaction of several different governments in Britain has to be explained. Their reasons for not acting were probably different, although interrelated. It is hard to know what evidence can be used to produce a reliable answer, given that the available testimony is very sparse.

None the less in two respects it is an interesting question to consider. It prompts one to ask what actually catalysed the convening of Lady Warnock's Committee, given the diversity of issues which that body eventually addressed. Moreover, the reluctance of the present government to act even now, except in specific areas, is likely to stem from the same inhibiting political factors that operated, earlier in, and prior to, the 1980s. This would imply that judgements about the need to act or to be seen to act, balanced against the complications of changing the law, have not shifted much, despite the campaigning of the 'moral Right'.

One claim that the three recent governments, one Labour and two Conservative, have been slow to act comes from Leo Abse. His political reputation rests on his constituency activities and his bizarre style of dress. He has never found particular favour with the Labour leadership, or been prominent in mainstream Labour or trade union politics, having pursued somewhat idiosyncratic campaigns over the years, of which his controversial support of fathers' rights is the most recent. It is hard to resist the view that his observations about governmental hesitancy are, in fact, complaints that he has been overlooked. Nevertheless, his comments are corroborated by the remarks of Mary Warnock, cited below. His first request to a minister for some action was addressed to Shirley Williams in the early summer of 1978. He asked that the Genetic Manipulation Advisory Group (GMAG), as it was then called, be required to broaden its interests from a concern with the safety of laboratories and industrial workplaces where genetic engineering experiments were conducted, to consider *in vitro* fertilisation. Given the controversy over the establishment of this novel regulatory body, on which scientific trade unions, industrial management and scientists were represented, it is not at all surprising that his request was turned down, since such a shift of agenda would have called the *raison d'être* of the GMAG into question (Bennett *et al.*, 1986).

Abse continued to ask for some official inquiry for the next four years, without significant success:

As late as February 1982 the Prime Minister gave me a dusty procrastinat-

ing reply when I urged the formation of a comprehensive interdepartmen-
tal interdisciplinary committee. I pressed the demand again in an
adjournment debate in March 1982, and then for the first time the Government began to falter. Hesitatingly the Under-Secretary of State for Health
and Social Security admitted the need for some enquiry. (Abse, 1986,
p. 209)

While the initial request was made to the Department of Education
and Science, the initiative was eventually taken by the Department of
Health and Social Security, in collaboration with other departments.
What was framed initially as a question relating to medical research
policy was later taken up as a question of health and social policy, a
considerable broadening of focus. In the meantime, three separate
committees had been set up by non-governmental organisations, the
Medical Research Council, the British Medical Association and the
Royal College of Obstetricians and Gynaecologists. With no organised political lobby pressing for examination of *in vitro* fertilisation,
as the best known form of 'artificial reproduction' then in use, it is not
surprising that government ministers were in no hurry to act, at least
while 'expert' committees considered their views. But this is a rather
weak explanation, which to some extent begs the question of why
aspects of this research were not seen as requiring urgent resolution.

There are real dangers, both logical and empirical, in making
inferences about the genesis of the Warnock Committee from the
evidence of its ultimate recommendations. But two features of the
Report are very striking in this connection. Firstly, it covers a much
wider range of different policy areas than any of the non-
governmental reports. This is not to deny that the *Report* also
contains some remarkable silences and omissions, or to imply that all
the areas discussed are dealt with adequately. It is tempting to
speculate that the breadth and complexity of the issues that would
need to be covered had been recognised for some while, and that the
work of a government committee would be eased by waiting for the
more specialised recommendations that would emerge from pro-
fession-based working parties. One can interpret a comment by Mary
Warnock in this way:

> None of the members of the Inquiry had any doubt that they were
> concerned with moral issues. But we were not perhaps all of us certain how
> such issues ought to be approached, and especially how they should be
> approached by a body set up by Parliament to make recommendations
> which might lead to legislation. Many of our critics . . . have not really

addressed themselves to this problem either: the problem of legislation, and its relation to morality, in such controversial fields. (Warnock, 1985, p. viii)

Later in her annotations to the re-issued version of her Committee's *Report* she says:

> It is often said that committees are set up only when Parliament wants to postpone legislation, to give themselves a breathing space. For it is very disagreeable to have to legislate on a controversial non-party matter which has wide public effects and the longer it can be put off the better. There is much truth in this. No government can look forward to legislating on matters in regard to which they know in advance that many voters will be outraged whatever they do. They may well wish to put off the evil hour. Nevertheless, on a more charitable view, it can be argued that if they did not establish a committee, Ministers would have to seek advice only from their own civil servants . . . A committee of inquiry, on the other hand, though not exactly accountable to the public, is nevertheless far more open in its work, and a great deal less anonymous than the civil service. (Warnock, 1985, p. 98)

This implies that, by 1982, the steadily ramifying questions posed by the new reproductive technologies were viewed by the government of the day as requiring attention from a body that could claim to have consulted public opinion. Moreover, the likelihood of strong moral disagreement is explicitly addressed by the report. It offers a distinctive consensual moral framework intended to help the formulation of policies and legislation in areas where disagreement on fundamental moral issues can be expected. This approach and the firm tone in which it is presented was obviously largely Mary Warnock's contribution, since she has both elaborated upon and defended it in several publications (Warnock, 1985; Warnock, 1987). She feels that, in promoting such a framework, the Committee actually addressed its difficult political task, whatever the more ambitious expectations of its sponsors:

> Equally, there must often be disappointment on the part of Ministers, who, understandably enough, may hope for a solution to a problem essentially insoluble. In the case of our committee, for example, it was hoped, I now see, that the cool and reasonable voice of philosophy would reconcile the irreconcilable, and find a compromise where none can exist. There may even have been a secret belief that there is a right solution which could be proved right if it were only found. But Ministers, like the rest of humanity, have to realise that in matters of morality this is not

possible. Society may value things, genuinely and quite properly, which are incompatible with each other. (Warnock, 1985, p. 99)

The example used to make this point, both here and in many other places, is the possible conflict between the value accorded to advances in medicine such as *in vitro* fertilisation and the value to be attached to the notion of the sanctity of human life. The much criticised reformulation of utilitarianism in the report, that figures into the calculus of utility the social harm of offending others' moral sentiments, was an attempt to indicate both how such conflicts could and should be solved in a pluralist society.

One of the more astute comments on the *Warnock Report* has come from Rosalind Pollack Petchesky, in the foreword to the British edition of her book, *Abortion and Woman's Choice*. It deals specifically with the question of the way issues are framed:

> The Warnock Report may be read as an ideological document that lays down the terms of a neo-liberal, utilitarian 'fertility contract'. Anticipating the inevitable attacks from conservatives for its basic acceptance of 'artificial' methods of reproduction, the Report adopts an evenhanded tone and a 'balancing interests' approach. Yet embedded in this very approach are fundamental assumptions about morality and family that undercut feminist understandings with respect to reproductive decisions, the position of women and alternative household arrangements. In its very title, 'A Question of Life', the Report overdetermines the issue of whether or not or how human beings ought to 'bring life into the world' or 'destroy life' as the central moral issue in fertility control debates. Other ways of framing what constitute 'the moral issues' – for example, the distribution of responsibility for children after birth, the distribution of power over reproductive decisions, the conditions of informed consent, the health needs of women – are nowhere considered. In particular, the Warnock Committee immediately reduces the 'morally relevant' question in reproductive decision-making to 'how to regard embryos' or 'the value of human life'. (Petchesky, 1986, pp. xv–xvi)

A government reluctant to take a position on controversial issues was thus offered a politically subtle, if philosophically questionable, formula for compromise.

Why has there been so little Government Action and Legislative Change since 1984?

The *Warnock Report* was published in July 1984, after extensive leaking of some of its conclusions and of the fact that on some issues, particularly human embryo research and surrogacy, the Committee had been unable to reach unanimity. It endorsed the two main novel reproductive technologies it has reviewed, artificial insemination and *in vitro* fertilisation, and made a large number of recommendations. These can be divided roughly into four groups: those relating to the routine practice of artificial insemination and *in vitro* fertilisation, to be overseen by a newly constituted Licensing Authority; those relating specifically to the use of human embryos, involving either immediate or delayed transfer to a woman's body or some research procedure; those relating to the law of legitimacy; and those relating to surrogacy.

On the last three there has been some action in Parliament since 1984, although in one case, that concerning human embryos, the government was not actively involved. A series of Private Members' Bills, of which Enoch Powell's was the most significant, have sought to prohibit research with human embryos and to introduce controls on the practice of *in vitro* fertilisation. These have not had government support in terms of Parliamentary time or significant ministerial endorsement.

On the other hand, Parliament has begun debating proposed government legislation to revise the law of legitimacy, stemming from the work of the Law Commission prior to the sitting of the Warnock Committee (Law Commission, 1982). And in 1985 the government adopted and modified a Private Member's Bill on commercial surrogacy, in a climate of 'moral panic' following several well-publicised surrogacy contracts in Britain. These included the contract arranged by an American businesswoman, Harriet Blankfeld, between Kim Cotton and an unnamed foreign couple. Kim Cotton's account of this arrangement, including the transfer of a baby in January 1985 to the commissioning couple, has been published as a book (Cotton, 1986). Both she and Harriet Blankfeld faced repeated vigorous criticism of their actions, whilst little attention was paid to the other adults involved. The passage of a Bill through Parliament in 1985 that sought to ban such activity was very rapid, despite some comment that the legislation ignored many psychological and moral subtleties involved (Morgan, 1985; Morgan, 1986; Payne, 1987; Zipper and Sevenhuijsen, 1987).

More strikingly, the government chose not to act on several occasions, despite evidence of strong concern in Parliament, in the area of human embryo research. The failure of Private Members' initiatives in this area is considered below. In the autumn of 1987, a White

Paper was published that offered alternative legislative proposals, one of which would ban such research and one of which would implement the Warnock Committee proposal of controlled experimentation up to a limit of fourteen days after fertilisation. The government has said that this issue will be treated as a 'non-party' question, allowing MPs to choose their preferred option. Debate began on these proposals in January 1988. The Earl of Lauderdale's comments cited above are from the debate in the House of Lords. More recently, the Duke of Norfolk's re-introduction of Enoch Powell's Bill to the House of Lords failed in April 1989. Further parliamentary debate on the proposed government legislation is expected in future sessions.

In 1985, a Voluntary (as opposed to statutory) Licensing Authority (VLA) was set up by the Medical Research Council and the Royal College of Obstetricians and Gynaecologists to regulate such human embryo research (see Price and Steinberg in this volume). It has already produced three reports. Its creation was clearly a prudential measure, intended to safeguard a controversial area of science by indicating that it was subject to some control. As Robert Edwards has recently pointed out, this is somewhat ironic, given the antipathy to *in vitro* fertilisation by the Medical Research Council in 1978, when he and his collaborator sought funds from them to continue their work (Edwards and Steptoe, 1980). Moreover, the limits of the power possessed by a voluntary body were clearly revealed in 1987, when a doctor specialising in IVF, Ian Craft, made it clear that he would continue his practice of selectively destroying foetuses *in utero*, after transferring as many embryos as possible to women in his IVF programme. This was despite strong criticism of this policy from the VLA, from other doctors involved with IVF, and from a range of public commentators (Craft, 1987). His stand came to appear even more intransigent and insensitive, both politically and emotionally, in the light of the highly publicised brief survival in the summer of 1987 of sextuplets, born to a woman in Liverpool, who had been given a fertility drug known to make multiple pregnancies likely.

The major political event linked to human embryo research in Britain has already been mentioned, namely the Bill introduced in Parliament by Enoch Powell in December 1984 and debated the following year. Since it did not receive government support, it is not surprising that it failed to reach the statute book, although it was said to command significant support outside Parliament. Its failure again points to the tension between different moral ideologies in British culture, which is a theme of this chapter.

The genesis of the principal Bill proposing to ban embryo research has already been described. It is important to remember that anti-abortion organisations, including the Society for the Protection of the Unborn Child, worked hard to mobilise support at the constituency and (parish level, once Enoch Powell's Unborn Children (Protection) Bill had been introduced to Parliament. But, Leo Abse has claimed, only when it attracted significant support, mainly from the Conservative backbenches, at its second reading did its opponents organise a serious response. The real prospect that it might become law within 1985 provoked some scientists, doctors, and MPs with a longstanding interest in abortion and reproductive rights to greater activity. Eventually this Bill, like most Private Members' Bills, was defeated by being talked out.

David Marsh and his colleagues have analysed the fate of Private Members' Bills over the last thirty years (Marsh *et al.*, 1986; Marsh *et al.*, 1987). Their conclusions suggest, firstly, that the chances of success without government support are extremely low, because the relevant rules of procedure allow even minimal objection to stop the bill. Secondly, they indicate that such unsupported initiatives can succeed none the less in circumstances where an atmosphere of 'moral panic' makes objection politically impossible. Thus, for example, Winston Churchill's attempt to extend the scope of the Obscene Publications Act in 1985 failed because it was opposed by important sections of the media. On the other hand, the Video Recordings Bill in the preceding year was passed into legislation, Marsh *et al.* argue, because of the moral panic created by the National Viewers and Listeners Association and the absence of a lobby with any political influence, able to mobilise opposition within Parliament. They argue generally that pornography is an area where there are no well-established liberal interest groups that can block well-drafted, narrowly focused legislation. Abortion-related issues, such as human embryo research, on the other hand, are different:

> The pro-abortion lobby is a skilled and knowledgeable one, and was well aware that if the [Powell] bill was passed it would provide a basis for an inevitable attack on the 1967 Abortion Act. For this reason a write-in campaign was organised which went some small way to counteracting the letters from the Powell supporters. (Marsh *et al.*, 1986, p. 195)

The implication is that, whereas in the case of surrogacy, legislation was passed through Parliament very rapidly because of an atmosphere of moral panic, this did not work with human embryo research, despite the efforts of a section of the 'moral Right' to present the need for a ban in similar terms. The effects of this failure by the anti-abortion lobby are likely to be twofold: firstly, any new attempts to get Parliament to prohibit research will fail, because sentiment against such controls is now organised; and, secondly, it would be difficult for a Conservative government to propose its own legislation, because this would only open up divisions amongst its own supporters. Indeed, the government has deliberately avoided taking a position on this issue by offering MPs a choice. Much may depend on the outcome of the debates generated in the wake of David Alton's unsuccessful attempt in 1988 to amend the 1967 Abortion Act. That initiative dominated the foreground of political debate about reproductive rights in Britain in a way that highlighted the fact that human embryo research is, in many ways, a side issue.

It remains to be seen whether the effective stalemate on the issues defined by the Warnock Committee as central to any moral or legislative response to reproductive technology will be affected by the ending of another round of conflict on abortion law reform. From 1984 to 1986 the desire of more liberally minded Conservative ministers, like Kenneth Clarke, who was then, and is again now, the Minister of Health, to act on the *Warnock Report*, was blocked by disquiet from colleagues much more sympathetic to the extreme demands of the 'moral Right'. At the same time, the possibility of highly restrictive legislation was also stopped by the solidity of liberal opinion within Parliament, which stood behind what Rosalind Pollack Petchesky has called the 'new utilitarian fertility contract' that guarantees to some women limited access to new forms of reproduction in return for acceptance of patriarchal moral norms (Petchesky, 1986). Whether the defeat of David Alton's Private Member's Bill in the 1987–8 session of Parliament will strengthen the hand of those who want legislation to regulate human embryo research, or whether this position will be the focus of displaced moral anger about abortion, remains to be seen. The recent use of foetal brain tissue obtained at abortion in experimental transplant operations intended to cure Parkinson's disease has lead to controversy and may lead to the banning of such use of foetal material. The use of foetal tissue is currently (May 1989) being reviewed by the Polkinghorne Committee.

Conclusion

This chapter is written from a conviction that research with human embryos is not *self-evidently* an issue of fundamental moral import-

ance, and certainly not the most important issue raised by reproductive technologies. In my view, the feelings and interests of women
involved in one way or another with such technologies should define
the central area of debate.

Yet some people clearly find embryos the primary concern. This
may be because of their view of the value of entities within the human
species, which derives from a particular world-view. Or they may
accept this focus on moral issues because they are provoked by others
to debate this question. This has had the effect of giving the whole
area of research with human embryos a particular salience in the
mass media since 1984. The emphasis has been on the supposed
rights that embryos do or do not possess, or on their value as 'life'. As
I have suggested, the framing and ordering of debate in this way is
not inevitable. It requires explanation. In approaching this task I
have explored a series of negative questions.

When one asks why this area did not surface earlier, given that in
some form such research has been going on since the 1940s, several
answers suggest themselves. It is possible that, until the full scale of
in vitro fertilisation became generally apparent, very few people took
any notice. On the other hand, those commentators who did discuss
this research rarely emphasised the question of the sanctity of embryonic life. They were more likely to raise the different but related
question of whether the handling of embryos in medical rather than
research procedures would cause unpredictable damage.

If one asks why such issues were not the concern of a government
inquiry in Britain at an earlier stage, a plausible answer seems to be
that the balance of political advantage lay in not tackling these
non-party issues, at least until the activity of professional bodies
made possible a more authoritative and general investigation. More
research is needed here to substantiate these claims. The testimony
of one idiosyncratic parliamentary crusader and the discreet retrospective comments of Mary Warnock are not quite enough. Since I
have argued that the activities of organisations now referred to as the
'moral Right' were generally important in drawing attention to the
moral implications of new modes of reproduction, and in shaping the
terms of the continuing debate, it would be important to know
whether these also catalysed the formation of a government working
party on these questions.

Certainly once the Warnock Inquiry was announced in July 1982,
groups from the 'moral Right', began to stress their view of the
sanctity of human life in embryonic form. This led some liberal

philosophers, Warnock among them, to challenge their use of language and their moral framework. It also led to the modification of utilitarianism in the *Warnock Report*, in an attempt to take account of the harm caused by an affront to some moral sentiments. This is a philosophy of compromise and political accommodation.

One of the key questions that has been raised here is why those groups pressing for a ban on human embryo research have failed thus far, albeit only narrowly. To say that their view is very much a minority one in Britain may be true, as Alder *et al.* (1986) have demonstrated. But the evidence available to MPs during their debates would have suggested something different – that some of their constituents were strongly opposed to such research, and that these views formed part of an ideological framework that re-emphasised the connections between morality and politics. In such a context, one might expect apparently small minorities to exert a large influence.

Enoch Powell's Bill is a case in point. It failed because of the way in which its opponents were able to use the rules of parliamentary procedure against it. To say that Private Members' Bills very rarely succeed without government support is also true, but this only shifts the question to be explained to the lack of government support. It suggests that, on some abortion-related issues, the present Conservative leadership accepts that they cannot endorse all the demands of the 'moral Right'. This seems to have been the case with David Alton's proposed amendment to the Abortion Act. In other areas, such as the debate over obscenity, they see things differently. The present situation is one of political stalemate over an issue that is, in large part, a proxy for debates about abortion. In late 1987 and early 1988 the terms on which abortions can be performed – the substantive rather than the proxy question – came to command much more attention.

Unless a ban is imposed, the use of human embryos for a variety of research purposes will expand. One source will be *in vitro* fertilisation programmes. A Licensing Authority could probably ensure that women gave informed consent to the use of embryos for research, but this kind of regulation leaves untouched the kind of indebtedness that people feel in such situations. Another source of embryos could be ova taken from women having hysterectomies. There are already indications that women agreeing to be superovulated and to act as ovum donors prior to sterilisation have their operations sooner than they would otherwise have done. In fact this is the deal they are often offered. This clearly violates the ideal of freely given consent, which is held to apply in medicine (see Price in this volume). However, it is not clear how such informal arrangements could be controlled. Examples like these suggest that focusing on the moral status of the human embryo *per se* – using an 'over-individualised conception of the embryo' – distracts attention from the more important questions of medical power and women's rights posed by reproductive technologies like *in vitro* fertilisation. This chapter constitutes an argument for attempting to analyse the political context within which research policy is made and implemented. Such analysis is a prerequisite for understanding how moral discourse is constructed and put to work, and what it achieves. It is also a prerequisite for being able to change it.

Notes

1. I have to acknowledge an intellectual debt to Rosalind Pollack Petchesky. In her article on the imagery of the foetus in anti-abortion literature, she writes of foeto-centric notions and representation, which suggest that the foetus is an independent entity, whereas biologically it is highly dependent upon and physically located within the body of a woman (Petchesky, 1987). Thus, the production of such an image photographically is very contrived and, in a serious sense, misleading. What I have to say concerning ideas about embryos is very similar.
2. For a more extensive discussion of the different meanings of 'public concern', see Yoxen, 1988.

8 Deconstructing 'Desperateness': The Social Construction of Infertility in Popular Representations of New Reproductive Technologies

Sarah Franklin

Introduction

NEW HOPE FOR THE CHILDLESS, COMFORT FOR THE CHILDLESS, JOY FOR
BABY HOPE COUPLES, CHILDLESS COUPLES GIVEN HOPE, INFERTILE COUPLES
GET HOPE FROM NEW METHOD, MOTHER'S JOY OVER 1000th TEST-TUBE BABY,
TEST-TUBE BOY FOR THRILLED PARENTS, TEST-TUBE TRIPLETS A CITY FIRST
FOR 'ECSTATIC' PARENTS.[1]

These are the headlines of a now familiar story of infertility and its
'treatment' via new reproductive technologies. The typical description of the infertile is one that emphasises their 'desperation', 'anguish'
and 'suffering' and refers to them as the 'victims of childlessness',
'unwillingly childless', 'involuntarily childless' or as the 'sufferers of
infertility'. Juxtaposed against these tales of 'desperateness' are the
stories of the 'happy couples' who have won their battle against
childlessness by producing a 'miracle baby' with the help of modern
medical science. Together, these two sets of stories, of happiness and
hopelessness, constitute the major frame of reference for discussions
of infertility.

In the decade since the birth of Louise Brown, 'test-tube baby'
clinics have been established in many parts of Britain, and *in vitro*
fertilisation has become widely practised in this country and abroad.[2]
Research into embryology and reproduction have both expanded

and become highly profitable medical and scientific specialities. Consequently, infertility and new reproductive technologies have become the subject of considerable media attention and public debate, culminating in Britain in proposed legislation currently before Parliament.[3]

Popular representations of infertility and its 'treatment' via new reproductive technologies have become regular media features, responding to the considerable public fascination with the unprecedented procreative arrangements made possible by these new techniques. These representations are an important public source of both formal knowledge and commonsense understandings of the experience of infertility and the rapidly expanding field of 'test-tube baby' science. Indeed, for many people, they are the *only* source of information. As such, they have considerable influence upon public opinion and parliamentary debate concerning the important issues of reproductive control which have emerged as a result of recent techno-scientific innovations.

What is at stake within current debates is no less than the redefinition of parenthood and procreation, of motherhood and fatherhood, of kinship and the family. This process of redefinition is taking place at many levels, from everyday assumptions about 'the facts of life' to medical, legal and religious constructions of human reproduction and parenting. Reproduction is becoming a commercial activity at the centre of a new market-place, in which reproductive services, such as surrogacy, can command a fee and reproductive tissues, such as eggs, sperm and embryos, are exchanged as commodities. New reproductive technologies have removed procreation from the protected realm of the private and the symbolic domain of the 'natural' and relocated it within the scientist's laboratory.

Central to this process of redefinition is the question of the extent to which both the products and the processes of procreation will become subject to state and legal control. Clearly this question will have substantial implications for women's reproductive rights, especially in a political climate marked by the rise of New Right moral conservatism (see Arditti, Klein and Minden, 1984b; Corea, 1984; Corea, 1985; Stanworth, 1987c; Spallone and Steinberg, 1987; Spallone, 1989). It is therefore disturbing to find that the question of women's reproductive rights is a consistent absence within both public and parliamentary debates about new reproductive technologies. Neither is there mention of women's reproductive rights within popular representations of infertility and new reproductive technologies, except in the feminist press. In fact the only mention made of women's interests is in terms of the putative *benefits* offered by these new technologies, their supposed *enhancement* of the reproductive choice and control they offer women, and the *new options* they are said to create for women who would 'otherwise remain childless'.

In this chapter I shall attempt to demonstrate how popular representations of infertility contribute to the formation and widespread acceptance of this now common myth of the benevolence of new reproductive technologies. The subject of this chapter is not only the exclusion of the issue of women's reproductive rights, but its *preclusion* by the very terms through which these debates are conducted.[4] In particular, it is the role of popular representations in the production of public knowledge about infertility and new reproductive technologies which is at stake here.

Methodology

Within cultural studies,[5] the influence of popular culture in the formation of public debates about sexuality, reproduction and the family is a subject which has received considerable attention. Of the many recent approaches to this subject, those which analyse narrative and discourse are two of the most widely used. Both emphasise the 'constructedness' of popular culture, and the extent to which it is both determining of, and determined by, prevailing social practices and beliefs. Both also stress the importance of understanding popular culture in terms of the social forces which inform its production and its consumption. In particular, these approaches have been helpful in demonstrating how social practices which are represented as 'natural' or as 'biologically determined' are, in fact, socially constructed.

In the first section of this chapter, extracts from a variety of sources are used to demonstrate the narrative construction of popular representations of infertility. Drawing upon a range of popular sources, including articles from the local and national press, infertility guidebooks and government documents, the social construction of infertility is analysed using approaches developed within cultural studies. Central to this analysis are questions of how descriptions of infertility and reproductive technology are constructed as stories, as linear progressions of events over time, structured by the emergence of a conflict or obstacle, and the subsequent need to provide a resolution. In the second section, the discursive construction of these accounts is the subject of discussion. Returning to the examples presented in the first section, suggestions are made about the ways in which these same accounts can be seen to operate discursively to produce a regime of medical and scientific 'truth' about the infertile body. Whilst the emphasis in both sections is upon the production of ideas in accordance with dominant social practices and beliefs, there are also many *discordances* evident within the examples discussed. Indeed, I have argued that one of the most important features of the accounts, both discursively and as narratives, is the way in which they *attempt* to mediate the tensions and contradictions posed by 'artificial conception'. The question of how these representations mediate certain salient contradictions, and the question of what these accounts obscure, are explored further in the conclusion.

The Desperate Infertile Couple Stories

The opening passage of a recent feature in *The Times* is typical of many media representations of the new reproductive technologies as treatments for infertility:

> The bright clusters of snapshots pinned to the memo board in a London clinic are a constant reminder that at least some dreams come true. Every picture of a new-born baby tells its own story of a successful fight against infertility.
> More than anything else in her life, Tessa Horton wants to add to that collection. But she is 38 now and after five years of disappointment, she knows the odds are against her.
> Neither she nor her husband Michael will surrender their dream while the doctors continue to offer them even a slender hope . . .
> For the Hortons, and an estimated one million other couples in Britain striving to overcome childlessness, doctors can resort to a remarkable and increasing number of treatments.
> Advances in the use of drugs, surgical techniques and *in vitro* fertilization mean that babies are now being born to couples who until quite recently would have been described as hopeless cases. (Prentice, 1986b, p. 10)

This story contains all of the standard components of the desperate infertile couple stories. The plot is structured around the tension between the desperate desire for a child and the biological inability to produce one. It is both an adventure story and a romance, in which a successful fight 'against the odds' may end in 'a dream come true'. It is an epic story of medical heroism in the face of human suffering and the forward march of scientific progress. It is a story of winners and losers, of happy endings for some and hopelessness for others. It is, in fact, many stories condensed into one, an over-determined story with several familiar themes. Most importantly, however, it is a story about 'desperateness'.

The representation of infertility in terms of desperateness is a subject which has been commented upon by other researchers (Pfeffer and Woollett, 1983; Pfeffer, 1987). Naomi Pfeffer has written extensively on the subject of the stigma that is attached to infertility as a result of representations such as this. She writes:

> Besides their involuntary childlessness there is one characteristic which the infertile are said to share, that of desperation. The word desperation or some such synonym appears so frequently in conjunction with infertility that sometimes it appears that what troubles infertile men and women is not the absence of a child as such but some form of emotional disorder related to their failure. Desperation combined with infertility appears to produce a particularly potent mix; one that forces fecund women to lease their womb, sends infertile men and women scouring the world for orphans to adopt and incites some doctors into developing new techniques that subject people to many indignities. (Pfeffer, 1987, p. 82)

Pfeffer's argument is that the highlighting of desperateness not only stigmatises the infertile but obscures the broader social context in which it must be understood. Moreover, she maintains, not all infertile couples are necessarily 'desperate' for children. To the contrary, she points out, there are, for many people, clear advantages to remaining 'child-free'.

Despite the fact that 'desperateness' need not necessarily result from infertility, it is consistently the primary frame of reference within popular representations of infertility. Pfeffer is concerned with the way this representation effects the infertile. However, the question here is how the focus on desperation affects the formation of public opinion and debate over reproductive technologies. Almost invariably, these stories revolve around two central questions: 'Why are they desperate?' and 'What are they desperate for?'. As a result, these representations proceed first in terms of *how the desperateness is accounted for*, and second, *how it can be resolved*. It is the need to account for the desperateness, and then to resolve it, which provides the central conflict structuring the narrative movement in these accounts.

Accounting for 'Desperateness': the Social Pressures to Conform

The accounting for, and the resolution of, desperateness are commonly presented through two explanatory systems: the social and the biological. These two systems work together in ways that are both complementary and contradictory. In the first part of this chapter, social and biological explanations drawn from popular texts are presented separately. Their relationship to one another is discussed later in the chapter.

Social pressures to conform to the conventional roles of adulthood are one of the most frequently encountered explanations for the emotional stress suffered by the infertile and their desperation to produce a child. According to such accounts, the stress of infertility derives from the sense of social failure or emotional loss it may cause an individual or couple. The inability to produce a biologically related child is represented in terms of a sense of exclusion, a lack of self-esteem or a loss of identity. In the article from *The Times* cited above, expert testimony from a psychiatrist is provided to explain this loss: 'They face not only the loss of self as the kind of person they would have become, but the loss of the imaginary family, and with it the kind of life they would have led' (Prentice, 1986a, p. 13).

The *Warnock Report*, the report of the government committee appointed in 1982 to investigate infertility 'treatments' in Britain, also refers to the loss of social identity and the sense of personal failure that may result from infertility: 'Childlessness can be a source of stress even to those who have deliberately chosen it . . . They may feel that they will be unable to fulfil their own or other people's expectations. They may feel excluded from a whole range of human activity and particularly the activities of their child-rearing contemporaries' (Warnock, 1985, p. 9).

These and many other examples demonstrate that the need for social approval is one of the major causes of the desperateness said to characterise the infertile within popular representations of infertility. It is their desperateness for social approval and their biological inability to achieve it which provides the central conflict within these representations.

In *Getting Pregnant in the 1980's*, a popular guide to *New Advances in Infertility Treatment and Sex Pre-Selection*, the authors, a doctor and a scientist, write:

For most individuals, life moves in a progression that is highlighted by the

> events of marriage and childbirth. When this progression is interrupted by infertility, it produces an effect beyond just the physical absence of a child. A couple may, for the first time, feel they have lost control over a significant part of their lives. Their own anxieties about infertility may be magnified by well-meaning, but unthinking, relatives and friends who continually ask about the prospects for pregnancy. (Glass and Ericsson, 1982, p. 11)

It is because 'life moves in a progression' that infertility poses an obstacle to happiness. It is the disruption of the normal progression in the lives of 'most individuals' which causes them to 'feel they have lost control' and to suffer from 'anxieties' about their infertility. In *New Conceptions: A Consumer's Guide to the Newest Infertility Treatments*, author Lori Andrews makes the same point, quoting from a psychiatric expert who claims that 'No one enters a marriage expecting to hear that they are infertile' (Andrews, 1984, p. 86). Socially and emotionally, the stress of childlessness is attributed to failure to fulfil conventional adult roles and to 'found a family'. The cause of desperateness, in other words, is an inability to conform to social norms.

However, the suggestion in these accounts of an inevitable trajectory from marriage to childbirth, in which infertility can only be understood as an obstacle to happiness, is both simplistic and reductive. For whom is childlessness unacceptable? Under what conditions? For whom is adoption problematic? Must infertility continually be reduced to desperateness? Because the narrative sequence of events begins with a desperate infertile couple, who already desire to conform to the traditional biological family, the inevitability of life's 'progression' along only one trajectory which ends in childbirth is repeatedly reinforced. As a result, alternative child-rearing practices are obscured. Couples or individuals not 'desperate' to conform, such as those who remain childless voluntarily, those who adopt, lesbian and gay parents, or others who parent children non-traditionally do not fit into the desperate infertile couple story, and are therefore not represented.

In sum, the narrative representation of the social pressures upon the desperate infertile couple offers only certain very specific positions to the reader. The reader is positioned so as to identify with the 'desperate desire' for conformity to the traditional nuclear family, for conventional social approval, and for biologically-related children. The experience of infertility does not, however, reduce to this. And the desire for a family or for children may be quite a different thing from the experience of actually having them. Thus the narrative representation of the desperate infertile couple limits the kinds of questions which might be asked to only one: how can a pregnancy be achieved?

'Natural' Pressures: The In-built Drive to Reproduce

In addition to social pressures, many popular representations of infertility also draw on the idea that there are natural, even biological, pressures to have children which cannot be suppressed. Thus, the desire to have a family is not only represented as a desire to conform to social expectations but as a natural or biological desire independent of a social context. The opening paragraph of *The Fertility Handbook*, a recently published, popular guide to infertility 'treatment' written by a doctor and a science journalist, reproduces this view precisely: 'Call it a cosmic spark or spiritual fulfilment, biological need or human destiny – the desire for a family rises unbidden from our genetic souls. In centuries past, to multiply was to prevail – the family was stronger, and better able to survive, than the individual' (Bellina and Wilson, 1986, p. xv). The conflation of the language of evolutionary genetics with the language of spiritual desire and personal fulfilment in this passage (for example, 'genetic souls') is revealing. It suggests that the desire to have a family is not merely social but also biological, genetically determined by our evolutionary heritage and essential to our survival both as individuals and as a species. This view is reiterated in the introduction to *The New Fertility*, another popular guide to infertility treatment, written by Dr Graham Barker. In the introduction, Barker describes the desire for parenthood as 'the natural product of pair bonding' and explains that 'the desire to produce children is deeply rooted in biological instinct . . . and a natural expression of love' (Barker, 1986, p. 9). Another example of this view is expressed by Lois Davitz, author of *Baby Hunger*: 'Baby hunger is powerful, defying all laws of logic. The drive to have a baby unleashes a whole range of obsessive emotions a woman may never have had to face. When a woman has baby hunger, nothing else is as important to her as this inner drive to bear a child' (Davitz, 1984, p. 1).

These views are also publicly expressed by 'test-tube baby' doctors such as the late Patrick Steptoe (who wrote the foreword to Barker's book). At a conference in Oxford in February 1987, Steptoe publicly stated that 'it is a fact that there is a biological drive to reproduce'.

He went on to claim that 'women who deny this drive, or in whom it is frustrated, show disturbances in other ways' (quoted in Stanworth, 1987a, p. 15). In each of these accounts, the existence of an instinctive biological urge to reproduce, which is independent of the social context, is presented as an explanation for the 'desperate' desires of the infertile to procreate successfully.

This view is not limited to popular representations of infertility or individual members of the medical profession. The Warnock Committee expressed a similar view in its report, stating explicitly that: 'In addition to social pressures to have children there is, for many, a powerful urge to perpetuate their genes through a new generation. This desire cannot be assuaged by adoption' (Warnock, 1985, p. 9). In this account, as in others, the argument that a sense of desperateness results from biological urges which cannot be suppressed is used to complement the argument that this desperateness is the result of social pressures. Indeed, these two arguments are used to reinforce one another and are obviously understood as complementary explanations for the desperate desire to reproduce biologically that couples feel. Not only are they desperate for social approval, these accounts suggest, but it is 'natural' they should feel a powerful urge to reproduce because it is a 'biological' drive.

However, if the drive to reproduce is biological, then everyone shares it, whereas, if it is a product of social expectations, then only people who desire to conform to convention will be 'desperate' to reproduce. In other words, although the social and the biological explanations are used in these accounts as if they complement one another, their premises may be contradictory. Patrick Steptoe, for example, simultaneously believed that all women have a biological drive to reproduce, and that it is immoral for lesbians or single women to have children. Thus, for socially acceptable women, biology should be destiny, whereas for socially unacceptable women, the demands of biology should be restricted by social sanctions.

This shifting use of social and biological explanations of reproductive 'drives' reveals how contradictory explanations can be adapted to the dictates of particular moral and political beliefs. Indeed these contradictions are necessary for this sort of moral argument. The same is true of many representations of sexuality, in which the relationship of heterosexuality to reproduction is depicted as 'natural' or as socially and morally determined, depending upon the circumstance. In the case of infertility, life is said to move in an inevitable progression, dictated by the forces of both social convention and biological urgency, for some but not for others.

Thus, in answering the question 'why are they desperate?', the desperate infertile couple stories provide two explanations. They are desperate because of social pressures to conform, and they are desperate because of biological pressures to reproduce. However these claims are used selectively, so as to produce explanations of the experience of infertility which reinforce social norms. Through familiar narrative mechanisms the contradictions between the social and biological explanations are obscured, and they are held together as mutually reinforcing explanations of the 'desperateness' of infertility. Examples which might suggest alternatives to existing social norms are excluded from these stories, indeed are precluded by the structural requirements of the narrative.

Resolution 1: Medical Experts and Scientific Progress

In addition to providing explanations of the cause of 'desperateness', it is also necessary within popular representations of infertility to provide resolutions to this dilemma. This too is accomplished through familiar narrative mechanisms. Moreover, like the narrative construction of the causes of infertility, narrative resolutions of the dilemma of infertility contain it forcefully within existing social institutions and practices.

One of the most important features of the desperate infertile couple stories is the way in which they directly link the 'desperate' desire for a child with the hope for a medical 'cure'. Physically there is only one possible resolution to the desperate infertile couple story, and that is a medical cure. The narrative movement from cause to effect here again obscures alternative options. Infertility having been constructed as a biological problem, there is no alternative to a biological resolution. In these stories it is the recently acquired capability of medical science to provide a child for infertile couples which provides *the only hope of resolution*. As a result, the difference between happiness and hopelessness rests entirely in the hands of medical experts. In the *The Times* article quoted above we read that: '*Their only hope* lies with the gynaecologists, andrologists, urologists, endocrinologists and others who specialise in treating infertility, including the growing number of experts in *in vitro* fertilisation – the so-called "test-tube baby" doctors' (Prentice, 1986b, p. 10, my emphasis). Thus within and framed by this tragic narrative of the desperate infertile couple is a catalogue of the latest discoveries of medical scientists in the laboratory. In the language of advancements, achievements and progress, we read descriptions of medical scientists who are striving to alleviate the condition of infertility. In the *The Times* article, we are informed that:

> [S]ome surgeons are now applying lasers to tubal surgery. Mr Simon Wood, a consultant gynaecologist at the Royal Devon and Exeter Hospital, has achieved a 33 per cent live birth rate in a small number of patients using a laser . . .
> Last November, Australian scientists announced they were the first team to successfully freeze and thaw human ova . . .
> Professor David Baird is trying to develop tests to identify which fertilized human eggs are healthy, and which are abnormal. They hope to exclude abnormal 'pre-embryos' from IVF treatment . . . (Prentice, 1986b, p. 10)

This glossy view of scientific progress is shared by many authors of infertility guidebooks. In *Miracle Babies and Other Happy Endings*, the authors write: 'Only a few years ago most couples with infertility problems had to turn to adoption or remain childless. But now, with advances in pharmaceuticals, micro-surgery, *in vitro* fertilization, and embryo transfer, many viable options have opened up to infertile couples – with the result that "miracle babies" are being born every day. *There is every reason for hope*' (Perloe and Christie, 1986, p. ix, original emphasis). A similar vision of scientific progress was espoused by the Warnock Committee, which described the development of *in vitro* fertilisation as 'a considerable achievement' which 'opened up new horizons in the alleviation of infertility'. In their report, the Committee claimed that advances in 'the science of embryology' have created 'hope of remedying defective embryos', 'pride in technological achievement' and 'pleasure at the new found means to relieve . . . the unhappiness of infertility' (Warnock, 1985, p. 4).

Enthusiastic representations such as these, uncritically depicting the 'achievements' of medical scientists in the 'battle' to overcome infertility, provide the adventure component of the desperate infertile couple story. It is important to emphasise the manner in which this component of the story is both introduced and framed by the hopes and desires of the infertile, such as Tessa Horton in the *The Times* article above. Just as it is the woman's body which, quite literally, contains the 'reproductive frontier' which is the subject of manipulation by the 'pioneering' medical scientists described in this account, so it is her emotions and her desires which contain these descriptions within the text itself. It is the narrative movement from conflict to resolution which makes this shift in perspective, from infertile woman to medical expert, appear 'logical' despite the fact that it involves a dramatic transition in point of view.

A related consequence of this narrative structure is that the woman who is used to frame the story suddenly disappears with the introduction of reproductive technologies. From being the subject of the text, she is transformed into its object as soon as the medical descriptions begin. Whereas her point of view begins the story (for example, 'Tessa Horton wants . . .'), she is eclipsed by the more privileged point of view of the medical/scientific 'expert' shortly thereafter. The transition in the language is dramatic. In the space of one paragraph we move from the description of Mrs Horton, who 'lives from one appointment to the next', to a description of ovulation and 'the complex interplay of the pituitary hormone FSH (follicle stimulating hormone) and the hormone oestrogen in the ovary'. The language shifts directly from the emotive description of 'slender hopes' and 'dreams come true' to the detached objective language of scientific description. 'Mrs. Horton' is replaced by parts of her anatomy: 'eggs', 'tubes', 'ovaries' and 'embryos'.

The focus shifts as well from a human drama to a techno-scientific one in which detailed descriptions of technique figure centrally. Thus we are led directly from the infertile woman who 'will not surrender [her] dream' to the 'small pumps placed beneath the skin, which release regulated pulses of hormones', and the 'hundreds of embryos . . . now stored in liquid nitrogen tanks at 200C below zero'. The infertile woman described in the first four paragraphs is displaced by ten scientists, five scientific teams and over a dozen techniques in the next forty paragraphs, which constitute the bulk of the story (Prentice, 1986b, p. 10).

Sometimes these accounts do not return to the infertile woman/ subject at all. In these cases, the stories simply become adventure stories about techno-pioneers on the frontiers of reproductive biology. This absence results from certain tensions in the relationship between infertility and new reproductive technology. Firstly, there is a tension between the assertion that medical technology is the 'only hope' for the infertile and the fact that medical technologies such as IVF have such low success rates.[6] Secondly, there is a tension between the representation of procreation as a 'natural' process, and the 'artificiality' of the technological means of intervening to 'treat' infertility. One of the most important features of *narrative* representations of infertility is the attempt to resolve these tensions through narrative closure.

**Resolution 2:   The 'Happy' and the 'Hopeless': Stories of
Heterosexual Romance**

The provision of a medical 'cure' provides the physical resolution to
the desperate infertile couple, but there is often an emotional resolution provided to complete the 'happy ending'. For this purpose, the
subjective point of view of the infertile is often reintroduced to
provide narrative closure. To achieve this closure, the familiar conventions of heterosexual romance are frequently invoked.

   In a conventional romantic fiction, a barrier to the shared happiness of the couple which must be overcome is the source of both
character motivation and narrative progression (Radway, 1984). We
see this convention being drawn upon in the representation of both
'happy' and 'desperate' stories of infertility. 'Happy' stories are often
accompanied by a photograph of the 'successful' couple, and/or their
much sought-after infant(s). The photograph serves as proof or
evidence of their happiness, and thus provides a visual signifier to
reinforce the narrative closure. The accompanying text includes
descriptions of the couple's relationship, family ties, professional/
work profile and other details in addition to the account of their
infertility and its treatment. The baby is typically described as a
'miracle' baby, or a 'precious' baby.

   Some recent examples, in this case from the Birmingham *Daily
News*, can be used to demonstrate the characteristic resolution of the
desperate infertile couple stories. In one example, the paper ran a
front page story of a 'happy' couple, parents of triplets, beneath the
banner headline: 'OUR GORGEOUS TINY WONDERS'. Above the
headline are photographs of all three babies attached to infant life
support systems. The couple are prominently pictured below, with
the caption: 'Delighted parents Mandy and Clint Baker: overjoyed
by their instant family.' At the end of the article we read that 'the
couple met at a Birmingham Kissogram agency where Mandy worked
when Clint joined as a "gorilla-gram". Now he runs his own garage
and says they will have to move from their two-bedroomed semi
[-detached house] into a bigger house' (Matthews and Jones, 1987,
p. 1).

   The second article, entitled 'TEST TUBE BOY FOR THRILLED
PARENTS', also received front-page coverage in the *Daily News* (29
March 1988). Described as 'A miracle of modern science' and as 'a
triumph for the team who pioneered Birmingham's IVF programme',
'test tube baby Samuel' is featured in the requisite photograph of the

happy couple with their longed-for progeny. In the accompanying text we read that:

> Proud parents Phil and Carol Goulding last night trembled with joy as they cradled their newborn son, Samuel . . .
> (. . .) for Carol and Phil, of Bewl Head, Bromsgrove, 9lb 5oz Samuel is nothing less than a miracle.
> 'We've been married 14 years, and trying for a baby for 12,' said 37-year old Carol. 'I still can't believe he's finally here.'
> Carol began treatment for infertility in 1977 in Bromsgrove and almost gave up hope of ever having a child when an operation to unblock her fallopian tubes failed . . .
> 'We were on holiday in Scotland when I realised I was pregnant, and we were just so happy.' (Cunningham, 1988, p. 1)

These personal details perform an important function in providing closure to the narrative. Their presence indicates the need for more than a medical resolution to the desperateness caused by infertility. Whereas the medical 'cure' provides a physical resolution, the details of the couple's lives fulfils the need for an emotional resolution by providing a recognisable and familiar 'happy ending' in which all the threads are tied together. In these examples from the Birmingham *Daily News*, the resolution of infertility is linked to heterosexual romance, 'successful' marriage, upward mobility and parental approval. The themes of hope, happiness and dreams-come-true are thus linked to the 'miracle of modern science', a test-tube baby.

In the reverse case of the 'unhappy' stories, the failure of a couple to conceive may become a metaphor for the relationship itself. In the *The Times* article mentioned above we read that: 'Sarah Browne and her husband are still solidly together, despite her ten miscarriages and seven operations. Others are less strong, *finding they cannot remain unified without a child*' (Prentice, 1986a, p. 13, my emphasis). Infertility guidebooks provide many similar examples of the effects of infertility on a couple's relationship. In her book *New Conceptions*, author Lori Andrews cites many experts on this subject: '"People have fantasies about having a child. . . . People become depressed, unhappy and wonder "What happened to our dreams?" says psychologist Aphrodite Clamar.' 'The couple that can't have children faces a philosophical crisis. They ask themselves "What am I on earth for? What will be left of me when I am gone?" declares psychiatrist E. James Lieberman' (Andrews, 1984, p. 86). Thus, in both the 'happy' and 'unhappy' stories, the resolution of infertility is closely linked to individual self-esteem and conjugal harmony, demonstrating the profound symbolic importance of successful procreation for social approval, acceptance and establishment.

Summary: The Narrative Construction of Desperateness

I have attempted thus far to identify some of the key ingredients and structures of popular representations of infertility and its treatment. Whilst it is important to recognise the different conditions in which these accounts were produced, varying from government documents to infertility handbooks to stories in the local and national press, the emphasis in this argument has been on their underlying similarities. Indeed, these similarities are all the more significant *because of the diversity* of social sites in which they were produced. Because of the apparent consensus within these, and many other, accounts, about what the experience of infertility involves and what to do about it, even accounts which are partial or incomplete partake in what might be described as the emergent popular 'myth' of infertility. Through its myriad enunciations and retellings, this popular 'myth' is established as a commonsense understanding of the relationship between infertility and reproductive technology. In turn, this understanding informs the consumption of further information, according to the narrative construction of a myth which has become commonsensical.

In writing of contemporary mythologies, Roland Barthes concludes that a myth is primarily defined by its form rather than its content. Myth, he argues, is essentially a form of communication: *a message* (Barthes, 1973). It is the form of the message, not its object, which makes of it a myth. To describe the formulaic, repeated, indeed ritualistic use of narrative structures in the desperate infertile couple story, this definition is certainly accurate.

The 'logic' of this mythic narrative is clear from the examples discussed. These stories revolve around the theme of desperateness: its 'causes' and 'effects'. Both the explanations and the resolutions of desperateness involve a combination of social and natural determinants, often used interchangeably. The need both to explain and to resolve the 'desperateness' of the infertile provides the plot structure for narratives which draw on familiar conventions of romance and adventure in representing the anguish of the infertile and the activities of medical scientists. These representations, I have argued, use the emotions of the couple, their 'longing' and 'hope' as a way into a discussion of medical achievements, thereby providing an apparently natural and obvious link between the 'hope for a medical cure' and the capability of medical science to provide one. Through the narrative mechanisms of selection, reduction, progression and closure, these stories mediate both the contradictions in the accounts of desperateness and the transgressive potential of new reproductive technologies.

In addition to providing a 'logic' of cause and effect, through which events are ordered and their interrelations established, narratives also function through the forms of identification and recognition they offer to the reader. Indeed, one might argue that the popularity of narrative as a form derives largely from this aspect of its construction. In this sense, narrative is similar to discourse as a form of representation which operates through the principle of inclusion and exclusion, constructing particular points of view that are accessible, often inviting, and excluding others. This feature of narrative allows us to see quite clearly how the desperate infertile couple stories 'work' as social constructions of infertility. The positions of identification and recognition established within these stories are very familiar: for example, the desire to create a family, the desire to restore conjugal harmony, the desire for social approval and acceptance, or the desire for a genetically related child. All of these desires are on offer as points of identification for the reader in the narratives of desperate infertile couples. They are not only recognisable desires but, of course, socially constructed desires, which correspond to established social practices and institutions.

These narratives also offer a wide range of possibilities for identification and recognition in terms of the points of view established within the stories. The pioneering medical scientists offer one set of readers (probably male) the pleasures of identification with a recognisable adventure hero. The infertile woman offers another set of readers (probably female) a different form of identification with an equally recognisable 'heroine': the woman who is devoted to motherhood at whatever cost. The possibility of identifying with the desire to create a family is a strong point of identification which is recognisable whether the reader is infertile or not, indeed whether or not he/she desires to have children at all.

The popularity of narrative, and the predominance of narrative format within popular media, derive from this quality of narrative, that it is open to various forms of simultaneous identification from a wide range of readers. Yet this openness goes only so far. Points of view which are not familiar or recognisable are less likely to be included in the range of identifications on offer. In this respect, *popular* narratives must, by definition, reinforce the *status quo* to a greater degree than other forms of representation. In the case of the narratives of infertility described above, this is clearly true, and has important implications for popular understandings of the experience of infertility.

It is through the establishment of a 'logic' of cause and effect, and of familiar points of identification and recognition that the narrative construction of representations of infertility structures commonsense understandings of the experience of infertility. The narrative mechanisms deployed in these accounts are a major means by which techniques such as IVF now appear the 'obvious' and even 'normal' means to 'cure' infertility, despite the fact that they are rarely successful, are costly and traumatic, contradict the supposed 'naturalness' of procreation, raise substantial moral and ethical questions, and do nothing to alleviate the condition of infertility itself. Such is the power of narrative that it can produce of these contradictions a coherent representation, in which the message that new reproductive technologies are the 'only hope' for desperate infertile couples becomes popular knowledge.

The Discursive Dimensions of Desperateness

It has been argued that the representation of the desperateness of infertility is framed in terms of loss and hope. The losses are described as both social and biological, the hope is described in terms of medical technology and scientific progress. It has been suggested that the framing of the representation of infertility in this way has a significant effect upon popular understandings of infertility and its treatment via new reproductive technologies. The emphasis upon the 'desperateness' of the infertile in these accounts provides the primary conflict or obstacle within the narrative; thus structuring the narrative trajectory along a particular sequence of causes and effects. The conventional points of identification and recognition on offer within these narratives contain them within the boundaries of the *status quo*. It has also been argued that these representations achieve narrative closure by presenting techno-scientific means of reproductive intervention as the only solution to the problem posed, and by providing a 'happy family' as a 'happy ending'. Lastly, it has been argued that, in this respect, popular representations of infertility, drawn from a wide variety of sources, demonstrate a remarkable degree of consistency.

These representations are analysed in terms of the concept of discourse, in order to draw attention to the construction of a regime of medical–scientific knowledge or 'truth' of infertility. In other words, it is argued that these representations can be understood in terms of a discursive 'logic' as well as a narrative one. It is also possible to suggest the ways in which discourse and narrative work together in the production of popular knowledge about infertility. For the purposes of this analysis, I have identified three discourses of infertility: the discourse of social loss, the discourse of biological destiny and the discourse of medical hope. Through the identification of these discourses, it is possible to map the production of the 'truth' of infertility across the many different sites in which it occurs. This is one of the several reasons why the concept of discourse is especially useful for an analysis of this sort.

Both narrative and discourse can be understood as essential to the mythic status of the desperate infertile couple stories, for both are structural forms of speech characteristic of myth as a form of communication, or as a message. There are, however, important differences between narrative and discourse in terms of the subject positions they construct, particularly in terms of their power to inscribe subject positions beyond the text itself. Whereas the relation of the subject, or reader, to narrative is comparatively open, inviting multiple possibilities for identification, engagement or resistance, the subject position inscribed by discourse is non-negotiable.[7] Discourse is the authoritative language of the expert, whereas narrative is the more popular language of the storyteller. Whereas narrative invites the subject/reader to engage with it personally and emotionally, in exchange for the pleasures of identification and recognition, discourse is non-inviting and non-reciprocal, naming and positioning both the subject and desire with forceful authority. Although the two forms of speech may easily coincide and overlap, the difference in their power to determine the position of the subject in social, as well as textual, locations is substantial.

The work of Michel Foucault, from which the concept of discourse is derived, has been particularly influential within studies linking the production of bodies of knowledge with the regulation of individual physical bodies (Foucault, 1973, 1976, 1980a). Historical studies, particularly those concerning sexuality, have demonstrated how knowledges about the body are produced in accordance with specific social formations involving medicine, religion and the law (see, for example, Walkowitz, 1980; Weeks, 1981, 1985). The current production of particular forms of knowledge about infertility, and its subsequent management via new technologies, provides a basis for a similar case study in discourse formation. The development and deployment of legislative measures to facilitate the control and 'treatment' of infertility based on this knowledge can thus be described as a discursive practice. The Foucauldian concept of discourse, with its emphasis upon the power relations implicit within the production and deployment of knowledges about the body, is especially useful in identifying the relationship between discursive knowledge and discursive practice. It is also helpful in providing a framework for demonstrating the relationship between the transformation of knowledges, the transformation of social practices (such as the law) and the transformation of physical bodies. The aim of using discourse theory in the present analysis is thus to delineate the particular formations of knowledge associated with recent 'treatments' for infertility, and their linkages to other social practices.[8]

The Discourse of Social Loss: 'The Kind of Life They Would Have Led'

As we have seen, the social losses suffered by 'the involuntarily childless' are represented as a major source of desperateness in popular representations of infertility. In the *Warnock Report*, for example, childlessness is said to result in a couple 'feeling excluded from a whole range of human activity' and to produce a sense of loss which 'cannot be assuaged by adoption'. Other accounts refer to 'the loss of self', and 'the loss of the imaginary family'. Couples are said to experience a loss of control over their lives, their individual identity, and their conjugal harmony. Couples are described in terms of existential loss, facing a 'philosophical crisis' as a result of their childlessness. They have lost the future they imagined and expected for themselves, their dreams and hopes for 'the kind of life they would have led'. It is said that 'life moves in a progression that is highlighted by the events of marriage and childbirth', and that the disruption of this progression causes anguish. It is said of infertile couples that: 'They may feel unable to fulfil their own or other people's expectations' and that this causes despair. It is the tremendous scope of their personal and social loss which is said to account for the 'desperateness' of infertility.

The logic of discourse operates differently within these accounts from the logic of narrative. The logic of narrative concerns the causes of conflict, the relationship between events, and the mechanisms of resolution of the story. It is a teleological logic, ordering the movement of events from a beginning, or origin, to an end point or closure. The logic of discourse is rather, as Foucault has described it, a logic of *enunciation*, defining the terms upon which knowledge is produced and deployed. It is a logic of inclusion and exclusion, of enhancement of some features and diminution of others. It is a logic which defines the positions from which legitimate knowledge is produced, thus delimiting the field of knowledge by establishing the definitive concepts and categories.

The way in which discourse is implicated in the exercise of power also differentiates it from narrative. The power of discourse is that of articulating the production of knowledge with existing social practices of regulation and control. This exercise of power is not dependent upon the active participation of the subjects of discourse. Conversely, narrative requires a more active subject who is willing to position him/herself within it. The power of narrative also lies in its ability to order and to relate events into a logical sequence, whereas the power of discourse is to define their meaning in terms of truth.

In the discourse of social loss, the features of infertility which are repeatedly enunciated are those which contain it within the institutions of marriage and the family. It is a discourse which enunciates a specific definition of acceptable parenthood, and defines a specific context for 'acceptable' procreation. Through the discourse of social loss, which is enunciated across a wide range of representations, knowledge about the experience of infertility is contained within the parameters of the dominant legal and social institutions which structure kinship: heterosexuality, marriage and the patriarchal nuclear family. It is in this way that the discourse articulates the production of knowledge about the body (infertility) with existing social institutions and practices which regulate and discipline bodily acts, such as procreation.

For example, the conflation of infertility with childlessness within the discourse of social loss is a means by which knowledge about infertility is restricted to a narrow frame of reference. Childlessness is only synonymous with infertility from the point of view of people medically diagnosed as infertile who want a biologically related child. However, these people represent only a tiny fraction of the number of people who are actually 'childless' in contemporary society. There are many people who are childless for reasons other than infertility. There are also people who are infertile who do not necessarily desire to have a biologically related child. If it were truly childlessness which was the major source of distress, as the headlines quoted at the beginning of this chapter suggest, then infertility would be only one of many causes for concern.

Discussions of infertility would be very different if they were not discursively constructed in terms of only one way to have children, and therefore only one way to be childless. It is claimed by the Warnock Committee that 'Childlessness may be a source of stress, even to those couples who have deliberately chosen it . . . They may feel excluded from a whole range of human activity . . .' (Warnock, 1985, p. 9). But if childlessness were itself the problem, if it were actually the difficulties of being excluded from parenting and the family that the Warnock Committee was concerned with, then the first question to ask would be: 'Who has access to children in this society and under what conditions?' In fact, these conditions are quite exclusive. Not everyone is equally positioned to 'choose' to have children or to participate in their upbringing. Rather than questioning these conditions, however, the Warnock Committee chose to reinforce their exclusive nature by validating only the needs of the 'acceptable' childless – those who are socially acceptable but physically incapable of producing a child. The Committee readily acknowledged that new reproductive technologies could increase the number of available options for parenting and procreative arrangements, and that they could increase the range of those who had the potential to parent. This, they stated openly, would not be desirable. The Committee was explicit in its conclusion that new reproductive technologies should only be used to enhance the reproductive capacity of people who intend to conform to the traditional nuclear family. 'It is better', they baldly state, 'for children to be born into a two-parent family, with both father and mother, although we recognise it is impossible to predict with any certainty how lasting such a relationship might be' (Warnock, 1985, pp. 11–12).

The unhappiness caused by childlessness is, thus, only recognised under certain conditions. As the *Report* clearly states, it is not of concern if one does not intend to conform to the traditional family. If one is a single parent, if one is not in a heterosexual relationship, or if one is intending to attempt any other 'pretended family relationship' (to borrow a phrase that is current), it is better that you should remain childless. Nor is your childlessness of concern if it is the result of unemployment, lack of day care facilities, disability, sexual preference, denial of citizenship or if, for any other reason, one is prevented from having children by law, by prejudice or by social circumstance.

Discursively, therefore, the conflation of infertility with childlessness, as if they were one and the same thing, narrowly restricts the frame of reference within which infertility is discussed. The problem is defined entirely within the parameters of the traditional nuclear family, with the result that the only knowledge available about the experience of infertility is that which reconciles it with the expectation of social conformity. This attempt to mediate the tension between the possibilities opened up by new reproductive technologies and the demands of the traditional nuclear family is particularly ironic given that the traditional nuclear family is less frequently the context for most parenting and procreation in contemporary British society.[9] It is only through rigid narrative and discursive conventions that the representation of infertility and new reproductive technologies can be contained within the frame of reference of desperate couples longing for a conventional happy family.

The Discourse of Biological Destiny: The 'Inner Drive' to Reproduce

Of particular importance is the relationship between the discourse of social loss and the discourse of biological destiny. As we have already seen, the 'desperateness' of infertility is explained in biological as well as social terms. The desire to biologically procreate is described as essential and innate. It is described as 'the natural product of pair-bonding', as 'deeply rooted in biological instinct' and as a 'natural expression of love'. Experts call it an 'inner drive', a 'biological need' and refer to it as instinctual. 'The desire for a family' is said to '[rise] unbidden from our genetic souls' as a result of 'human destiny' and the 'powerful urge to perpetuate [our] genes through a new generation'.

The discourse of biological destiny, which is also enunciated across a wide range of representations, invokes the authority of the sciences, specifically of evolution, embryology and genetics. These powerful scientific knowledges already play important roles in the legitimation of extisting kinship beliefs and practices. In particular, beliefs about the *naturalness* of heterosexuality and the nuclear family (also known as the 'biological family') derive their authority from the biological sciences. Defining infertility in accordance with the dictates of science further locates it within the domain of the natural family.

This has a particular significance when we consider the specific constellation of beliefs and practices which make up the prevailing kinship system. In British culture, as in most contemporary western cultures, kinship ties are legitimated in two ways: through law (producing 'in-laws') and through genetics (producing 'blood' ties). Biological procreation through heterosexual intercourse in the context of marriage is the exclusive means of establishing 'legitimate' parenthood. Both the biological and the legal requirements of parenthood must be established in order for parenthood to be legitimate and 'true'.[10] Without marriage, parenthood is illegitimate. Without shared biogenetic substance, kinship ties are incomplete, as evidenced by the statement by the Warnock Committee, for example, that the losses posed by infertility cannot be assuaged by adoption.

Thus, shared biogenetic substance is the 'true' basis for kinship ties, but it must be legitimated by the institution of marriage. Therefore, according to the conventional trajectory of life's 'progression', marriage should be consummated by procreation which should result in childbirth. Thus the legal (social) and 'natural' requirements of 'true' and legitimate parenthood should be sequenced as one, unified trajectory. Like all kinship beliefs, this sequence and trajectory are considered normal, 'obvious' and even 'natural' despite the fact that exceptions abound. Both the unity and the sequence of this trajectory are protected. Violations, such as illegitimacy, adultery, single-parent families, 'pretended family relationships' and childlessness are named and stigmatised. In short, child-rearing arrangements which do not reflect the protected unity of the conjugal and procreative function are, in this society, regarded as lesser forms of parenthood, at best, and as immoral or even perverse in some cases.[11]

It is, of course, precisely the unity of the procreative and the conjugal function which is so profoundly disrupted by the new reproductive technologies. Not only do many techniques require third-party donations of what might be described as extra-conjugal gametes, but many are also non-procreative, by any conventional sense of the term. In addition, the 'naturalness' of procreation and the 'biological' family are thrown into question by new reproductive technologies through which an unprecedented degree of 'artifice' has been introduced into the procreative process. Thus, the belief that the unity of the conjugal and procreative function is protected by the dictates of our evolutionary heritage, our 'selfish genes' and the 'natural' relationship of heterosexuality to procreation is also transgressed by these technologies. This poses a contradiction which must be resolved or, at least, contained. Indeed, it is this difficulty, of mediating the contradiction between the existing kinship system and the unprecedented 'artificial' procreative arrangements made possible by new reproductive technologies which, in part, explains the persistence of certain rigidly specific narrative and discursive mechanisms in the representation of infertility.

Genetic science not only plays a role in providing the language of 'true' kinship ties ('blood' ties) but in defining many aspects of personhood and inter-generational continuity. It is, after all, the inability to produce a *genetically related* child which is at issue in the discourse of biological destiny evident in representations of infertility. Genetic science provides the 'truth' of kinship in terms of inheritance and descent, shared substance, parenthood and procreation. The importance of this language is further demonstrated by its central place within dominant cultural understandings of human origins (genetic selection) and human conception (genetic recombination). The language of genetics is also important in the construction of personhood, as it is genetic inheritance which is said to make each individual both unique and like his/her parents.

All of this is lost to couples who cannot biologically procreate, and it is to this loss that the discourse of biological destiny refers. The importance of this discourse thus lies in the specific definitions of 'true' parenthood, personhood and procreation it constructs, in which genetic continuity is privileged above all other forms of parent–child ties. Not surprisingly, therefore, since the desired kinship bond is defined in terms of biological science, the 'treatment' of infertility must be provided by biological science, and infertility is primarily defined as a biological condition.

The Discourse of Medical Hope: 'Their Only Hope'

According to these accounts, there was a time when the victims of infertility had little choice but to suffer the stigma and unhappiness of barren wedlock. Now, thanks to scientific progress and the miracles of modern medicine, we need no longer endure the random injustices nature bestows upon us. Reproduction, it is said, is no longer the dark continent of medical knowledge, but a new frontier for the enterprising pioneers of modern medical science. We now have greater reproductive choice than ever before, and our choices are rapidly expanding. With greater reproductive choice we also gain greater reproductive control. Today we are increasingly capable not only of choosing when we reproduce, but how we reproduce, and even what we reproduce by testing and selecting and even genetically engineering the embryos we choose to nurture to viability. Or so would seem to be the story according to the popular press, the television news and the reports of government committees.

The discourse of medical hope at work in this version of infertility and its treatment is defined by several features: a belief in scientific progress and the ability to control and manipulate 'nature' for the greater benefit of 'man'; an objective, clinical definiton of human reproduction as a 'biological' process; and an emphasis upon the capability of medical scientists to increase reproductive choice through reproductive intervention. All of these features which characterise this discourse appear with regularity in media representations of infertility and its treatment.

These media stories about the miraculous achievements of doctors limit the kinds of questions that can be asked about infertility and its treatment through a characteristic fascination for details: why the embryo did not implant, what the woman wore at the insemination, how the doctor could not find the egg, and so forth. It is as if, given the biological urge to propagate and the capability of modern science to improve the process, no more need be said. This marriage of natural urges and scientific progress has been pre-eminently portrayed by the media as a beneficent union.

As a result of the medicalisation of infertility, a privileged and disproportionate authority is conferred upon representatives of the medical and scientific profession in public debates about the control of reproduction. Framed by the subjective hopes and desires of the infertile, media representations of infertility uncritically present medical science as the obvious solution to the problem. This, in turn, reinforces the view of medical science, as occupying a neutral position of objectivity and detached, clinical logic.

However, as many feminists have demonstrated, the objective gaze of science is not neutral, especially when it is focused upon women's reproductive organs (see Ehrenreich and English, 1976a, 1976b, 1979; Gordon 1977; Oakley 1980, 1984). Historically the perspectives of both medicine and science emerged as specific discursive formations in which the articulation of power and knowledge are clearly evident. The language of clinical objectivity is not the language of neutrality, but of detached surveillance, through which the discipline of rationality is imposed upon the unruly body in the name of therapeutic obligation (see Foucault, 1973). It is the discourse of medical hope which defines this position as the legitimate position from which to speak about infertility and its 'management' via new medical technologies.

We have already seen how, within descriptions of medical management of infertility, reproductive bodies – almost always women's bodies – are constructed as the site of physiological functions and dysfunctions requiring therapeutic technological intervention. In this process, the woman–subject of medical therapy becomes the woman–object of scientific scrutiny. This shift occurs both narratively and discursively. There is a convergence between the narrative movement from infertile woman as subject of the text to infertile woman as object of the text and the discursive mechanisms which legitimate this transition.

Although the narrative positioning of women may be seen as a textual process, the discursive positioning of woman-as-object of the scientific gaze is not confined to the text itself. The discursive positioning of women's reproductive capacity, of women's bodies, within representations of infertility, is a process that exists in social, as well as textual, practice (see Crowe, Price and Steinberg, this volume). The subject positions produced by the discourse in the text are also subject positions inhabited by women in actual medical practices. The medical definition of women's reproductive capacity, for example, has a privileged role in the formation of legal definitions of reproductive products and processes. It is the medical–scientific expert whose definition of reproduction wields greatest authority in both the public and parliamentary arena. Because it is seen as rational, detached and objective, the expertise of medical and scientific professionals is regarded as 'balanced' and 'factual' in legal and political debates, as if it did not represent a particular point of view.

Conclusion: Reproductive Control in the Late 1980s

In the current political climate, in which reproduction, sexuality and the family are prime targets on the moral agenda of the New Right, the implications of current public debates about state regulation of new reproductive technologies are far-reaching indeed. The establishment of legal protections for eggs, sperm and embryos cannot be separated from the current attempts by anti-abortionists to establish state protection for the foetus. Both the debate about abortion and that about new reproductive technologies are shaped by the power of medical discourse to enunciate the 'truth' of reproductive processes. Likewise, the establishment of legal restrictions upon eligibility for infertility treatment, in the name of 'protecting the children', is an attempt to regulate parenthood and procreation which cannot be separated from the current attack on the 'pretended family relationships' of lesbians and gay men.[12]

In sum, what is at stake in popular representations of infertility, and the current public and parliamentary debates, is not only the condition of 'involuntary' childlessness. Neither is it merely the 'treatment' of infertility. Nor is it simply the provision of 'medical miracles' for desperate couples mired in the hopelessness, the helplessness and the unhappiness of having lost 'the kind of life they would have led'. Rather, these representations must be seen as constructions built on the occasion of these dilemmas which open up a space for the narrative and discursive negotiation of a much broader range of concerns. In these accounts, infertility has become an over-determined signifier of the need to reconstruct traditional kinship beliefs and practices in the face of disruption, not only by new reproductive technologies, but by the rise of single-parent families, illegitimacy and other 'pretended families' (Stanworth, 1987b). In short, an analysis of the narrative and discursive construction of these accounts reveals that there is more than one reproductive dilemma at stake: not only the biological capacity of couples to reproduce, but the necessity for the social and cultural reproduction of specific definitions of parenthood and procreation, of traditional family values and of conventional sexual arrangements. By limiting discussion of childlessness to that of heterosexual, married couples who cannot biologically procreate, representations of infertility narrowly restrict the kinds of questions that can be asked within current public debates. Moreover, this discursive construction of reproduction in popular representations of infertility is also evident in the discursive practices of medicine and the law through which reproduction and parenting are regulated.

It remains, of course, an open question as to how successful either popular representations or legislation will be in containing the transgressive potential implicit in the very existence of reproductive technologies. The contradiction between the 'unnaturalness' of test-tube conception, and the supposed 'naturalness' of the institutions these techniques are meant to perpetuate can never be resolved, but only contained. Moreover, the representation of techniques such as IVF as 'the only hope' for the 'desperate infertile couples' will continue to be an unstable equation as long as IVF success rates remain in the rather dim vicinity of 5–10 per cent.

In the meantime, however, it is clear that public debate about infertility and new reproductive technologies needs to be greatly widened, to encompass the long-term social implications of techno-scientific reproductive intervention. These implications are too important to be considered merely in terms of medical 'treatment' of infertility and the provision of 'happy families' for 'desperate infertile couples'. As we move into the era of biotechnology and genetic engineering, control over the means of reproduction is destined to be an increasingly important arena of political and legislative dispute. The stake women have in the outcome of this process of redefining reproductive control cannot be overestimated.

The question for feminists is not only that of introducing women's sex-specific interests into the existing debate, but of challenging the narrow terms upon which these debates are at present conducted. As I have attempted to demonstrate in this chapter, such a challenge requires careful analysis of existing representations in terms both of their structure and of their content. As other feminists have also argued, popular representations are a powerful force in the social and cultural construction of reproduction (Petchesky, 1987). The need to address this dimension of current public debate is therefore paramount in the struggle over reproductive control currently occurring in relation to new reproductive technologies.

Notes

Several people were instrumental in the production of this chapter. I would especially like to thank the members of the Women Thesis Writers' Group connected to the Department of Cultural Studies at the University of Birmingham for their constructive criticisms and support. Richard Johnson also provided many useful criticisms and suggestions. Jackie Stacey provided invaluable assistance in the restructuring of this paper from its original form into a finished piece. Finally, thanks to Maureen McNeil for consistently detailed and thoughtful feedback on this paper throughout the seemingly interminable process of revision.

  1. *Choice* reporter, 1987; 'Comfort for the Childless', letters page, *The Times*, 11 April 1983; Newbold, 1987; correspondent, the *Guardian*, 1986; Morris, 1987; correspondent, *Yorkshire Post*, 1987; Cunningham, 1988; Matthews and Jones, 1987.

228   *The Social Construction of Infertility*

2. According to the most recent figures of the Voluntary Licensing Authority for Human *In Vitro* Fertilisation and Embryology in Britain, there are currently thirty-four 'approved' IVF centres in Britain. An additional ten centres are in the process of being established, and forty-one 'approved' research projects involving human embryos are currently in progress (Voluntary Licensing Authority, 1988, pp. 24–7).
3. On 4 February 1988, Members of the British Parliament began debate on proposed legislation on 'Human Fertilisation and Embryology'. The aims and scope of this legislation, which closely follows the recommendations of the *Warnock Report*, is outlined in a series of government documents, beginning with the *Warnock Report*, published in 1984 (*Report of the Committee of Inquiry into Human Fertilisation and Embryology*). In December 1986, the Department of Health and Social Security (DHSS) published a consultation ('white') paper entitled *Legislation on Human Infertility Services and Embryo Research: A Consultative Paper*. This was followed in March of 1987 by another DHSS White Paper entitled *Human Fertilisation and Embryology: A Framework for Legislation*. Further information is also available in the three published reports of the Voluntary Licensing Authority (VLA) established by the Medical Research Council (MRC) and the Royal College of Obstetricians and Gynaecologists (RCOG) in response to the suggestion of the *Warnock Report* that such a body be established to regulate IVF and embryo research. The substantive proposals within the legislation are to give the VLA statutory powers, and to put a 'conscience' vote before parliament on the question of whether embryo research should be banned or continue to be subject to the guidelines proposed by the VLA. For further details, see Voluntary Licensing Authority, 1986, 1987, 1988.
4. It is difficult to separate 'reproductive rights' from other rights, such as the right to health, the right to work, or the right to bodily integrity. Moreover the politics of reproduction, and particularly the place of reproductive activity in the maintenance of sexual inequality, can hardly be described adequately in the simple language of 'rights'. However, despite the limitations of the term 'women's reproductive rights', it continues to serve as the most recognisable gloss for that dimension of women's subjection most directly tied to reproductive practices.
5. For an introduction to approaches developed within cultural studies, see Johnson, 1983.
6. According to the third report of the VLA (VLA, 1988), the current overall success rate of IVF centres in Great Britain is 8.6 per cent.
7. I would like to acknowledge the help of Richard Johnson in formulating these distinctions between narrative and discourse.
8. The main problem of borrowing from discourse theory for the purposes of a feminist analysis is, of course, the fact that it is gender-blind. In addition, as Donna Haraway has written: 'This is the main feminist criticism of Michel Foucault's work: by highlighting the ubiquitous microcirculations of domination in his masterful analysis of the *capillarity* of power relations, that is the constitution of resistance by power in a never-ending dialectic and the demonstration of the impossibility of acquiring space without reproducing the domination named, he threatens

to make the grand circulations of power invisible' (Haraway, 1981, p. 480).

9. According to recent figures released by the Office of Population Censuses and Surveys, nearly one-quarter of children born in England and Wales last year were illegitimate. Whereas, in 1950, the proportion of children born to unmarried mothers was down to 4 per cent, it has since risen rapidly, and is now approaching 23 per cent. These figures reflect a trend towards cohabitation rather than marriage, as reported in the latest edition of *Social Trends* (1988).

10. For further discussion of the role of genetics in kinship beliefs, see Schneider, 1968.

11. For a comparative historical perspective on kinship beliefs, see Collier, Rosaldo and Yanagisako, 1982.

12. In the spring of 1988, the British Parliament passed into law a section of the Local Government Bill which prohibits local authorities from 'promoting' either homosexuality or the 'pretended family relationships' of lesbian and gay people.

Bibliography

ABSE, L. (1986) 'The Politics of In Vitro Fertilisation in Britain', in S. Fishel and E. M. Symonds (eds), *In Vitro Fertilisation: Past, Present and Future* (Oxford: IRL Press).

AKHTER, F. (1987) 'Wheat for Statistics: A Case Study of Relief Wheat for Attaining Sterilisation Targets in Bangladesh', in P. Spallone and D. L. Steinberg (eds), *Made to Order: The Myth of Reproductive and Genetic Progress* (Oxford: Pergamon).

ALDER, E. M. (1984) 'Psychological Aspects of Treatment by AID and IVF' (paper presented to the Society for Reproductive and Infant Psychology Annual Conference, Warwick).

ALDER, E. M. and A. A. TEMPLETON (1985) 'Patient Reaction to IVF Treatment', *Lancet*, i, p. 168.

ALDER, E. M., D. T. BARIA, M. M. LEES, D. W. LINCOLN, N. B. LUDON and A. A. TEMPLETON (1986) 'Attitudes of Women of Reproductive Age to In Vitro Fertilisation and Embryo Research', *Journal of Biosocial Sciences*, 18, pp. 155–67.

ANDERSON, D. C. (1987) 'Licensing Work on IVF and Related Procedures', *Lancet*, i, p. 1373.

ANDERSON, M. (1987) *Infertility: A Guide for the Anxious Couple* (London: Faber and Faber).

ANDREWS, L. (1984) *New Conceptions: A Consumer's Guide to the Newest Infertility Treatments* (New York: Ballantine Books).

ANDREWS, M., M. WEBSTER, J. E. E. FLEMING and M. B. McNAY (1987) 'Ultrasound Exposure Time in Routine Obstetric Screening', *British Journal of Obstetrics and Gynaecology*, 94, pp. 843–6.

ANGELL, R. R., R. J. AITKEN, P. F. A. VAN LOOK, M. A. LUMSDEN and A. A. TEMPLETON (1983) 'Chromosome Abnormality in Human Embryos after In Vitro Fertilisation', *Nature*, 303, pp. 336–8.

ARAL, S. and W. CATES (1983) 'The Increasing Concern with Infertility: Why Now?', *Journal of the American Medical Association*, 250, pp. 2327–31.

ARDITTI, R., R. DUELLI KLEIN and S. MINDEN (1984a) 'Introduction', in R. Arditti, R. Duelli Klein and S. Minden (eds), *Test-Tube Women: What Future for Motherhood?* (London: Pandora).

ARDITTI, R., R. DUELLI KLEIN and S. MINDEN (eds) (1984b) *Test-Tube Women: What Future for Motherhood?* (London: Pandora).

'Ares-Serono Has Announced it is to Spend 100 Billion Lire on Research into Genetic Engineering', *24 Ores* (Italian financial newspaper), 7 October 1984.

'Ares-Serono Pharma Sales', *CRNR*, 4 April 1986.

BADHAM, R. (1984) 'The Sociology of Industrial and Post-Industrial Society', *Current Sociology*, 32, pp. 1–94.

BARKER, G. H. (1981) *Your Search for Fertility: A Sympathetic Guide to Achieving Pregnancy for Childless Couples* (New York: William Morrow & Company).

BARKER, G. (1986) *The New Fertility: A Guide to Modern Medical Treatment for Childless Couples* (London: Adamson Books).

BARKER, J. and H. DOWNING (1980) 'Word Processing and the Transformation of Patriarchal Relations of Control in the Office', *Capital and Class*, 10, pp. 64–99.

BARNES, B. (1982) *T. S. Kuhn and Social Science* (London: Macmillan).

BARNES, B. (1983) 'On the Conventional Character of Knowledge and Cognition', in K. D. Knorr-Cetina and M. Mulkay (eds), *Science Observed* (London: Sage).

BARTHES, R. (1973) *Mythologies* (trans. Annette Lavers) (St. Albans: Paladin).

BEAUVOIR, S. DE (1952) *The Second Sex* (trans. and ed. H. M. Parshley) (London: Jonathan Cape).

BELL, D. (1973) *The Coming of Post-Industrial Society: A Venture in Social Forecasting* (New York: Basic Books).

BELLINA, J. and J. WILSON (1986) *The Fertility Handbook: A Positive and Practical Guide* (Harmondsworth: Penguin).

BENNETT, D., P. GLASNER and D. TRAVIS (1986) *The Politics of Uncertainty: Regulating Recombinant DNA Research in Britain* (London: Routledge & Kegan Paul).

BERAL, V. (1986) 'Assessment of the Safety of In-Utero Exposure to Ultrasound in Humans', in Medical Research Council, *Report of An Ad Hoc Meeting to Discuss the Risks and Benefits of Obstetric Ultrasound* (London: MRC).

BERER, M. (1985) 'Infertility: A Suitable Case for Treatment', *Marxism Today* 29, 6, pp. 29–31.

BERNSTINE, R. L. (1969) 'Safety Studies with Ultrasound Doppler Technique: A Clinical Follow Up of Patients and Tissue Culture Study', *Obstetric Gynaecology*, 34, pp. 707–9.

BERWICK, D. M. and M. C. WEINSTEIN (1985) 'What Do Patients Value? Willingness to Pay for Ultrasound in Normal Pregnancy', *Medical Care*, 23, pp. 881–93.

BIGGERS, J. D. (1981) 'In Vitro Fertilisation and Embryo Transfer in Human Beings', *New England Journal of Medicine*, 304, pp. 336–42.

BIJKER, W. E., T. P. HUGHES and T. J. PINCH (eds) (1987) *The Social Construction of Technological Systems* (Cambridge, Mass.: MIT Press).

BIRKE, L. (1986) *Women, Feminism and Biology: The Feminist Challenge* (Brighton: Harvester).

BLACKWELL, R. E., B. R. CARR, R. J. CHANG, A. N. DE CHERNEY, A. F. HANEY, W. R. KEYE, Jr., R. W. REBAR, J. A. ROCK, Z. ROSENWAKS, M. M. SEIBEL and N. R. SOULES (1987) 'Are We Exploiting the Infertile Couple?', *Fertility and Sterility*, 48, pp. 735–9.

BLAND, L. (1981) 'The Domain of the Sexual: A Response', *Screen Education*, 39, pp. 56–67.

BLAND, L. (1985) 'Sex and Morals: Re-arming the Left', *Marxism Today*, 29, 6, pp. 21–4.

BLANK, R. (1984) *Redefining Human Life* (Boulder, Colorado: Westview Press).

BLYTH, E. (1987) 'Wanted: A Modern Day Solomon', *Community Care*, 23 April, pp. 22–4.

BOARD FOR SOCIAL RESPONSIBILITY (1984) *Human Fertilisation and Embryology* (London: BSR).

BOARD FOR SOCIAL RESPONSIBILITY (1985) *Personal Origins* (London: CIO Publishing).

BOCK, G. and M. O'CONNOR (eds) (1986) *Human Embryo Research: Yes or No?* (London: Tavistock).

'Bolam v. Friern Hospital Management Committee' (1957) *Weekly Law Reports*, 1, p. 582.

BOSTON WOMEN'S HEALTH COLLECTIVE (1978) *Our Bodies Ourselves: A Health Book By and For Women*, British edition, A. Phillips and J. Rakusen (eds) (Harmondsworth: Penguin).

BRAHAMS, D. (1987) 'Assisted Reproduction and Selective Reduction of Pregnancy', *Lancet*, ii, pp. 1409–10.

BRANDON, J. and J. WARNER (1977) 'AID and Adoption: Some Comparisons', *British Journal of Social Work*, 7, pp. 335–41.

BRAVERMAN, H. (1974) *Labor and Monopoly Capital: The Degradation of Work in the Twentieth Century* (London: Monthly Review Press).

BRIGHTON WOMEN AND SCIENCE GROUP (1980) 'Technology in the Lying-in-Room', in Brighton Women and Science Group (eds), *Alice Through the Microscope* (London: Virago).

BRITISH AGENCIES FOR ADOPTION AND FOSTERING (1984) *AID and After* (London: BAAF Discussion Series, no. 4).

BROWN, P. and L. J. JORDANOVA (1981) 'Oppressive Dichotomies: The Nature/Culture Debate', in Cambridge Women's Studies Group (ed.), *Women in Society: Interdisciplinary Essays* (London: Virago).

BRUEL and KJAER UK Ltd (1986) 'A Bridge To New Life' (Publicity brochure published in the UK).

BUNKLE, P. (1984) 'Calling the Shots? The International Politics of Depo-provera', in R. Arditti, R. Duelli Klein and S. Minden (eds), *Test-Tube Women: What Future for Motherhood?* (London: Pandora).

'By a Correspondent', 'Childless Couples Given Hope By Sperm Process', *Guardian*, 12 May 1986.

CALLAHAN, D. (1986) 'Abortion: The New Debate', *Primary Care*, 13, (June) pp. 255–62.

CAMPBELL, S., A. E. READING, D. N. COX, C. M. SLEDMORE, R. MOONEY, P. CHUDLEIGH, J. BEEDLE and H. RUDDICK (1982) 'Ultrasound Scanning in Pregnancy: The Short-term Psychological Effects of Early Real-Time Scans', *Journal of Psychosomatic Obstetric Gynaecology*, 1, pp. 57–61.

CAMPBELL, S., J. DIAZ-RECASENS, D. R. GRIFFIN, T. E. COHEN-OVERBECK, J. M. PEARCE, K. WILLSON and M. J. TEAGUE (1983) 'New Doppler Technique for Assessing Uteroplacental Blood Flow', *Lancet*, i, pp. 675–7.

CAMPBELL, S., A. E. READING, D. N. COX, C. M. F. WIRTH, N. MORIN, D. JOHNSON, M. FRANK, H. PRESBERG, V. VAN DE WATER and J. MILLS (1987) 'Follow-up Study of Children Born as a Result of IVF' (paper presented to the Fifth World Congress on In Vitro

Fertilisation and Embryo Transfer, Norfolk, Virginia).
CANTACUZINO, M. (1986) 'It's Early Days Yet', *The Sunday Times*, 26 January.
CHALMERS, I. (1984) 'Confronting Cochrane's Challenge to Obstetrics', *British Journal of Obstetric Gynaecology*, 91, p. 722.
CHALMERS, I. (1986) 'Minimizing Harm and Maximizing Benefit During Innovation in Health Care: Controlled or Uncontrolled Experimentation', *Birth*, 13, pp. 155–67.
'Choice Reporter', 'New Hope for the Childless', *Birmingham Choice*, 20 March 1987.
CLARKE, A. (1984) 'Subtle Forms of Sterilisation Abuse', in R. Arditti, R. Duelli Klein and S. Minden (eds), *Test-Tube Women: What Future for Motherhood?* (London: Pandora).
CLARKE, M. (1985) 'Chances of Legislation Fade', *Nature*, 318, p. 197.
COCHRANE, A. L. (1979) '1931–1971: A Critical Review With Particular Reference to the Medical Profession', in *Medicine for the Year 2000* (London: Office of Health Economics).
COCKBURN, C. (1981) 'The Material of Male Power', *Feminist Review*, 9, pp. 41–58.
COCKBURN, C. (1983) *Brothers: Male Dominance and Technological Change* (London: Pluto).
COCKBURN, C. (1985) *Machinery of Dominance: Women, Men and Technical Know-How* (London: Pluto Press).
COHEN, H. (1986) 'Pregnancy, Abortion and Birth after In Vitro Fertilisation', in S. Fishel and E. M. Symonds (eds), *In Vitro Fertilisation: Past, Present and Future* (Oxford: IRL Press).
COLLIER, J., M. Z. ROSALDO and S. YANAGISAKO (1982) 'Is There a Family: New Anthropological Views', in B. Thorne with M. Yalom (ed.), *Rethinking the Family: Some Feminist Questions* (New York: Longman).
COREA, G. (1979) *The Hidden Malpractice: How American Medicine Mistreats Women* (New York: Harper & Row).
COREA, G. (1984) 'Egg Snatchers', in R. Arditti, R. Duelli Klein and S. Minden (eds), *Test-Tube Women: What Future for Motherhood?* (London: Pandora).
COREA, G. (1985) *The Mother-Machine: Reproductive Technologies from Artificial Insemination to Artificial Wombs* (New York: Harper & Row).
COREA, G., R. DUELLI KLEIN, J. HANMER, H. B. HOLMES, B. HOSKINS, M. KISHWAR, J. RAYMOND, R. ROWLAND and R. STEINBACHER (1985) *Man-Made Women: How New Reproductive Technologies Affect Women* (London: Hutchinson).
COREA, G. and S. INCE (1987) 'Report of a Survey of IVF Clinics in the USA', in P. Spallone and D. Steinberg (eds), *Made to Order: The Myth of Reproductive and Genetic Engineering Progress* (London: Pergamon).
COREA, G., J. HANMER, R. D. KLEIN, J. G. RAYMOND and R. ROWLAND (1987) 'Prologue', in P. Spallone and D. L. Steinberg (eds), *Made to Order: The Myth of Reproductive and Genetic Progress* (Oxford: Pergamon Press).
COTTON, K. (1986) *For Love and Money* (London: Dorling Kinnersly).
COUNCIL FOR SCIENCE AND SOCIETY (1984) *Human Procreation*

(Oxford: Oxford University Press).

COWAN, R. S. (1979) 'From Virginia Dare to Virginia Slims: Women and Technology in American Life', *Technology and Culture*, 20, pp. 51–63.

COWAN, R. S. (1976) 'The "Industrial Revolution" in the Home: Household Technology and Social Change in the Twentieth Century', *Technology and Culture*, 17, pp. 1–23.

COWAN, R. S. (1983) *More Work for Mother: The Ironies of Household Technology from the Open Hearth to the Microwave* (New York: Basic Books).

'CP Ventures Goes Straight to the High Tech Flyers', *Australian Financial Review*, 18 July 1985.

CRAFT, I. (1987) 'Voluntary Licensing and IVF/ET', *Lancet*, i, p. 1148.

CRAFT, I., M. AH-MOYE, T. AL-SHAWAF, W. FIAMANYA, P. LEWIS, D. ROBERTSON, P. SERHAL, P. SHRIVASTAV, E. SIMONS and P. BRINSDEN (1988) 'Analysis of 1071 GIFT Procedures – the Case of a Flexible Approach to Treatment', *Lancet*, i, pp. 1094–8.

CRAFT, I., P. R. BRINSDEN and E. G. SIMONS (1987a) 'How Many Oocytes/Embryos Should Be Transferred?', *Lancet*, ii, p. 109.

CRAFT, I., P. R. BRINSDEN and E. G. SIMONS (1987b) 'Licensing Work on IVF and Related Procedures', *Lancet*, i, p. 1373.

CROOKS, N. A. (1986) *DES Action/Toronto: Fact Sheet* (Toronto: DES).

CROWE, C. (1987) 'Women Want It: IVF and Women's Motivations for Participation', in P. Spallone and D. L. Steinberg (eds), *Made To Order: The Myth of Reproductive and Genetic Progress* (London: Pergamon).

CROWE, C. (1988) 'Bearing the Consequences: Women Experiencing IVF', in J. Scutt (ed.), *The Baby Machine: The Commercialisation of Motherhood* (Melbourne: McCulloch).

CUNHA, G. R., O. TAGUCHI, R. NAMIKAWA, Y. NISHIZUKA and S. J. ROBBEY (1987) 'Teratogenic Effects of Clomiphene, Tamoxifen and Diethylstilbestrol on the Developing Human Female Genital Tract', *Human Pathology*, 18, pp. 1132–43.

CUNNINGHAM, A. (1988) 'Test-tube Boy for Thrilled Parents', *Birmingham Daily News*, 29 March.

DALY, M. (1979) *Gyn/Ecology: The Metaethics of Radical Feminism* (London: The Women's Press).

DAVID, M. E. (1983) 'The New Right in the USA and Britain: A New Anti-Feminist Moral Economy', *Critical Social Policy*, 2, pp. 31–45.

DAVIDSON, C. (1986) *A Woman's Work is Never Done: A History of Housework in the British Isles* (London: Chatto & Windus).

DAVIES, D. (1986) 'Embryo Research' (Correspondence), *Nature*, 320, p. 570.

DAVITZ, L. (1984) *Baby Hunger: Every Woman's Longing for a Baby* (Minneapolis, Minnesota: Winston Press).

DEPARTMENT OF HEALTH AND SOCIAL SECURITY (1984) *Report of the Committee of Inquiry into Human Fertilisation and Embryology*, CmnD 9314 (London: HMSO).

DEPARTMENT OF HEALTH AND SOCIAL SECURITY (1986) *Legislation on Human Infertility Services and Embryo Research: A Consultative Paper*, Cm 46 (London: HMSO).

DEPARTMENT OF HEALTH AND SOCIAL SECURITY (1987) *Human Fertilisation and Embryology: A Framework for Legislation*, Cm 259 (London: HMSO).

DINGWALL, R., J. EEKELAAR and T. MURRAY (1983) *The Protection of Children* (Oxford: Basil Blackwell).

DIRECKS, A. (1987) 'Has the Lesson Been Learned?: The DES Story and IVF', in P. Spallone and D. L. Steinberg (eds), *Made to Order: The Myth of Reproductive and Genetic Progress* (Oxford: Pergamon).

DIRECKS, A. and H. BAQUAERT HOLMES (1986) 'Miracle Drug, Miracle Baby', *New Scientist*, 112, pp. 53–5.

DOBBS, R. H. and D. GAIRDNER (1966) 'Foetal Medicine – Who is to Practise It?', *Archives of Diseases in Childhood*, 41, p. 453.

DONNISON, J. (1977) *Midwives and Medical Men: A History of Inter-Professional Rivalries and Women's Rights* (London: Heinemann).

DONOVAN, P. (1976) 'Sterilizing the Poor and Incompetent', *Hastings Centre Report* 6.

DORLAND, W. A. N. and M. J. HUBENY (1926) *The X-ray in Embryology and Obstetrics* (London: Henry Kimpton).

DOUGLAS, M. (1984) *Purity and Danger*, 1st edn, 1966 (London: Ark Paperbacks).

DOYAL, L. (1987) 'Infertility – a Life Sentence?, in M. Stanworth (ed.), *Reproductive Technologies: Gender, Motherhood and Medicine* (Cambridge: Polity Press).

DUELLI KLEIN, R. (1985) 'What's "New" about the "New" Reproductive Technologies?', in G. Corea, R. Duelli Klein, J. Hanmer, H. B. Holmes, B. Hoskins, M. Kishwar, J. Raymond, R. Rowland and R. Steinbacher, *Man-Made Women: How New Reproductive Technologies Affect Women* (London: Hutchinson).

DUNN, E. (1984) 'Meddling with the Conceptus', *The Sunday Times*, 25 November.

DURHAM, M. (1985) 'Family, Morality and the New Right', *Parliamentary Affairs*, 38, pp. 180–91.

DWORKIN, A. (1974) *Woman Hating* (New York: E. P. Dutton).

EASLEA , B. (1980) *Witch-Hunting, Magic and the New Philosophy* (Brighton: Harvester).

EASLEA, B. (1981) *Science and Sexual Oppression: Patriarchy's Confrontation with Woman and Nature* (London: Weidenfeld & Nicolson).

EDWARDS, R. G. (1965) 'Maturation In Vitro of Human Ovarian Oocytes', *Lancet*, ii, pp. 926–9.

EDWARDS, R. G. (1983) 'Chromosomal Abnormalities in Human Embryos', *Nature,* 303, p. 283.

EDWARDS, R. G., B. D. BAVISTER and P. C. STEPTOE (1969) 'Early Stages of Fertilisation in Vitro of Human Oocytes Matured in Vitro', *Nature,* 221, pp. 632–5.

EDWARDS, R. G., P. C. STEPTOE and J. M. PURDY (1970) 'Fertilisation and Cleavage in Vitro of Preovulatory Human Oocytes', *Nature,* 227, pp. 1307–10.

EDWARDS, R. G. and P. C. STEPTOE (1980) *A Matter of Life: The Story of a Medical Breakthrough* (London: Hutchinson).

EDWARDS, R. G., S. B. FISHEL, J. COHEN, C. B. FEHILLY, J. M. PURDY, J. M. SLATER, P. C. STEPTOE and J. M. WEBSTER, (1984) 'Factors Influencing the Success of In Vitro Fertilisation for Alleviating Human Infertility', *Journal of In Vitro Fertilisation and Embryo Transfer*, 1, pp. 3–23.

EEKELAAR J. and R. DINGWALL (1984) 'Some Legal Issues in Obstetric Practice', *Journal of Social Welfare Law*, pp. 258–70.

EHRENREICH, B. and D. ENGLISH (1976a) *Complaints and Disorders: The Sexual Politics of Sickness,* first published in 1973 (London: Writers and Readers Publishing Cooperative).

EHRENREICH, B. and D. ENGLISH (1976b) *Witches, Midwives and Nurses: A History of Women Healers,* first published in 1973 (London: Writers and Readers Publishing Cooperative).

EHRENREICH, B. and D. ENGLISH (1979) *For Her Own Good: 150 Years of Experts' Advice to Women* (London: Pluto).

ELIAS, N. (1985) *The Loneliness of the Dying* (Oxford: Basil Blackwell).

EUROPEAN SOCIETY OF HUMAN REPRODUCTION AND EMBRYOLOGY (ESHRE) (1986) 'Brussels Conference Abstracts; June 22–25, 1986', *Human Reproduction*, 1.

FERRIMAN, A. (1987) 'Better We Have Just One Baby Than None', *Observer*, 1 November.

FINNRET (1984) *Reproductive Wrongs* (London: Finnret).

FISHEL, S. (1986) 'IVF–Historical Perspectives', in S. Fishel and E. M. Symonds (eds), *In Vitro Fertilisation: Past, Present and Future* (Oxford: IRL Press).

FISHEL, S., J. WEBSTER, P. JACKSON and B. FARATION (1986) 'Presentation Of Information On In Vitro Fertilisation', *Lancet*, ii, p. 1444.

FISHEL, S. and J. WEBSTER (1987) 'IVF and Associated Techniques: Whom Can We Believe?', *Lancet*, ii, p. 273.

FISHER, B., M. BAUER, R. MARGOLESE, R. POISSON, Y. PILCH, C. REDMOND, E. FISHER, N. WOLMARK, M. DEUTSCH, E. MONTAGUE, E. SAFFER, L. WICKERHAM, H. LERNER, A. GLASS, H. SHIBATA, P. DECKERS, A. KETCHAM, R. OISHI and I. RUSSELL (1985) 'Five Year Results of a Randomized Clinical Trial Comparing Total Mastectomy and Segmental Mastectomy With or Without Radiation in the Treatment of Breast Cancer', *New England Journal of Medicine*, 312, pp. 665–73.

FLEMING, L. (1988) 'The Moral Status of the Foetus: A Reappraisal', *Bioethics*, 1, pp. 15–34.

FLETCHER, J. C. (1985) 'Fetal Research: The State of the Question', *Hastings Center Report* 15, pp. 6–12.

FOUCAULT, M. (1970) *The Order of Things: An Archaeology of the Human Sciences,* (London: Tavistock).

FOUCAULT, M. (1972) *The Archaeology of Knowledge,* translated from the French by A. M. Sheridan Smith (London: Tavistock).

FOUCAULT, M. (1973) *The Birth of the Clinic,* translated from the French by A. M. Sheridan Smith (London: Tavistock).

FOUCAULT, M. (1976) *The History of Sexuality,* vol. 1, translated from the French by Robert Hurley (Harmondsworth: Penguin).

FOUCAULT, M. (1980a) *Herculine Barbin*, translated from th French by Richard McDougall (Brighton: The Harvester Press).

FOUCAULT, M. (1980b) *Power/Knowledge: Selected Interview and Other Writings 1972–1977*, edited by C. Gordon, (Brighton: The Harvester Press).

FOUCAULT, M. (1982) *Discipline and Punish: The Birth of the Prison*, translated from the French by A. Sheridan (Harmondsworth: Penguin).

FOX-KELLER, E. (1985) *Reflections on Gender and Science* (New Haven, Conn: Yale University Press).

FRASER, L. (1987) 'Sisters Share Test Tube Joy of Twin Girls', *Mail on Sunday*, 8 November.

FRENCH, M. (1986) *Beyond Power: Women, Men and Morals* (London: Butler and Tanner Ltd.).

FRYE, M. (1983) *The Politics of Reality: Essays in Feminist Theory* (Trumansburg, New York: Crossing Press).

FURNESS, M. E. (1987) 'Reporting Obstetric Ultrasound', *Lancet*, i, p. 675.

FRIZZELL, L. A. (1986) 'Dosage Specifications for Ultrasound Equipment', *Medical Biology*, 12, pp. 707–8.

GILLIE, O. (1987) 'Test-Tube Baby Hospital Denies Abortion Claim', *The Independent* 10 March.

GLASS, R. and R. ERICSSON (1982) *Getting Pregnant in the 1980's: New Advances in Infertility Treatment and Sex Pre-Selection* (Harmondsworth: Penguin Books).

GLENDINNING, C. (1983) *Unshared Care* (London: Routledge & Kegan Paul).

GOFFMAN, E. (1968) *Stigma* (Harmondsworth: Penguin).

GORDON, L. (1977) *Woman's Body, Woman's Right: A Social History of Birth Control in America* (Harmondsworth: Penguin Books).

GORZ, A. (1982) *Farewell to the Working Class: An Essay on Post-Industrial Socialism*, translated by Michael Sonenscher (London: Pluto Press).

GREENWOOD K. and L. KING (1981) 'Contraception and Abortion', in Cambridge Women's Studies Group (eds), *Women in Society* (London: Virago).

GREENWOOD V. and J. YOUNG (1976) *Abortion on Demand* (London: Pluto).

GROBSTEIN C., M. FLOWER and J. MENDELOFF et al. (1983) 'External Human Fertilisation: An Evaluation of Policy', *Science*, 222, pp. 127–33.

GROBSTEIN C. and M. FLOWER (1985) 'Current Ethical Issues', *Clinics in Obstetrics and Gynaecology*, 12, pp. 887–91.

GUSFIELD, J. (1975) 'Categories of Ownership and Responsibility in Social Issues', *Journal of Drug Issues*, no. 5.

HAIMES, E. (1986a) 'What Can the Creation of Families through Artificial Means of Reproduction Learn from Adoption?' (paper presented to the Society for Reproductive and Infant Psychology Annual Conference, Bristol).

HAIMES, E. (1986b) 'Regulating the Family: Natural and Social Relationships in Adoption and AID' (paper presented to the BSA Medical Sociology Conference, York).

238 *Bibliography*

HAIMES, E. (1988) 'Secrecy: What can Artificial Reproduction Learn from Adoption?', *International Journal of Law and the Family*, 2, pp. 46–61.

HAIMES, E. and N. TIMMS (1985) *Adoption Identity and Social Policy* (Aldershot: Gower).

HANMER, J. (1981) 'Sex Predetermination, Artificial Insemination and the Maintenance of Male-Dominated Culture', in H. Roberts (ed.), *Women, Health and Reproduction* (London: Routledge & Kegan Paul).

HANMER, J. (1983) 'Reproductive Technology: The Future for Women', in J. Rothschild (ed.), *Machina Ex Dea: Feminist Perspectives on Technology* (Oxford: Pergamon).

HANMER, J. and P. ALLEN (1980) 'Reproductive Engineering: The Final Solution?', in Brighton Women and Science Group (eds), *Alice Through the Microscope* (London: Virago).

HANMER, J. and M. MAYNARD (eds) (1987) *Women, Violence and Social Control*, (London: Macmillan).

HANMER, J. and S. SAUNDERS (1984) *Well Founded Fear: A Community Study of Violence Toward Women* (London: Hutchinson).

HARAWAY, D. (1981) 'In the Beginning was the Word: The Genesis of Biological Theory', *Signs*, 6, pp. 469–81.

HARDING, S. (1986) *The Science Question in Feminism* (Milton Keynes: Open University Press).

HARRIS, C. (1983) *The Family and Industrial Society* (London: George Allen & Unwin).

HARRISON, M. (1982) *A Woman in Residence: A Doctor's Personal and Professional Battles Against an Insensitive Medical System* (Harmondsworth: Penguin).

HELLMAN, L. M., G. M. DUFFUS, I. DONALD and B. SUDÉN (1970) 'Safety of Diagnostic Ultrasound in Obstetrics', *Lancet*, i, pp. 1133–5.

HIBBARD, B. M., C. J. ROBERTS, G. H. ELDER, K. T. EVANS and K. M. LAURENCE (1985) 'Can We Afford Screening for Neural Tube Defects?: The Southern Wales Experience', *British Medical Journal*, 290, pp. 293–5.

HIMES, N. E. (1970) *Medical History of Contraception*, first published 1936 (New York: Schocken Books).

HOMANS, H. (ed.) (1985) *The Sexual Politics of Reproduction* (Aldershot: Gower).

HULL, M. G. R., G. M. A. GLAZENER, N. J. KELLY, D. I. CONWAY, P. A. FOSTER, R. A. HINTON, C. COULSON, P. A. LAMBERT, E. M. WATT and K. M. DESAI (1985) 'Population Study of Causes, Treatment and Outcome of Infertility', *British Medical Journal*, 291, pp. 1693–7.

HUMPHREY, M. (1984) 'Parenthood through Donor Insemination' (paper presented to the Society for Reproductive and Infant Psychology, Annual Conference, Warwick).

HUXLEY, A. (1985) 'Research and the Embryo', *New Scientist*, 106 p. 2.

HYDE, B. (1986) 'An Interview Study of Pregnant Women's Attitudes to Ultrasound Scanning', *Social Science and Medicine*, 22, pp. 586–92.

IGLESIAS, T. (1985) 'Social and Ethical Aspects of IVF', in *Test Tube Babies: A Christian View*, first published 1984 (London: Unity Press).

ILLICH, I. (1985) *Limits to Medicine: Medical Nemesis: The Expropriation of Health* (Harmondsworth: Penguin).

INSEMINATION COMMITTEE SWEDEN (1983) *Children Conceived by Artificial Insemination*, Summary Report (Statens Offentliga Utredningar: 43).

IRONSIDE, V. (1985) 'How To Breed Healthy Babies', *Guardian*, 18 November.

JOHNSON G., D. ROBERTS, R. BROWN, E. COX, Z. EVERSHED, P. GOUTAM, P. HASSAN, R. ROBINSON, A. SAHDEV, K. SWAN and C. SYKES (1987) 'Infertile or Childless by Choice? A Multi-practice Survey of Women aged 35 and 50', *British Medical Journal*, 294, pp. 804–6.

JOHNSON, R. (1983) 'What is Cultural Studies Anyway?' (Stencilled Paper no. 74, Centre for Contemporary Cultural Studies, University of Birmingham).

JOHNSTON, M., R. SHAW and D. BIRD (1987) 'Test-Tube Baby Procedures: Stress and Judgements under Uncertainty', *Psychology and Health*, 1, pp. 25–38.

JORDANOVA, L. (ed.) (1986) *Languages of Nature* (London: Free Association Books).

KAMAL, S. (1987) 'Seizure of Reproductive Rights? A Discussion on Population Control in the Third World and the Emergence of the New Reproductive Technologies in the West', in P. Spallone and D. L. Steinberg (eds), *Made to Order: The Myth of Reproductive and Genetic Progress* (Oxford: Pergamon).

KANHAI, H. H. H., E. J. C. VAN RIJSSEL, R. J. MEERMAN and J. BENNERBROEK GRAVENBORST (1986) 'Selective Terminations in Quintuplet Pregnancy During First Trimester', *Lancet*, i, p. 1447.

KANTER, H., S. LEFANU, S. SHAN and C. SPEDDING (eds) (1984) *Sweeping Statements: Writing from the Women's Liberation Movement 1981–83* (London: The Women's Press).

KEOWN, J. (1987) 'Selective Reduction of Multiple Pregnancy', *New Law Journal*, 137, pp. 1165–6.

KENNEDY, I. (1986) 'A Survey of the Year I: The Doctor-Patient Relationship', in P. Byrne (ed.), *Rights and Wrongs in Medicine: King's College Studies, 1985–6* (London: King's Fund).

KEVLES, D. J. (1986) *In the Name of Eugenics: Genetics and the Uses of Human Heredity* (Berkeley and Los Angeles: University of California Press).

KITZINGER, S. (1987) *Freedom and Choice in Childbirth: Making Pregnancy Decisions* (Harmondsworth: Penguin).

KLEIN, R. (ed) (1989) *Infertility: Women Speak Out about Their Experiences of Reproductive Medicine* (London: Pandora Press).

KLEIN, R. and R. ROWLAND (1988) 'Women as Test-Sites for Fertility Drugs: Clomiphene Citrate and Hormonal Cocktails', *Reproductive and Genetic Engineering*, 1, pp. 251–374.

KOSSOFF, G. (1986) 'President's Address: Ultrasound 1985: Challenges and Opportunities', *Ultrasound in Medicine and Biology*, 12, pp. 3–4.

KOSSOFF, G. and S. B. BARNETT (eds) (1986) 'Proceedings of First

Symposium on Safety and Standardisation of Ultrasound in Obstretics', *Ultrasound in Medicine and Biology*, 12, pp. 673–724.

KUHN, T. *The Structure of Scientific Revolutions* (1970) (2nd ed) (London, Chicago: University of Chicago Press).

KUMAR, K. (1986) *Prophecy and Progress: The Sociology of Industrial and Post-Industrial Society*, revised edition with new Preface (Harmondsworth: Penguin).

LABORIE, F. (1987) 'Looking For Mothers You Only Find Fetuses', in P. Spallone and D. L. Steinberg (eds), *Made To Order: The Myth of Reproductive and Genetic Progress* (London: Pergamon).

LANCASTER, P. A. L. (1987a) 'Congenital Malformations after In Vitro Fertilisation', *Lancet*, ii, pp. 1392–3.

LANCASTER, P. A. L. (1987b) 'How Many Oocytes/Embryos Should be Transferred?', *Lancet*, ii, p. 109.

LAND, H. and R. PARKER (1978) 'United Kingdom', in S. B. Kamerman and A. J. Kahn (eds), *Family Policy: Government and Families in Fourteen Countries* (New York: Columbia University Press).

LAUDERDALE, EARL OF (1988) 'Human Fertilisation and Embryology' (Speech in House of Lords Debate, 15 January, *Hansard*, 491 cols 1450–88.

LAURANCE, J. (1987) 'The Test-Tube Dilemma', *New Society*, 82, pp. 19–20.

LAW COMMISSION (1982) *Family Law: Illegitimacy* (London: HMSO).

LEATHARD, A. (1986) 'Reproductive Technologies: The Reality of Choice for Women' (paper presented to the BSA Medical Sociology Conference, York).

LEESE, H. (1981) 'An Analysis of Embryos by Non-Invasive Methods', *Human Reproduction*, 2, pp. 37–40.

LEIBLUM, S. R., E. KEMMANN and L. TASKA (1989) 'Attitudes Toward Multiple Births and Pregnancy Concerns in Infertile and Fertile Women' (paper to be presented to the 9th International Congress of Psychosomatic Obstetrics and Gynaecology, Amsterdam.

LIEBESKIND, D., R. BASES, F. MENDEZ, F. ELEQUIN, M. KOENIGSBERG (1979) 'Sister Chromatid Exchanges in Human Lymphocytes after Exposure to Diagnostic Ultrasound', *Science*, 205, pp. 1273–5.

LILFORD, R. J. and T. CHARD (1985) 'The Routine Use of Ultrasound', *British Journal of Obstetric Gynaecology*, 92, pp. 434–6.

LILFORD, R. J. and M. E. DALTON (1987) 'Effectiveness of Treatment of Infertility', *British Medical Journal*, 195, pp. 155–6.

LINN, P. (1987) 'Gender Stereotypes, Technology Stereotypes', in M. McNeil (ed.), *Gender and Expertise* (London: Free Association Press).

LOVENDUSKI, J. and J. OUTSHOORN (eds) (1986) *The New Politics of Abortion* (London: Sage).

LYNCH, M. (1985) 'Discipline and the Material Form of Images: An Analysis of Scientific Visibility', *Social Studies of Science*, 15, pp. 37–66.

MACINTOSH, I. J. C. and D. A. DAVEY (1970) 'Chromosome Aberrations Induced by and Ultrasonic Fetal Pulse Detector', *British Medical Journal*, 4, pp. 92–3.

MACINTYRE, S. (1977) *Single and Pregnant* (London: Croom Helm).

MACKENZIE, D. and J. WAJCMAN (eds) (1985) *The Social Shaping of Technology: How the Refrigerator Got its Hum* (Milton Keynes: Open University).

McLAREN, A. (1984) *Reproductive Rituals: The Perception of Fertility in England from the Sixteenth Century to the Nineteenth Century* (London: Methuen).

McLAREN, A. (1986) 'Embryo Research', Correspondence, *Nature*, 320, p. 570.

McLAREN, A. (1986b) 'Why Study Early Human Development?' *New Scientist*, 110, pp. 49–53.

R. MACKLIN and W. GAYLIN (eds) (1981) *Medical Retardation and Sterilisation: A Problem of Competency and Paternalism* (New York: Plenum).

McLOUGHLIN, L. (1982) *The Pill, John Rock and the Church: The Biography of a Revolution* (Boston: Little and Brown).

McNEIL, M. (1987a) 'Being Reasonable Feminists', in M. McNeil (ed.), *Gender and Expertise* (London: Free Association Press).

McNEIL, M. (1987b) *Gender and Expertise* (London: Free Association Books).

MAHOWALD, M. B. (1987) 'The Ethical Options in Transplanting Fetal Tissue', *Hastings Center Report*, 17, pp. 9–15.

MAHOWALD, M. B. (1987) 'The Transplantation of Neural Tissue from Fetuses', Correspondence, *Science*, 225, pp. 1307–8.

MALOS, E. (1980) *The Politics of Housework* (London: Allison and Busby).

MAO, K. and L. WOOD (1984) 'Barriers to Treatment of Infertility by In-Vitro Fertilisation and Embryo Transfer', *Medical Journal of Australia*, 140, p. 532.

MARSH, D., P. GOWIN and M. READ (1986) 'Private Members Bills and Moral Panic: Video Recordings', *Parliamentary Affairs*, 39 pp. 179–98.

MARSH, D., M. READ and B. MYERS (1987) 'Don't Panic: The Obscene Publications (Protection of Children, etc.) Amendment Bill' (1985), *Parliamentary Affairs*, 40, pp. 73–9.

MARTIN, E. (1987) *The Woman in the Body: A Cultural Analysis of Reproduction* (Boston: Beacon Press).

MATHIESON, D. (1986) *Infertility Services in the NHS: What's Going On?* (report prepared for Frank Dobson, MP, House of Commons).

MATTHEWS, L. and G. JONES (1987) 'Our Gorgeous Tiny Wonders', *Birmingham Daily News*, 3 December.

MEDICAL RESEARCH COUNCIL (1985a) *Report of Inquiry into Human Fertilisation and Embryology: Medical Research Council Response* (London: MRC).

MEDICAL RESEARCH COUNCIL (1985b) 'Research Related to Human Fertilisation and Embryology', *British Medical Journal*, 285, p. 1480.

MEDICAL RESEARCH COUNCIL (1986) *Report of An Ad Hoc Meeting to Discuss the Risks and Benefits of Obstetric Ultrasound* (London: MRC).

MEIRE, H. B. (1987) 'The Safety of Diagnostic Ultrasound', *British Journal of Obstetrics and Gynaecology*, 94, p. 1122.

MERCHANT, C. (1980) *The Death Nature: Women, Ecology and the*

Scientific Revolution (London: Harper & Row).

MIES, M. (1987) 'Why Do We Need All This? A Call Against Genetic Engineering and Reproductive Technology', in P. Spallone and D. L. Steinberg (eds), *Made to Order: The Myth of Reproductive and Genetic Progress* (Oxford: Pergamon Press).

MINDEN, S. (1984) 'Designer Genes: A View from the Factory', in R. Arditti, R. Duelli Klein and S. Minden (eds), *Test-Tube Women: What Future for Motherhood?* (London: Pandora).

MOLD, J. W. and H. F. STEIN (1986) 'The Cascade Effect in the Clinical Care of Patients', *New England Journal of Medicine*, 314, pp. 512–14.

MOLE , R. (1986) 'Possible Hazards of Imaging and Doppler Ultrasound in Obstetrics', *Birth*, 13, pp. 29–37.

MORGAN, D. H. J. (1985) *The Family, Politics and Social Theory* (London: Routledge & Kegan Paul).

MORGAN, D. (1985) 'Making Motherhood Male: Surrogacy and the Moral Economy of Women', *Journal of Law and Society*, 12, pp. 219–38.

MORGAN, D. (1986) 'Who to Be or Not to Be: The Surrogacy Story', *Modern Law Review*, 49, pp. 358–68.

MORI (1985) *Public Attitudes to New Technology* (London: MORI).

MORRIS, M. (1987) 'Infertile Couples Get Hope From New Method', *Guardian*, 27 November.

MORT, F. (1980) 'The Domain of the Sexual', *Screen Education*, 36, pp. 65–84.

MOSHER, W. D. and W. F. PRATT (1985) 'Fecundity and Infertility in the United States, 1965–1982', *National Center for Health Statistics, Advance Data*, no. 104.

MUASHER, S. J., C. WILKINS, J. E. GARCIA, Z. ROSENWALES and H. W. JONES (1984) 'Benefits and Risks of Multiple Transfer with In Vitro Fertilisation', *Lancet*, i, p. 570.

MUASHER, S. J. and J. E. GARCIA (1986) 'Pregnancy and its Outcome', in H. W. Jones *et al.* (eds), *In Vitro Fertilisation* (Baltimore: Williams and Wilkins).

MUMFORD, L. (1967) *Technics and Human Development*, Vol. 1, first published in 1930 (London: Harvester).

MURPHY, K. (1984) 'From Mice to Men? Implications of Progress in Cloning Research', in R. Arditti, R. Duelli Klein and S. Minden (eds), *Test-Tube Women: What Future for Motherhood* (London: Pandora).

MUSHIN, D. N., M. C. BARRECK-HANSON and Y. C. SPENSLEY (1986) 'In Vitro Fertilisation Children: Early Psychosocial Development', *Journal of In Vitro Fertilisation and Embryo Transfer*, 3, pp. 247–57.

NATIONAL COUNCIL ON RADIATION PROTECTION AND MEASUREMENTS (1983) *Biological Effects of Ultrasound: Mechanisms and Clinical Implications* (Bethesda: National Council on Radiation Protection and Measurements, Report no. 74).

NATIONAL INSTITUTES OF HEALTH CONSENSUS DEVELOPMENT CONFERENCE (1984) *Consensus Statement: Diagnostic Ultrasound in Pregnancy* (US Government Printing Office: Washington DC).

NEAD, L. (1987) *Myths of Sexuality* (Oxford: Basil Blackwell).

NELKIN, D. (ed.) (1979) *Controversy: Politics of Technical Decisions* (London: Sage).

NELKIN, D. (1984) *Science as Intellectual Property: Who Controls Research* (London: Collier Macmillan).

NELKIN, D. and J. P. SWAZEY (1979) 'Science and Social Control: Controversies over Research on Violence', in H. Skoie (ed.), 'Scientific Expertise and the Public: Conference Proceedings', *Studies in Research and Higher Education*, 5, pp. 2098–222.

NEWBOLD, A. (1987) 'Joy For Baby Hope Couples', *Birmingham Daily News*, 19 March.

NEWILL, R. (1974) *Infertile Marriage* (Harmondsworth: Penguin).

OAKLEY, A. (1976) 'Wisewoman and Medicine Man: Changes in the Management of Childbirth', in J. Mitchell and A. Oakley (eds), *The Rights and Wrongs of Women* (Harmondsworth: Penguin).

OAKLEY, A. (1979) *Becoming a Mother* (Oxford: Martin Robertson).

OAKLEY, A. (1980) *Women Confined: Towards a Sociology of Childbirth* (Oxford: Martin Robertson, 1980).

OAKLEY, A. (1981a) *From Here to Maternity* (Harmondsworth: Pelican).

OAKLEY, A. (1981b) 'Interviewing Women: A Contradiction in Terms', in H. Roberts (ed.), *Doing Feminist Research* (London: Routledge & Kegan Paul).

OAKLEY, A. (1984) *The Captured Womb: A History of the Medical Care of Pregnant Women* (Oxford: Basil Blackwell).

O'BRIEN, B. (1986) *What Are My Chances Doctor? A Review of Clinical Risks* (London: Office of Health Economics).

O'BRIEN, M. (1981) *Politics of Reproduction* (London: Routledge & Kegan Paul).

O'BRIEN, W. D. (1983) 'Dose-Dependent Effect of Ultrasound on Fetal Weight in Mice', *Journal of Ultrasound Medicine*, 2, pp. 531–2.

O'SULLIVAN, S. (ed.) (1987) *Women's Health: A Spare Rib Reader* (London: Pandora).

OVERALL, C. (1987) *Ethics and Human Reproduction: A Feminist Analysis* (Boston: George Allen & Unwin).

OWENS, D. (1982/3) 'Artificial Insemination by Donor: Members' Views', *NACK: Journal for the National Association for the Childless* (Winter).

OWENS, D. (1984) 'Attitudes of the Involuntarily Childless to Artificial Insemination by Donor' (paper presented to the Society for Reproductive and Infant Psychology Annual Conference, Warwick).

PAIGE, C. and E. B. KARNOFSKY (1986) 'The Anti-abortion Movement and Baby Jane Doe', *Journal of Health Politics, Policy and Law*, 11, pp. 255–69.

PANORAMA (1988) 'The Agony and the Ecstasy' (screened on BBC 1).

PARTON, N. (1985) *The Politics of Child Abuse* (London: Macmillan).

PAYNE, V. L. (1987) 'The Regulation of Surrogate Motherhood', *Family Law*, 17, pp. 168–71.

PEEL REPORT: DEPARTMENT OF HEALTH AND SOCIAL SECURITY (1972) *The Use of Fetuses and Fetal Material for Research: Report of the Advisory Group* (London: HMSO).

PERLOE, M. and L. G. CHRISTIE (1986) *Miracle Babies and Other Happy Endings: How Modern Medical Advances Can Help Couples Conceive* (New York: Rawson Associates).

PETCHESKY, R. P. (1986) *Abortion and Woman's Choice: The State, Sexuality and Reproductive Freedom*, first published in 1985 (London: Verso).

PETCHESKY, R. P. (1987) 'Foetal Images: The Power of Visual Culture in the Politics of Reproduction', in M. Stanworth (ed.), *Reproductive Technologies: Gender, Motherhood and Medicine* (Cambridge: Polity Press).

PFEFFER, N. (1987) 'Artificial Insemination, *In Vitro* Fertilisation and the Stigma of Infertility', in M. Stanworth (ed.), *Reproductive Technologies: Gender, Motherhood and Medicine* (Cambridge: Polity Press).

PFEFFER, N. and A. QUICK (1988) *Infertility Services – A Desperate Case* (London: Greater London Association of Community Health Councils).

PFEFFER, N. and A. WOOLLETT (1983) *The Experience of Infertility* (London: Virago).

POLLARD, S. (1968) *The Idea of Progress: History and Society* (London: C. A. Watts).

PRENTICE, T. (1984) 'Pioneers Defend Embryo Research', *The Times*, 19 December.

PRENTICE, T. (1986a) 'Living in Limbo, Longing for Life', *The Times*, 8 April.

PRENTICE, T. (1986b) 'The Test-tube Maybe. . . . .', *The Times*, 9 April.

PRESTON, R. C. (1986) 'Measurement and Characterisation of Acoustic Output of Medical Ultrasound Equipment, Pt. 1', *Medicine, Biology, Engineering and Computing*, 24, pp. 113–20.

PRICE, F. V. (1988) 'Establishing Guidelines: Regulation and the Medical Management of Infertility', in R. Lee and D. Morgan (eds), *Birthrights: Law and Ethics at the Beginnings of Life* (London: Routledge & Kegan Paul).

PROGRESS (CAMPAIGN FOR RESEARCH INTO REPRODUCTION) (1986) Information Sheet (printed in UK).

RADWAY, J. A. (1984) *Reading the Romance: Women, Patriarchy and Popular Literature* (Chapel Hill: University of North Carolina Press).

RAKUSEN, J. and N. DAVIDSON (1982) *Out of Our Hands: What Technology Does to Pregnancy* (London: Pan).

RAVETZ, A. (1965) 'Modern Technology and an Ancient Occupation: Housework in Present-Day Society', *Technology and Culture*, 6, pp. 256–60.

RAYNER, J. (1986) 'Philosophy into Dogma: The Revival of Cultural Conservatism', *British Journal of Political Science*, 16, pp. 455–74.

READING, A. E., S. CAMPBELL, D. N. COX and C. M. SLEDMERE (1982) 'Health Beliefs and Health Care Behaviour in Pregnancy', *Psychological Medicine*, 12, pp. 379–83.

REILLY, P. (1977) *Genetics, Law and Social Policy* (London: Harvard University Press).

RHODES, S. and S. McNEILL (eds) (1985) *Women Against Violence Against Women* (London: Onlywomen Press).

RICH, A. (1977) *Of Woman Born: Motherhood as Experience and Insti-*

tution, first published 1976 (London: Virago).

RICHARDS, M. and F. PRICE (1987) 'Licensing Work on IVF and Related Procedures', *Lancet*, i, pp. 1373–4.

ROBERTS, C. J., K. T. EVANS, B. M. HIBBARD, K. M. LAURENCE, E. E. ROBERTS and I. B. ROBERTSON (1983) 'Diagnostic Effectiveness of Ultrasound in Detection of Neural Tube Defect', *Lancet*, ii, pp. 1068–9.

ROBERTS, H. (ed.) (1981a) *Doing Feminist Research* (London: Routledge & Kegan Paul).

ROBERTS, H. (ed.) (1981b) 'Women and their Doctors: Power and Powerlessness in the Research Process', in H. Roberts (ed.), *Doing Feminist Research* (London: Routledge & Kegan Paul).

ROBERTS, H. (ed.) (1981c) *Women, Health and Reproduction* (London: Routledge & Kegan Paul).

ROCK, J. and M. MENKIN (1944) 'In Vitro Fertilisation and Cleavage of Human Ovarian Eggs', *Science*, 100, pp. 105–7.

ROSSER, S. V. (ed.) (1988) *Feminism within the Science and Health Care Professions: Overcoming Resistance* (Oxford: Pergamon).

ROTHMAN, B. K. (1982) *In Labour: Women and Power in the Birth-Place* (London: Junction Books).

ROTHMAN, B. K. (1984) 'The Meaning of Choice in Reproductive Technology', in R. Arditti, R. Duelli Klein and S. Minden (eds), *Test-Tube Women: What Future for Motherhood?* (London: Pandora).

ROTHMAN, B. K. (1985) 'The Products of Conception: The Social Context of Reproductive Choices', *Journal of Medical Ethics*, 11, pp. 188–92.

ROTHMAN, B. K. (1987) *The Tentative Pregnancy: Prenatal Diagnosis and the Future of Motherhood* (New York: Penguin).

ROWLAND, R. (1985) 'Motherhood, Patriarchal Power, Alienation and the Issue of "Choice" in Sex Preselection', in G. Corea *et al*, *Man-Made Women: How New Reproductive Technologies Affect Women* (London: Hutchinson).

ROWLAND, R. (1987) 'Of Woman Born, But for How Long? The Relationship of Women to the New Reproductive Technologies and the Issue of Choice', in P. Spallone and D. L. Steinberg (eds), *Made to Order: The Myth of Reproductive and Genetic Progress* (Oxford: Pergamon Press).

ROWLAND, R. (1988) 'Making Women Visible in the Embryo Experimentation Debate', *Bioethics* 2, pp. 179–89.

ROYAL COLLEGE OF OBSTETRICIANS AND GYNAECOLOGISTS (1983) *Report of the Royal College of Obstetricians and Gynaecologists Ethics Committee on In Vitro Fertilisation and Embryo Replacement or Transfer* (London: Royal College of Obstetricians and Gynaecologists).

ROYAL COLLEGE OF OBSTETRICIANS AND GYNAECOLOGISTS (1984) *Royal College of Obstetricians and Gynaecologists Working Party on Routine Ultrasound Examination in Pregnancy Report* (London: Royal College of Obstetricians and Gynaecologists).

THE ROYAL SOCIETY (1983a) *Human Fertilisation and Embryology* (submission to DHSS Committee of Inquiry).

THE ROYAL SOCIETY (1983b) *Risk Assessment: Report of a Royal Society Working Party* (London: Royal Society).

SALING, E. and B. ARABIN (1988) 'Historic Landmarks of Perinatal Medicine in Obstetrics', *Journal of Perinatal Medicine*, 16, pp. 5–12.

SAVAGE, W. (1986) *A Savage Enquiry: Who Controls Childbirth?* (London: Virago).

SAYERS, J. (1982) *Biological Politics: Feminist and Anti-feminist Perspectives* (London: Tavistock).

SCHAFER, A. (1982) 'The Ethics of the Randomized Clinical Trial', *New England Journal of Medicine*, 307, pp. 719–24.

SCHNEIDER, D. (1968) *American Kinship: A Cultural Account* (Englewood Cliffs, NJ: Prentice Hall).

SCI JOURNAL CITATION REPORTS (1986) (Philadelphia: Institute for Scientific Information).

SCI SCIENCE CITATION INDEX: Citations vols 1975–1979, 1980, 1981, 1982, 1983, 1984, 1985, 1986 (Philadelphia: Institute for Scientific Information).

SEPPALA M. (1985) 'The World Collaborative Report on *In Vitro* Fertilisation and Embryo Replacement: Current State of the Art in January 1984', in M. Seppala and R. G. Edwards (eds), *In Vitro Fertilisation and Embryo Transfer Annals of the New York Academy of Sciences*, 442, pp. 558–63.

SHAPIRO, R. (1985) 'Britain's Sexual Counter-Revolutionaries' *Marxism Today*, 29, pp. 7–10.

SHAW, P. and M. JOHNSTON (1987) 'Couples Awaiting IVF: Counselling Needs, Emotional and Relational Problems' (paper presented to the Society for Reproductive and Infant Psychology Annual Conference. Edinburgh).

'Sidaway v. Gov. of Bethlem Royal Hospital, 2, *The Weekly Law Reports*, pp. 480–50.

SINGER, P. and D. WELLS (1984) *The Reproduction Revolution* (Oxford: Oxford University Press).

SKLAIR, L. (1973) *Organised Knowledge: A Sociological View of Science and Technology* (London: MacGibbon).

SMART, C. (1984) *The Ties That Bind* (London: Routledge & Kegan Paul).

SMART, C. (1987) 'There is of Course the Distinction Dictated by Nature: Law and the Problem of Paternity', in M. Stanworth (ed.), *Reproductive Technologies: Gender, Motherhood and Medicine* (Cambridge: Polity Press).

SMITH, B. (1985) 'NCT Ultrasound Survey – Results', *New Generation*, 4, pp. 5–6.

SNOWDEN, R. and G. D. MITCHELL (1981) *The Artificial Family* (London: George Allen & Unwin).

SNOWDEN, R., G. D. MITCHELL and E. SNOWDEN (1983) *Artificial Reproduction* (London: George Allen & Unwin).

SOUTH, J. (1985) 'And at the End of the Day Who is Holding the Baby?', *New Statesman*, 15 November, pp. 10–12.

SPALLONE, P. (1985) 'The Politics of Reproductive Technology: A Study in Repression' (MA thesis, University of York).

SPALLONE, P. (1989) *Beyond Conception: The New Politics of Reproduction* (London: Macmillan).

SPALLONE, P. and D. L. STEINBERG (eds) (1987) *Made to Order: The Myth of Reproductive and Genetic Progress* (London: Pergamon Press).

SPELMAN, E. V. (1978) 'On Treating Persons As Persons', *Ethics*, 88, pp. 150–61.

SQUIRE, J. (1984) 'Ultrasound', *AIMS Quarterly Journal*, Summer.

STACEY, M. (1988) 'The Manipulation of the Birth Process: Research Implications' (paper presented at Feb. 1987 meeting of the WHO European Advisory Committee for Health Resources, mimeo).

STANLEY, L. and S. WISE (1983) *Breaking Out: Feminist Consciousness and Feminist Research* (London: Routledge & Keagan Paul).

STANWORTH, M. (1987a) 'Deconstruction of Motherhood', in M. Stanworth (ed.), *Reproductive Technologies: Gender, Motherhood and Medicine* (Cambridge: Polity Press).

STANWORTH, M. (1987b) 'Editor's Introduction', in M. Stanworth (ed.), *Reproductive Technologies: Gender, Motherhood and Medicine* (Cambridge: Polity Press).

STANWORTH, M. (ed.) (1987c) *Reproductive Technologies: Gender, Motherhood and Medicine* (Cambridge: Polity Press).

STEEL BANK FILM CO-OP (1988) 'Soft Cell: A Feminist Analysis of Genetic Engineering' (film screened on British Channel 4).

STEINBERG, D. L. (1986) 'On the Question of Being Heard: Legal Protection and Legal Remedies for Women', (MA thesis, University of Kent).

STEVEN, C. (1987a) 'The First Glimpse of Your Baby', *Mother and Baby* (July) pp. 18–20.

STEVEN, C. (1987b) 'Test-Tube Sisters', *The Independent*, 29 September.

STEWART, A., J. WEBB and D. HEWITT (1958) 'A Survey of Childhood Malignancies', *British Medical Journal*, i, pp. 1495–1508.

STEWART, N. (1986) 'Women's Views of Ultrasonography in Obstetrics', *Birth*, 13, pp. 39–43.

STOPFORD, J. M. (1982) *The World of Multinational Enterprises* (London: Macmillan).

STRATHERN, M. (1980) 'No Nature, No Culture: The Hagen Case', in C. MacCormack and M. Strathern (eds), *Nature, Culture and Gender* (Cambridge: Cambridge University Press).

TAKABAYASHI, T., T. ABE, S. SATO and M. SUZUKI (1981) 'Study of Pulsewave Ultrasonic Irradiation on Mouse Embryos', *Medical Ultrasound*, pp. 286–8.

TEN TUSSCHER, T. (1986) 'Patriarchy, Capitalism and the New Right', in J. Evans *et al.* (eds), *Feminism and Political Theory* (London: Sage).

TESTART, J., B. LASALLE, J. BELAISCH-ALLART, R. FORNAN, A. HAZOUT, M. VOLANTE and R. FRYDMAN (1987) 'Human Embryo Viability Related to Freezing and Thawing Procedures', *American Journal of Obstetric Gynaecology*, 157, pp. 668–71.

THACKER, S. B. (1985) 'Quality of Controlled Clinical Trials. The Case of Imaging Ultrasound in Obstetrics: A Review', *British Journal of Obstetric Gynaecology*, 92, pp. 437–44.

TIMPANARO, S. (1980) *On Materialism* (London: Verso).

TORMEY, J. F. (1976) 'Exploitation, Oppression and Self-Sacrifice', in C. Gould, *Women and Philosophy: Toward a Theory of Liberation* (New York: G. P. Putnam and Sons).

TOURAINE, A. (1971) *The Post-Industrial Society* (New York: Random House).

TROUNSON, A. O. (1986) 'The Need for Appropriate Controls in Studies on Human in Vitro Fertilisation', *Journal of In Vitro Fertilisation and Embryo Transfer*, 3, p. 258.

TURNER, B. (1984) *The Body and Society* (Oxford: Basil Blackwell).

TURNEY, J. W. (1978) 'Public Responses to Experimental Biology' (unpublished PhD thesis, University of Manchester).

TURNEY, J. W. (1985) 'Embryo Guidelines Set Out', *Times Higher Education Supplement*, 658, p. 4.

'US Inquiries Inspire Initiative: Australian Technique Licensed to the US', *Australia Financial Review*, 12 April, 1985.

VEITCH, A. (1987) 'Three Became Mothers with Eggs from Sisters', *Guardian*, 5 May, p. 3.

THE VOLUNTARY LICENSING AUTHORITY (1986) *The First Report of the Voluntary Licensing Authority for Human 'In Vitro' Fertilisation and Embryology* (London: VLA).

THE VOLUNTARY LICENSING AUTHORITY (1987) *The Second Report of the Voluntary Licensing Authority for Human 'In Vitro' Fertilisation and Embryology* (London: VLA).

THE VOLUNTARY LICENSING AUTHORITY (1988) *The Third Report of the Voluntary Licensing Authority for Human 'In Vitro' Fertilisation and Embryology* (London: VLA).

WALKOWITZ, J. R. (1980) *Prostitution and Victorian Society: Women, Class and the State* (Cambridge: Cambridge University Press).

WALTERS, W. and W. SINGER (eds) (1984) *Test-Tube Babies: A Guide to Moral Questions, Present Techniques and Future Possibilities* (Oxford: Oxford University Press).

WARNOCK COMMITTEE (1984) *The Warnock Report* (Dame Mary Warnock, Chairman) (London: HMSO).

WARNOCK, M. (1985) *A Question of Life: The Warnock Report on Human Fertilisation and Embryology* (Oxford: Basil Blackwell).

WARNOCK, M. (1987) 'Do Human Cells Have Rights?', *Bioethics*, 1, pp. 1–14.

WEBSTER, J. (1986) 'Embryo Replacement, in S. Fishel and E. M. Symonds (eds), *In Vitro Fertilisation: Past, Present and Future* (Oxford: IRL Press).

WEEKS, J. (1981) *Sexuality and its Discontents* (London: Routledge & Kegan Paul).

WELLS, P. N. T. (1986) 'The Prudent Use of Diagnostic Ultrasound' (British Institute of Radiology Presidential Address 1986), *British Journal of Radiology*, 59, p. 708.

WELLS, P. N. T. (1987) *The Safety of Diagnostic Ultrasound* (Report of a British Institute of Radiology Working Group), *British Journal of Radiology Supplement*, 20, pp. 1–43.

WHITEHEAD, A. N. (1975) *Science and the Modern World*, first published in 1925 (Glasgow: Fontana Books).

WILLIAMS, L. S. (1988) 'It's Going to Work for Me: Responses to Failures of IVF', *Birth*, 15, pp. 153–6.

WILSON, R. W. and B. S. SCHIFRIN (1980) 'Is Any Pregnancy Low Risk?', *Obstetrics and Gynaecology*, 55, pp. 653–6.

WINSTON, R. and R. MARGARA (1987) 'Effectiveness of Treatment for Infertility', *British Medical Journal*, 195, p. 608.

WIRTH, F., N. MORIN, D. JOHNSON, M. FRANK, H. PRESBERG, V. VANDEWATER and J. MILLS (1987) 'Follow-up Study of Children Born As a Result of IVF' (paper given at the Fifth World Congress on In Vitro Fertilisation and Embryo Transfer, Norfolk, Virginia).

WITCOMBE, J. B. and A. RADFORD (1986) 'Obstetric Ultrasonography: Wider Role for Radiographers?', *British Medical Journal*, 292, pp. 113–55.

Who Owns Whom: Continental Europe (1986), Dun and Bradstreet (eds) (Oldworking: The Gresham Press).

WOLFE, A. (1981) 'Sociology, Liberalism and the New Right', *New Left Review*, 128, pp. 3–27.

WOOD, C. and A. WESTMORE (1984) *Test-tube Conception* (London: George Allen & Unwin).

WOOD, J. (1982) 'Criteria for Selection of Couples', in *Proceedings of the Conference on In Vitro Fertilisation: Problems and Possibilites* (Victoria, Australia: Monash University).

WOOLGAR, S. (1988) *Science: The Very Idea* (London: Tavistock).

WYNNE, B. (1987) *Risk Management and Hazardous Waste: Implementations and the Dialectics of Credibility* (Berlin: Springer-Verlag).

'Yorkshire Post Correspondent', 'Mother's Joy Over 1000th Test-Tube Baby', *Yorkshire Post*, 30 December, 1987.

YOXEN, E. (1988) *Public Concern and the Steering of Science* (Science Policy Steering Group Concept Paper, no.7 (London: Science Policy Steering Group).

ZANER, R. M. (1984) 'A Criticism of Moral Conservatism's View of IVF and ET', *Perspectives on Biology and Medicine*, 27, pp. 200–12.

ZIMMERMAN, J. (ed.) (1983) *The Technological Woman: Interfacing with Tomorrow* (New York: Praeger).

ZIMMERMAN, J. (1986) *Once Upon the Future: A Woman's Guide to Tomorrow's Technology* (London: Pandora).

ZIPPER, J. and S. SEVENHUIJSEN (1987) 'Surrogacy: Feminist Notions of Motherhood Reconsidered', in M. Stanworth (ed.), *Reproductive Technologies: Gender, Motherhood and Medicine* (Cambridge: Polity Press).

Index

abortion, 7, 9, 23, 121, 176, 183, 184, 185, 186, 187–8, 195–6, 198, 255–6
Abortion Act (British, 1967), 146, 195–6
Abse, Leo, 186–8, 189–90
accountability, of medical and scientific community, 100, 112–13, 124–5
Adler, Elizabeth, 182–3, 198
adoption, 23, 155–6, 161–2, 170, 171, 206, 208, 218, 222
adventure story, 203, 210–11, 214
AI, see artificial insemination
AID, see artificial insemination by donor
AIH, see artificial insemination by husband
AIMS, see Association for Improvements in Maternity Services
AKZO, N.V., 69–70
Alder, Elizabeth, 143, 162
Alton Bill (1987–8), 196, 198
Alton, David, 196
amniocentesis, 19, 22, 151
Anderson, Mary, 80, 81, 83, 90, 91, 94, 115, 117, 146
Andrews, Lori, 206, 213
anti-nuclear movement, 4
artificial insemination (AI), 19, 31–2, 156–7, 193
  by donor (AID), 95, 159–72
  by husband (AIH), 162, 163
Association for Improvements in Maternity Services (AIMS), 140

BAAF, see British Agencies for Adoption and Fostering
baby bottle, 6
Baird, David, 210
Barker, Graham, 96, 115, 117, 207
Barnes, Barry, 49, 50, 52
Barthes, Roland, 214

Bavister, David, 180
BBC, see British Broadcasting Corporation
Beauvoir, Simone de, 90
Beral, Val, 134
Bhophal, 4, 124
Bioethics, 176
biology, 13–6, 45
BMA, see British Medical Association
Board for Social Responsibility, 155, 160, 169, 172
body, the concept of, 15–16
Bolham v. Friern Hospital Management Committee, 128
Boston Women's Health Collective, 15
Braverman, Harry, 5, 6
Brighton Women and Science Group, 7
British Agencies for Adoption and Fostering (BAAF), 156, 157, 167
British Association of Perinatal Medicine, 153
British Broadcasting Corporation, 173
British Humanities Index, 177, 181
British Journal of Obstetrics and Gynaecology, 66, 67
British Medical Association, 190
British Medical Journal, 141
British Sociological Association 1987 Conference, ix
Bromocriptine, 115
Brown, Leslie, 35, 127
Brown, Louise, 59, 62, 68, 127, 148
Bruel and Kjaer (UK Ltd), 29, 82, 116
BSA, see British Sociological Association

Caesarean sections, 22
CARE (formerly Festival of Light), 41, 186

Centre for Social Ethics and Policy
    (University of Manchester), 176
Challenger (the space-craft), 124
Chernobyl, 4, 124
childlessness, 11, 114, 127, 159
    concept of, 37–8, 56, 90–3, 95,
        117
    depiction of, 70–1, 200, 201, 226
    'desperateness', 204, 206
    discourse of loss, 218–22
    see also couples
Chlamydia, 94
choice, 9–13, 25, 26, 113–14, 122,
    220, 224
chorionic villus sampling (CVS),
    19, 134, 136
Churchill, Winston, 195
Ciba Foundation, 176
citation index analysis, 18, 22, 24,
    61–8, 72
Clarke, Kenneth, 196
Clarke, Maxine, 47, 48
Clamar, Aphrodite, 213
Cleveland cases (of child abuse,
    1987), x
Clomid, *see* clomiphene citrate
clomiphene citrate, 29, 55, 79–80
Cochrane, Archibald, 129
Cockburn, Cynthia, 6, 58, 59
Committee on Safety of Medicines,
    128
commodification, 10, 24–5, 201
compulsiveness (in medical
    treatment), 26
concern, the sociology of, 176–99
consent, 108–11, 119, 120, 122,
    126, 127, 128, 130, 131, 143,
    198–9
Conservative Party (British), 184,
    185
consumerism, 10
content analysis, 24, 177–8
contracts (IVF), 108–11, 121–2
Cotton, Kim, 193
Council for the Professions
    Supplementary to Medicine,
    138
Council for Science and Society,
    155, 158, 159, 160, 163, 172

counselling, 105, 119–20, 127
couples, 70–2, 155, 161–2, 163, 175
    childless, 200, 203–4, 206, 208,
        209, 210, 212, 213, 214, 218,
        223, 226
    erasure of women, 14–15, 78–9,
        88, 92, 94, 95, 109, 115, 117,
        118, 120
CP Ventures, 70
cultural studies, 202, 228
culture medium (in IVF), 31, 32,
    34, 174
CVS, *see* chorionic villus sampling

Daily News (Birmingham), 212–13
Daily Telegraph, 177
Daly, Mary, 8, 75, 76, 115
David, Miriam, 184
Davies, David, 49, 57
demography, 7
Department of Education and
    Science (DES), 190
Department of Health and Social
    Security (DHSS), 118, 124,
    133, 153, 157, 158, 170, 190,
    228
Depo Provera, 21, 94
DES, *see either* Department of
    Education and Science *or*
    Diethylstibestrol
desperateness, 39–40, 200–29
DHSS, *see* Department of Health
    and Social Security
Diethylstibestrol (DES), 80, 100
discourse analysis, 15, 18, 23, 24,
    202, 215–26, 228–9
disembody, 108, 121
division of labour
    in science and medicine, 139,
        149–50
    in sociology of technology, 4–5,
        23
    see also midwifery
Dobson, Frank, 181
doctor–patient relationship, 98,
    125, 128–9, 148–9
domestic labour, 26
Donaldson, Mary, 102
donation of gametes and embryos,

36, 109, 130, 147–8, 198
anonymity (of donors), 23,
154–72
double standard
in regulating technology, 128–9,
150
of accountability in IVF, 112–13
Doyal, Lesley, 182

ecology movement, 4, 15
ectopic pregnancies, 127, 142
Edwards, Robert, 18, 29, 31–5, 39,
44, 56, 59, 61–8, 72, 73, 95,
126–7, 142, 180, 181, 194
eggs (*ova*)
collection of, 40, 81–2, 116
freezing of, 19, 20, 56, 58, 73
'harvesting' of, 81
'recovery' of, 81–2
term, 55
embryo transfer (ET), 19, 20, 22,
31, 125, 141, 162, 180, 210
embryology, 177, 200, 210
embryos
haploid, 31–2, 56
individualised notion of, 88,
106–8, 110–11, 120–1, 175,
176, 199
lavage, 162, 163, 164
'pre-embryo', 45–50, 61, 120–1
protectors, 108
research, *see in vitro* fertilisation,
embryo research;
experimentation on women
'spare', 36, 60, 61
status of, 41–2
epic, 204
ESHRE, *see* European Society of
Human Reproduction
ET, *see* embryo transfer
ethical committees, *see* local ethical
committees
ethnography, xi, 24
eugenics, 26, 110
European Society of Human
Reproduction, 60, 62, 68–70,
72, 73, 80, 115
experimentation, 6, 32, 33, 37, 53,
54, 55, 56, 60

see also in vitro fertilisation,
embryo research;
experimentation on women
expertise, ix, x, xi, 13, 18, 20–1,
59, 72, 123–4, 128, 130, 225

families, x, 9, 23, 37, 184, 206
gay and lesbian, 220, 222, 226,
229
'imaginary', 218, 219
'normal', 154–72
'pretended', 220, 222, 226
'the family', 220, 221
fatherhood (paternity), 37, 72, 130,
201
feminism, 4, 7, 8, 10, 13, 15, 16,
25, 26, 124, 182, 183, 185, 201,
227, 228–9
Festival of Light, 185
see also CARE
foetus
images of, 123, 125–7
use in transplants, 196
follicle stimulating hormone (FSH),
55, 69, 211
see also Metrodin
Foucault, Michel, 15–16, 217–18,
225, 228–9
FSH, *see* follicle stimulating
hormone
Galton, Francis, 26
gamete intra-fallopian transfer
(GIFT), 19, 58, 121, 127, 134,
141, 145–6, 149, 151
genetic engineering, 24, 69
Genetic Research, Cambridge, 73
genetics, 221, 223
GIFT, *see* gamete intra-fallopian
transfer
GnRH, Gonadotrophin Releasing
Hormone
Gonadotrophin Releasing Hormone
(GnRH), 115
Grobstein, Clifford, 180

hairdressing, 6
Hargreaves, Kenneth, 120
HGC, *see* human chorionic
gonadotrophin

heterosexuality, 9, 38–9, 208, 212–4, 219, 220, 223, 226
history of medicine and medical technology, 7, 76
HMG, *see* human menopausal gonadotrophin
homosexuality, 229
Humana Hospital, Wellington, 145, 149
human chorionic gonadotrophin (HCG), 30, 35, 55, 79
human menopausal gonadotrophin (HMG), 55, 115
human pituitary gonadotrophin (HCG), 79, 80, 115, 117
Human Population, 73
Hume, Basil (Cardinal), 177
Huxley, Andrew, 46, 49, 57
hydatiform mole (molar pregnancy), 115
Hyde, Beverley, 131–2, 138
hyperovulation, *see* superovulation
hysterectomies, 32, 34, 198

Iglesias, Teresa, 186
illegitimacy, *see* legitimacy
impact factor (of journals), 63, 64–66, 73
individualism, 9–13, 25, 165
  see also embryo, individualised notion of
infertility, 9, 11, 14, 28, 38, 44, 56, 57, 61, 70, 71, 115, 127, 161, 181–3, 187
  classification of, 90–100
  iatrogenic, 94
  idiopathic, 40, 93–5
  representations of, 200–229
innovations, *see* technologies, innovations in
in vitro fertilisation (IVF), 18, 19–20, 21, 22, 23, 163, 164, 167, 174, 178, 179, 180, 181, 190, 192, 193, 194, 197, 198, 200, 203, 210, 211, 216
  commercialisation of, 68–72
  couples, *see separate entry*
  criteria for selection for treatment, 39–40

depersonalisation of women in treatment, 74–122
embryo research, 23, 27, 40–45, 46–7, 52, 53, 54, 56–7, 68, 69, 120–1, 173–99, 196–7,
  experimentation on women, 28–37, 105–13, 119, 122
  history of development, 28, 31–6, 68, 126–7
  normalisation of, 58–73
  procedures, 28–31, 55, 56, 60, 74, 77–85
  provision of, 140
  regulation of, *see* Voluntary Licensing Authority
  risk and uncertainty in, 125, 126, 140–8
  scientific knowledge in, 27–57
  success rates of, 30–1, 56, 83–4, 99, 118, 120, 127, 211, 227, 228
  terminology, 77–8
In-Vitro Fertilisation Register (of the MRC), 142–3
IVF, *see in vitro* fertilisation
IVF Australia Ltd, 70

Johnson, Paul, 177
Johnson, Richard, 228
Journal of Endrocrinology, 64, 65
Journal of Experimental Zoology, 73
Journal of Obstetrics and Gynaecology, 66
Journal of Reproduction and Fertility, 66, 67
Journal of Reproduction and Fertility Supplement, 73

King's Fund Centre, 148
kinship, 222, 226
Kitzinger, Sheila, 8
Klein, Renate Duelli, 8, 14, 19, 20, 21, 29, 30, 55, 56, 84, 115, 118, 201
knitting, 6
knowledge, scientific, 27–57
Kuhn, Thomas, 59

Laborie, Francoise, 22, 30, 40, 94, 95
labour process analyses, 5
Lancet, 18, 64, 65, 66, 67, 73, 177
laparoscopy (laparoscopic procedure), 19, 20, 29–30, 34, 35, 36, 81–2
Lauderdale, Earl of, 173, 194
Law Commission (1982), 193
legitimacy, 160, 161, 193, 226, 229
leisure society, *see* post-industrial thesis
LH, *see* lutenizing hormone
licensing authority (for IVF), 193, 198
    see also Voluntary Licensing Authority
LIFE, 41, 186
linguistic analyses, 22, 24, 77–85
local ethical committees (of VLA, 103, 144
Longford, Lord, 173
lutenizing hormone (LH), 55, 56

manual labour, 4
Martin, Emily, 26
Marx, Karl, 5, 6
Marxism Today, 17–18
mass media, ix, x, 3, 16–19, 23, 143, 182, 184, 185, 195, 197, 224
    representations of IVF, 200–29
McLaren, Anne, 47, 49, 50
medical community, 18, 75, 100–1
    see also scientific community
medical ethics, 149
medical profession, 127–8, 132, 134, 178, 181, 208, 224, 225
    private medicine, 24, 141
    see also doctor–patient relationship
Medical Research Council (MRC), 43–4, 47, 48, 101, 102, 103, 119, 126–7, 132, 144, 148, 180, 190, 194, 228
    ad hoc meeting on ultrasound (March 1985), 133–4, 140
    Cell Biology and Disorders Board, 132–3

committee on ethics of IVF, 148
medicine, institutions of
Meire, Hylton, 140, 151
Metrodin, 69
microelectronics, 17
midwifery, 7, 130
Monash University, 70
Moral Majority, 185
    see also right-wing groups
Morgan, David H., 170
Mother and Baby, 136
motherhood, 14, 20, 30, 37–8, 40, 130, 163, 166, 201, 215
    lesbian, 38, 208, 215
    single, 208 (*see also* parenthood, single)
MRC, *see* Medical Research Council
multiple births and pregnancies, 30, 56, 115, 121, 142, 145, 146, 194
    see also superovulation
Mumford, Lewis, 5, 6, 58, 59
myth, 214, 217

narrative, 18, 23, 24, 26, 202–19, 225
National Association of Freedom, 185
National Childbirth Trust (NCT), 139, 140
National Council on Radiation Protection and Measurements, 132
National Health Service (NHS), 140, 141, 145–6
National Institutes of Health, 133
nationalism, 187
National Physical Laboratory, 135
National Viewers and Listeners Association, 185, 195
Nature, 57, 64, 65, 66, 67, 73
nature–culture dichotomy, 16
NCT, *see* National Childbirth Trust
Nelkin, Dorothy, 124
neonatal nurses and units, 146
NHS, *see* National Health Service
Neuberger, Julia (Rabbi), 144
Norfolk, Duke of, 194

normalisation of technological
intervention, *see in vitro*
fertilisation, normalisation of;
technologies, normalisation of

Oakley, Ann, 7
Obscene Publications Act (1985),
195
obstetrics, 123–5, 129–31, 136, 137
OCU, *see* Order of Christine Unity
Oldham (IVF) Clinic, 126–7
Order of Christine Unity (OCU),
186
Organon, 61, 69–72
Osborne, Sir John, 144
ovariectomies, 32
Oxford Survey of Childhood
Cancer, 126

Panorama, 17, 82
parenthood, 23, 163, 165, 169, 201,
206, 219, 220, 222, 223, 226
single parenthood, 163, 172, 222,
226
paramedicals, 140, 150, 151
patent analysis, 62
patriarchy, 8, 185
Pelvic Inflamatory Disease (PID),
94, 95, 117
Perganol, 69
Petchesky, Rosalind Pollack, 7, 9,
12, 17–8, 23–4, 192, 196, 199
Pfeffer, Naomi, 128, 182, 204
pharmaceutical industry, 24, 58, 61,
69–71
PID, *see* Pelvic Inflamatory Disease
policies (on new reproductive
technologies in Britain),
154–72, 173–99
political economy, 24–5
Polkinghorne Committee, 196
popular culture, 17–19
pornography, 195
post-industrial thesis, 1–5
Powell, Enoch, 121, 177, 178, 186,
187–8
Powell Bill, *see* Unborn Children
Protection Bill (1984–5)

pre-embryo, 21, 27, 28, 40, 45–53,
61, 106–7, 111–12, 120–1, 122,
210
pregnancy
definitions and meanings of, 22,
30, 51, 121
nature of, 130
press (popular), 24, 200–29
presumptive endangerment, 121
primitive streak, 45–51, 54
Private Members' Bills, 195, 198
PROGRESS (Campaign for
Research into Reproduction),
47–8, 51, 60
progress (scientific), 1–2, 36, 104,
113, 204, 209–11, 216, 223, 224
Purdy, Jean, 67, 126–7

radiation, 126
radiographer, 137–40, 150, 151
Radiographers' Board, Disciplinary
Committee of, 138
radiography, 126
randomised controlled trials
(RCTs), 129, 132–3, 142
Rantzen, Esther, 173
RCOG, *see* Royal College of
Gynaecologists
RCTs, *see* randomised controlled
trials
reflexivity in sociology, xi
representations, 17, 18, 23, 200–29
reproductive rights, 9–13, 201, 228
Responsible Society, 186
Rich, Adrienne, 11, 37
right-wing groups
'Moral Right', 183–9, 195–8, 201
'New Right', 176, 179, 184–5,
225
theorists of, 10
right to life (doctrine of), 53, 185,
192
risks (technological), ix, 18, 87, 99,
121, 123–53, 163
Rock, John, 179–80
romance, 203, 212–14
Rothman, Barbara Katz, 11
Royal College of General
Practitioners, 133

Royal College of Gynaecologists (RCOG), 43, 48, 101, 102, 103, 119, 132, 133, 137, 154, 155, 156–7, 160, 162–3, 190, 194, 228
Royal Society, 44, 46, 57, 124
Royal Society of Medicine, 186

Savage, Wendy, 8, 130
Sayers, Janet, 13
scanning, 134, 137–40
science fiction, 2
scientific community, 44, 47–54, 59–60
self-insemination, 20
Serono, 61, 69–70, 73
sex pre-selection, 19
Sidaway v. *Gov. of Bethlem Royal Hospital* (1984), 128
Smart, Carol, 139
Social Sciences Index, 181
Society for the Protection of the Unborn Child (SPUC), 41, 186, 195
sociology of technology, ix–x, 1–26
Soft Cell (film), *see* Steel Bank Film Co-operative
spare embryos, *see* embryos, spare
SPUC, *see* Society for the Protection of the Unborn Child
Stanworth, Michelle, 8, 9, 11, 13, 14
state regulation of technology, *see* technologies, state regulation of
Steel Bank Film Co-operative, 116
Steptoe, Patrick, 29, 31–5, 39, 44, 62, 67, 126–7, 180, 207–8
Sun, 17
superovulation, 32, 34, 35, 56, 60, 61, 69, 79–81, 83, 115, 198
see also multiple births and pregnancies
surrogacy, 14, 20, 71, 130, 162, 163, 165, 166–7, 180, 193, 195, 201
suspect classification, 90, 116
see also infertility, classification of

Sweden, policy on AID donors, 158–60, 162

technologies
childbirth, 7–8
determinism of, 4
disasters of, 124
domestic, 7
future orientation of, 1–3
inner and outer space, 3
innovations in, ix–x, 5, 18, 128–9
normalisation of, 58–73
productive, 3–9
state regulation of, ix, x
tension in scientific terminology, 49, 51
ten Tusscher, Tessa, 184–5
teratogenic malformations, 80
test-tube babies, 1, 17, 25, 68, 78, 127, 200, 201, 207, 209, 212, 213
Thalidomide, 80, 100
Thatcherism, 184
Times, The, 177–8, 203, 205, 209–10, 213
transducer, 116
Turney, Jon, 180

Unborn Children (Protection) Bill (the Powell Bill) (1984–5), 46–7, 52, 60, 120, 177, 179, 183, 186–8, 193–5, 198
uncertainty, 123–53
ultrasonography, 9, 19, 20, 22, 29
calibration of equipment in, 135–6
description of, 125–6
in egg recovery, 81–2
mechanical (caviation) mechanisms in, 132
population exposed, 133
risks of, 125–7, 131–40, 151
routinisation of, 126
thermal (heating) mechanisms in, 132
uncertainty in, 125–7, 131–40, 151
uses of, 136
ultrasound beam calibrator (of

National Physical Laboratory), 135

utilitarianism, 192, 196, 198

vagueness and overbreadth (in terms), 90, 116

Varcoe, Ian, 25

Video Recordings Bill, 195

videos, 69, 70–72

violence against women, 76, 87

visual images, 18, 137

VLA, *see* Voluntary Licensing Authority

Voluntary Licensing Authority, 24, 30, 48–9, 51, 61, 101–11, 118, 119–20, 121, 122, 127, 144, 145, 146, 148, 149, 194, 228

Warnock Committee (Committee of Inquiry into Human Fertilisation and Embryology, established in 1982), 20, 24, 40–7, 52, 54, 56, 61, 101–2, 144, 154, 155, 156, 157, 158, 159, 160, 161, 162, 163, 165, 166, 168, 170, 172, 174, 178, 179, 186, 187, 190–4, 197–8, 205, 208, 210, 218, 222, 228

Warnock, Mary, 41, 44, 154, 174, 176, 178, 187, 189, 190–1, 197, 198

Whitehouse, Mary, 185

Williams, Shirley, 189

WISE, *see* Women into Science and Technology programme

women
depersonalisation in IVF, 74–122
erasure of, 22, 56, 71, 77, 85, 89, 97, 104–8, 114–15, 116 (*see also* couples)
reproductive freedom and rights, 72, 88–9, 199, 201, 202, 227
research on, *see in vitro* fertilisation, exprimentation on women; embryos research
visibility of in IVF, 86–7, 88

Women into Science and Engineering (WISE) (1984), 59

women's health movement, 15

women's magazines, 19

women's movement, *see* feminism

Woolett, Anne, 182

Woolgar, 26

X-radiology, 126

Yearley, Steven, 26

Zimmerman, Jan, 12, 25